# Nogier's Arterial Reflex

Discover the profound connection between the autonomic nervous system and the art of clinical observation in *Nogier's Arterial Reflex: The Vascular Autonomic Signal.* This groundbreaking book explores Paul Nogier's revolutionary discovery—the arterial reflex (RAC) and its role as a diagnostic tool with a wide scope of possibilities for clinical exploration.

Through detailed methods, measurements, and tests, the authors present RAC as a simple yet powerful diagnostic approach, capable of unlocking the complexities of the neurovegetative system. By emphasising direct clinical observation over technology, this work reaffirms the importance of intuition, empathy, and the art of medicine.

Whether you are a medical professional, a student, or simply curious about the intersection of science and the art of medicine, *Nogier's Arterial Reflex* invites you to explore a transformative perspective on health and healing.

# Nogier's Arterial Reflex

## The Vascular Autonomic Signal

Raphaël Nogier MD
Anthony de Sousa MD

Translated from French by
Bo Kähler and Anthony de Sousa

CRC Press
Taylor & Francis Group
Boca Raton London New York

CRC Press is an imprint of the
Taylor & Francis Group, an **informa** business

First published in English 2027
by CRC Press
2385 NW Executive Center Drive, Suite 320, Boca Raton FL 33431

and by CRC Press
4 Park Square, Milton Park, Abingdon, Oxon, OX14 4RN

*CRC Press is an imprint of Taylor & Francis Group, LLC*



Published in French by Sauramps Medical, 2022



Library of Congress Control Number: 2026904464

ISBN: 9781041272823 (hbk)
ISBN: 9781041272779 (pbk)
ISBN: 9781003753629 (ebk)

DOI: 10.1201/9781003753629

Typeset in Times
by KnowledgeWorks Global Ltd.

# Dedication

*In memory of Dr Paul Nogier*

*In memory of Professor Pierre Magnin*

*In memory of Dr René Bourdiol*

*In memory of Dr Michel Marignan*

*To Astrid, Christian, Valentin and Ophelie*

*- With affection and gratitude for their relentless patience*

—**AS**

*- To Eloi, Colombe, Josephine, and those who will follow*

*May wisdom, courage and humility be with them throughout their lives. With my affection*

—**RN**

# Contents

# List of Protocols

# Preface to the English Edition

With the aim of better understanding the significance and scope of Paul Nogier's arterial reflex, which we call RAC, it may be of interest to take a brief look at the historical background of modern medicine.

Throughout the ages, medicine has been influenced by many cultures, such as Egypt, Ancient Greece, Rome, and especially the Judeo-Christian civilisation. In the 4th century AD, the Roman Emperor Constantine was the first to have officially adopted Christian religion in the Roman Empire. From then on, religious authorities imposed a strictly dualistic vision of Man, thereby splitting the individual into two entities having very different natures [2]. On one side, *the physical body* regarded as inferior, despicable, and responsible for passing down original sin across the generations. On the other side, *the soul*, of immaterial essence, akin to the divine and charged with imposing its power over the body. Thus, for many centuries, physicians have had to cope with the unending debate between spirit and matter, although their profession must have long since led them to perceive some degree of unity between body, emotion, and spirit. Many philosophers challenged the dualistic view, often at great risk, in favour of a more unitarian view, known as *monism*. Descartes is a well-known example: with a touch of malice, he argued that the soul penetrates the physical body through the pineal gland (epiphysis), specifically designed for that purpose.

From the Renaissance onwards, between the early 15th and late 16th centuries, medical thinking began to change drastically. Dualism and the notion of soul gradually faded from the field of medicine, and a new paradigm took shape, predominantly materialistic and based on analytical thought. Following the rhythm of scientific discovery, medicine acquired the opportunity to make rapid progress, eventually leading to the evidence-based medicine we know today.

But the trend has undoubtedly gone far in this direction. If the aim of medicine today is rightly concerned with efficiency, the drive towards materialistic modernity has become so powerful that it sometimes comes at the cost of neglecting the empathy we owe to our patients, to the extent that one may wonder whether present-day medicine is not gradually "losing its soul". Another consequence of the spirit of conquest in present-day medical technology is the risk of making us physicians over-confident, losing sight of *the clinical sense* that our original training meant to instil as the core of our profession. The power and efficiency of imagery, biochemistry, and computers would have us forget the outstanding diagnostic abilities the masters who taught us medicine possessed only a few decades ago, simply by dint of dialogue, direct physical examination, and little more technology than a stethoscope and a hammer.

The predominantly scientific approach to contemporary medicine has, of course, had its critics, such as the 20th century French physician and epistemologist Georges Canguilhem [1] who, during the last century, declared: *"Medicine is an art, at the crossroads between several sciences",* implying that a practising physician should naturally be a good scientist, yet at the same time be a competent clinician and a creative artist, duly concerned with the subtler aspects of the patient's psyche.

This leads to the question of how modern medicine can bridge the growing rift between intuition and clinical sense on the one side and scientific evidence and technology on the other.

*Michel Onfray*, a French philosopher, made an interesting comment on the evolution of medicine [3] at a medical congress in 2016. Focusing his talk on ***the neurovegetative, or autonomous nervous system*** (*hereafter the **ANS***), he unexpectedly mentioned that this system was the only one not to have yet given rise to an organised medical speciality, with its own body of knowledge and specialized physicians, as is the case for all other branches of medicine. In addition, Onfray pointed out that medical technology in general has undoubtedly brought dramatic progress to diagnosis and treatment in all branches of medicine, here again with the exception of the ANS, for which standard medical technologies such as imagery, chemistry, or electrophysiological methods are poorly effective, as opposed to the cerebrospinal nervous system, for example.

Yet historically, the basic structure and functions of the ANS have been extensively explored and well described by anatomists and physiologists since the second half of the 19th century. The properties of both its sympathetic and parasympathetic divisions are well known today, and their importance is widely demonstrated. The ANS, especially the sympathetic part, is present in virtually all parts of the body, directing it as if it were a conductor with his musicians. The astonishing diversity of functions that it regulates can be seen as materialising the essence of living processes. Beyond our control, the neurovegetative adapts us to the incessant variations of the outside and inside worlds. It controls homeostasis, metabolism, as well as the harmonious unity of our physiologic functions. Furthermore, it acts as a kind of psychosomatic interface that transduces our emotions into physiological expressions and vice versa. It will have us sweat through emotion; it will make Pavlov's dog salivate, just as it will have a youngster's heart throb when confronted with the loved one…

So great is the importance of the neurovegetative system that the philosopher Onfray ended his talk by suggesting to his medical audience that the ANS could, *in fine*, be regarded as a modern biological substrate of the *soul.* Of course, we understand this notion very differently from the time when it was thought of as an immaterial substance. The soul now simply refers to the deeper and more subtle aspects of the organism, which we think of intuitively as close to the mysterious concept of life. Although unexpected, the idea that the ANS and the concept of soul both evoke the same biological reality is well-thought, subtle, and perhaps not so surprising.

By contrast, however, it remains a disturbing fact that medical technologies are not as efficient when applied to the ANS than to other types of pathologies, and consequently remain so often unresolved.

If this, unfortunately, is the case, we have good reason here to finish on a more positive note. It is at this point indeed that Paul Nogier's discovery of the arterial reflex comes into play. Since the mid-sixties of the last century, we have gained a great deal of evidence showing beyond doubt that the ANS *responds remarkably well to the use of the arterial reflex, which we call the RAC.* Thus, Paul Nogier's research has provided us with a virtually royal access to the autonomic nervous system, as well as to a great many other aspects of the organism.

This book is all about the discovery of the RAC and its applications. It describes a wide range of related techniques for diagnosis and treatment in general and endeavours to show how this new approach harmoniously fits in as part of classical medicine. As a team, we have endeavoured to provide an overview of the principal methods, measurements, and tests made possible by the arterial reflex. We hope it will be of interest not only as general medical information but especially to those who wish to train as practitioners in these promising new prospects.

Finally, it is perhaps reasonable to hope that with time, this new clinical approach will contribute to bringing back a glimmer of Hippocratic spirit to the field of medicine.

**Anthony de Sousa**

# Acknowledgements

*Individual chapter authors:*

Michel Marignan, Jean-Luc Vigneron, and Chantal Vulliez

Dr Bernard Bricot
Dr Bernard Deffontaines
Mr Jean Girardot
Dr Bernard Julienne
Dr Françoise Petitjean
Professor Pierre Rabischong
Dr Yves Rouxeville
Dr Claudie Terral

All have made important contributions to the understanding of the RAC and for the most part, have collaborated with Paul Nogier.

## WE ALSO WISH TO THANK

- Our patients and our students, who constantly give us the opportunity for a better understanding of medicine

*Those who have made the original French version possible:*

- Yves Lefrand, editor
- Myriam Malvaut, editor
- Gerard Thiollay, computer scientist
- Alexia van Moorsel, graphics
- Cécile Bergeron, graphics

*Those who have made the English version possible:*

- Bo Kähler, computer scientist
- Miranda Bromage, editor
- Hudson Greig, assistant editor
- Bendik Johannesen, creator of 3D ear models
- Ronald de Sousa, philosopher

# About the Authors

**Raphaël Nogier**, born in 1953, is a physician in Lyon, France, where he has practiced auriculotherapy exclusively since 1985. Author of several books on auriculotherapy and on nutrition, he has taught in twenty-five countries, mainly in Germany, Scandinavia, Italy, the USA, Algeria, South America, New Zealand, and Japan. He has participated in several meetings organised by the World Health Organization for the standardisation of the nomenclature and practice of auriculotherapy. He belongs to the French medical school for which semiology remains the irreplaceable framework of the art of diagnosis in medicine.

**Anthony de Sousa**, born in 1943, is a physician in Geneva, Switzerland, and has been practising auriculotherapy since 1983. He trained at the GLEM (Lyon Group for Medical Studies) from 1979 and collaborated with Paul Nogier in his research group in Lyon until 1996. He has been teaching RAC techniques for more than 30 years at the GLEM and at the AGMAR (French Swiss Acupuncture Association) in Geneva and has also had the opportunity to teach in Australia, New Zealand, and Norway. He was an expert at the WHO meeting (World Health Organization) on auriculotherapy in 1990 in Lyon.

# Notice

This book is about a sympathetic arterial reflex perceptible when taking the radial pulse of our patients, called RAC. It was discovered in 1966 by Paul Nogier, who elaborated a new method for diagnosis and treatment, based on this reflex. The method is largely—but not only—an extension of auriculotherapy.

The reader will discover a new way of considering the patient.

Throughout the book, our aim was to provide answers to the many questions put to us by students.

Anthony de Sousa explains the original techniques taught by Paul Nogier, while Raphaël Nogier describes his own, more recent techniques. Such a synthesis had never been undertaken before.

We are conscious of the fact that the evolution of medicine implies many changes, so that what appears obvious today might not have been so evident during the past. This is particularly the case of the autonomous nervous system, of which we have a better understanding today, compared to some years ago.

With respect to the fact that the different techniques described were elaborated at different periods, it might occasionally appear to the reader that the two authors do not have an identical approach to the arterial reflex and its applications. Nevertheless, we consider it important to provide the reader with a richer scope of analysis by describing both the original and the more recent techniques, even at the cost of possible contradictions.

We hope you will enjoy reading about this very promising outlook.

**Raphaël Nogier and Anthony de Sousa**

***Medicine has three goals***
***Preventing diseases***
***Restoring the body's altered functions***
***Fighting pain***

CHAPTER 1

# Introduction and Background

**Raphaël Nogier**

## 1.1 HISTORY

When, in 1966, Paul Nogier (1908–1996), a general practitioner established in Lyon, discovered what he was later going to name the auriculo-cardiac reflex, also known as the RAC, VAS or vascular signal, he probably had no idea of its implications.

Paul Nogier began by acquiring a scientific background. He initially studied physics at the Ecole Centrale de Lyon under the influence of his father Thomas, an associate professor of medical physics, who aroused his interest in research and observation. After that, it was in 1931 that Paul Nogier began his medical career.

In those days, therapeutics were based solely on chemistry. Each disease had its own chemical molecule, and every symptom had its drug.

Paul Nogier's originality consisted of breaking free from this paradigm. Largely influenced by the ideas of Claude Bernard and by experimental medicine, he intuitively referred to several simple ideas to develop a new method of treatment:

- Chemistry is not the only solution for the treatment of diseases.
- Organic disease is often preceded by functional disorders.
- It is possible to influence the function of the organs by physically stimulating the skin.

Throughout his life, Paul Nogier endeavoured to treat his patients by developing techniques based on these three principles.

After completing his medical studies, he began studying homoeopathy. He understood that a homoeopathic granule, although it may not contain any active chemical molecule, probably carries physical, electromagnetic information that could explain its mode of action. His master in homeopathy was Dr Pierre Schmidt from Geneva.

Later, he studied acupuncture with Dr Jacques Niboyet in Marseille. This thousand-year-old Chinese method, hardly known of at the time, had only barely been introduced into France. It was even laughed at by the mainstream medical community of the time, unable to understand that for treating a patient, it was possible to take a step back from sacrosanct pharmacology.

DOI: 10.1201/9781003753629-1

At the same time, Paul Nogier also studied methods of osteopathic manipulation. With Dr Ammathieu, he learned how to reposition vertebrae. With Monneyron, he understood that vertebral repositioning can be carried out without brutality, in a reflex manner.

In 1951, Paul Nogier got an opportunity to begin his research on the auricle. Two of his patients suffering from intractable sciatica had travelled all the way to Marseille to consult a healer, Madame Barrin. This lady, well known for having successfully treated many celebrities, specialised in treating lower back pain and sciatic neuralgia by way of a very simple technique her father had taught her, consisting of cauterising a precise point located on the anthelix of the ear. To do this, she used a metal rod, tapered and heated to white at one end, which was then applied to the ear point to be treated. This somewhat crude method was nevertheless effective, as indeed, both patients were cured when returning from Marseille.

These two observations intrigued Paul Nogier and were the starting point that brought him to research the yet unexplored properties of the auricle. It dawned upon him that, considering sciatica is related to a problem on the L5 and S1 vertebrae, the fact that treating a precise point on the ear can alleviate the pain must imply the existence of a correspondence of some kind between the L5-S1 vertebrae and this "Barrin point" on the ear. Furthermore, if that were the case, it would be unlikely for this point to be just an isolated connection between the spine and the ear, and consequently, one could expect the entire spine to be "represented" on the ear. This reasoning led Nogier to formulate a basic hypothesis on the existence of a coherent mapping system inherent to the auricle. From then on, other points were to be found, such as a shoulder point, a knee point, a stomach point, and a pancreas point. Indeed, all the organs and parts of the body are represented in the ear. A mapping of the human body can be drawn on the auricle and used to treat functional disorders and pain. Thus, being trained as an acupuncturist, Paul Nogier, when he began treating auricular points, used gold and silver needles. He named the method he had developed "auriculotherapy".

It took Nogier several years to lay the foundations of this method. What appears obvious today was largely a mystery in the 1950s. For his research, Paul Nogier used a simple procedure. He assumed that pain located in a limb, or an organ would cause a specific point to appear on the ear and that this point would itself become painful when pressed with a rod. With statistical methods, one could show a correlation between the anatomic structures of the body and the various auricular points. Every time a new point was discovered, it would be submitted to numerous verifications and would then be published. But the exploration of the auricle was hampered by doubts, errors, and animated scientific discussions. Nevertheless, after 15 years of research, Paul Nogier succeeded in producing a very precise map containing points representing the spine, the upper and lower limbs, the abdominal and thoracic viscera, and the endocrine glands. This was a great achievement. The only thing missing was the location of the central nervous system.

And then in 1966, 15 years after the onset of his research on the ear, Paul Nogier discovered a new phenomenon, of which the wide scope of applications eventually led to a better understanding of the body's adaptation to a non-specific stimulation. When applying pressure to certain points on the ear, he simultaneously perceived a tactile variation of the radial pulse, which became stronger or weaker without affecting the heart rate. After many trials, he became convinced that there must be a link between the ear and the heart, an analogue to that existing between the eye and the heart (*Oculo-Cardiac-Reflex*). He, therefore, called this new phenomenon the *Auricular-Cardiac-Reflex* (in French *Réflexe Auriculo-Cardiaque RAC*) and later introduced an English name: *Vascular Autonomic Signal VAS*.

This arterial reflex enabled Nogier to explore the points on the ear and assess the reactions of each patient when stimulating the ear. Does the pulse become stronger or weaker? This evaluation of points allowed him to select the type of metal to treat points: gold or silver.

Initially seen as a means for improving detection of points in auriculotherapy, the arterial reflex is, in fact, a very general phenomenon that clearly goes beyond the scope of the ear and the heart. In 1943, an illustrious French surgeon, René Leriche, had observed in a patient he had operated for an aneurysm of the thigh, a phenomenon resembling that discovered by Paul Nogier (see Chapter 2.4.2). Leriche had found that touching the thigh caused an unusual "beat" on the femoral artery. He interpreted this as a local cutaneous-vascular phenomenon and did not pursue this observation any further.

Paul Nogier's originality consisted in understanding the arterial reflex as a general phenomenon and not as a local one so that it could be used to measure the adaptation of the organism to the various stresses to which it can be exposed. Arteries are innervated by the autonomic nervous system, particularly by the sympathetic system. By placing one's finger on an artery, one can, therefore, evaluate the tone of the artery with each pulse and so indirectly measure the activity of the sympathetic system. In short, the arterial reflex measures the body's ability to react to a stimulus.

Without knowing it, Paul Nogier had discovered a new clinical method of exploring the neuro-vegetative autonomous system. As we will see later, this system is involved in defence mechanisms, adaptation, and, ultimately, the maintenance of homeostasis.

Paul Nogier used the RAC for 30 years on all his patients. He initially studied the effect of stimulating ear points and, in a second stage, the effect of stimulating the skin in general. This enabled him to develop a method that one of his students misnamed "auriculomedicine" on the grounds that it uses the vascular signal for diagnosis and auriculotherapy for treatment (see Chapter 2.5).

## 1.2 DIFFUSION OF PAUL NOGIER'S METHOD

The term "auriculomedicine" was unfortunate because it suggested that the method was only concerned with the auricle, which is not the case. It was a poorly chosen term that undoubtedly contributed to maintaining at a distance valuable scientists who would have been able to contribute substantial elements to the understanding of this brilliant discipline. These scientists perhaps also feared a sectarian drift due to the ambiguity of the word auriculomedicine. I understand them. Paul Nogier himself disapproved of the term, and in 1983, in Montreal, proposed to replace "auriculomedicine" by the expression "*signal medicine*", which indeed appears much more logical. Today, however, it would prove difficult to abolish the term "auriculomedicine" altogether because it is still widely used by many who practice the method.

Imprecision of language was and remains one of the drawbacks of the method developed by Paul Nogier. The term "auriculomedicine" is an example. Many other terms have been and still are confusing. Paul Nogier, in the process of discovering new phenomena, often invented terms that were remote from classical medicine. He did not take time to give these new words a precise definition to the extent that some of his many students believed they understood concepts that he himself did not imagine. Imprecision of language has led to confusion, waste of time, and unfortunate drifts.

In the field of medicine, all hypotheses are acceptable so long as the language used to describe them is common to everyone and does not become hermetic. The words used must be simple and perfectly defined. One cannot discuss a scientific issue without a language shared by all. Medicine is a unity and cannot be divided into chapels. It is an art that calls upon many techniques and many specialties, each having a precise indication. Auriculotherapy and vascular signal research are disciplines, amongst others. A common language brings them together and unites them (see Epilogue).

Whenever Paul Nogier published papers on auriculotherapy, he had to face considerable criticism. Inserting a needle into an ear to alleviate pain was not an easily acceptable gesture within the scientific community. Yet, this was by no means comparable to the criticism he endured when he came out with his discovery of the vascular signal.

Since clinical use of the vascular signal depends solely on the practitioner's skill and experience, the measurement is subjective. It is therefore important to always refer to the physiological and pathological aspects, assessing the results obtained by means of the vascular signal according to their true value. It is necessary to denounce unscrupulous practitioners who have misused the vascular signal by misinterpreting it. Unfortunately, this has led the method to regrettable drifts, making us forget its brilliant and physiological aspects.

Paul Nogier taught his method mainly on frequent conference weekends, both at the medical association that he had founded in Lyon, France (GLEM: Groupe Lyonnais d'Études Médicales) and at his Advanced Course (Cours Supérieur). Facing large audiences composed of loyal students, he produced a truly original medical method based on the vascular signal and the ear. His very particular manner of approaching medical issues came up against preconceived ideas. By and large, he created a genuine school of thought.

Paul Nogier wrote little. His first book, written at the age of 61, *A Treatise of Auriculotherapy*, was published by Maisonneuve in 1969. The drawings were made by Dr. René Bourdiol, a neurophysiologist with whom he worked closely from 1966 to 1981. Both had strong personalities, complementary to each other, and were passionately interested in medicine. Their collaboration gave rise to criticism, contradiction, and positive emulation. René Bourdiol was, in my opinion, one of the great French physicians of the 20th century. An outstanding speaker and author, he left us with exceptional publications such as "*Elements of Auriculotherapy*" or "*Pied et Statique*", a genuine treasure for understanding back pain.

By 1975, Paul Nogier had launched a quarterly journal, "*Auriculomédecine*", in which he discussed his theories and observations. This journal had a few contributors. Professor Pierre Magnin, Dean of the Faculty of Medicine in Besançon, France, set the tone: "Auriculomedicine will be scientific, or it will not be". René Bourdiol produced general papers on auriculotherapy, but it was Paul Nogier who wrote most of the articles. The journal would contain the results of certain important discoveries and throughout the series of articles, one could follow the evolution of auriculomedicine techniques.

In 1981, Paul Nogier and René Bourdiol split apart and carried on with their work separately. As a result, at the age of 73, Paul Nogier no longer had a talented contradictor by his side and so lost his alter ego. This had a negative influence on the clarity of the method.

Shortly after, he published "From Auriculotherapy to Auriculomedicine". Written somewhat hurriedly to meet his publisher's repeated demands, this book is understandable for those who are already familiar with the method but totally obscure for those who are not. From 1981 to 1996, Paul Nogier carried on his research and teaching, but the fundamental aspects of his method had already been laid.

## 1.3 PAUL NOGIER'S METHOD TODAY

Auriculotherapy brings together a wide range of techniques part of which requires the vascular signal (RAC) and mainly the auricle as a reflex site.

Today, various approaches exist, several ways of proceeding and several "sub-schools" all in line with each other. These disparities, however, are a source of confusion for those who wish to be informed about the method.

Basically, these different approaches can be divided as follows:

*Paul Nogier's original method* is now taught by students who were close to Paul Nogier, such as Dr Anthony de Sousa, Dr Chantal Vulliez, Dr Jean-Luc Vigneron, Dr Bernard Julienne, Dr Bernard Deffonfaines, Dr Yves Rouxeville, Dr Jean Girardot, and many others, who were trained at the Advanced course. The method is based on auricular reflexotherapy, the RAC, frequencies, phases, and other techniques, which we will discuss later. Nevertheless, although efficient, the method remains complex because the terms were not clearly defined. It always comes up against the same problem of language. What was true in 1980 is still true today. A discipline that is not based on precise language is difficult to transmit. In this book, we will attempt to describe the techniques used by Paul Nogier by placing them in their historical and scientific context.

*Dr Frank Bahr's method* has the same basic aspects as Paul Nogier's method: auricular somatotopy, RAC, frequencies, etc., but it differs in spirit. Frank Bahr, a physician from Munich, comes up with notions of energy, yin, and yang. Referring to the name of Paul Nogier, he spread throughout Germany a set of techniques to which he gave names different from those given by Paul Nogier when he initially discovered them. Nogier's auriculotherapy in Germany is known as "Nogier/Bahr ear acupuncture"; the vascular signal became "the dynamic pulse", the frequencies discovered by Paul Nogier were revised and called "Bahr's frequencies", etc. Furthermore, Frank Bahr developed techniques, against which the creator of auriculotherapy was vigorously opposed. Dr. Bahr was a pupil of Paul Nogier and René Bourdiol in 1973 and 1974, 22 years after the discovery of auriculotherapy and six years after the discovery of the RAC. He worked mainly as an assistant to Paul Nogier in 1974 during the revision of auricular mapping using the RAC.

*Professor Pierre Magnin's approach:* Pierre Magnin, although younger than Paul Nogier, was the godfather, the good fairy who supervised the development of signal medicine. A brilliant academic, former Dean, and former rector of the Faculty of Medicine in Besançon, he became interested in the RAC for two reasons. The first is that he had always been aware of the importance of the neurovegetative system in the onset of diseases. For him, the study of the RAC is the only proper way of assessing how this system functions. The second reason implies his personal history and goes back to his childhood. When he was about 12 years old, one of his sisters, who had fallen seriously ill, was saved by a healer. The healer applied a therapy based on the action of crystals of different colours. Thus, having graduated as a doctor, Pierre Magnin became interested in colour therapy. Throughout his life, he had the same idea in mind: how to use photons for the process of healing. When he met Paul Nogier at the end of the 1960s, he realised that the RAC could help him in his research. So, he learned the technique of taking the pulse in search of the RAC and used it to treat his patients by projecting coloured lights on the body and on the ear. Pierre Magnin used the ear points only with punctual photonic stimulations while controlling the patient's reaction by means of the RAC.

In the last years of his life, Pierre Magnin spoke of *photonic medicine* to describe the technique he had developed. His method is based on the fundamentals of auriculotherapy: the use of the properties of the auricle, the RAC, and the use of photonic stimulation on the body and on the ear. It does not differ in substance from the method that Paul Nogier had developed. Moreover, Pierre Magnin has always referred to Paul Nogier's work. Personally, I do not advocate creating new terms when they are redundant. They can, in fact, lead to unnecessary questioning. The term photonic medicine suggests that this technique is not part of auriculotherapy, which is not the case. Pierre Magnin died in November 2020.

*The approach I developed myself.* It is a simplified technique. I rapidly understood that Paul Nogier's method could not be easily transmitted due to the vagueness of the terms used. My numerous trips abroad made me come across auriculomedicine techniques that were different from one country to another. In the United States, South America, Japan, Italy, and New Zealand, each one trimmed the method in their own manner. This can be explained by the fact that Paul Nogier did not teach according to a standard curriculum. He often proceeded by abandoning the ideas and techniques he had previously recommended, and when starting his classes, would warn the audience, saying: "Forget everything I told you last time, I was mistaken". One technique chased away the next; for example, those who had heard him in the United States in 1984 still scrupulously applied methods that the creator of signal medicine had abandoned entirely by 1985.

Despite the number of different techniques discovered during the 30 years of Paul Nogier's research with the RAC, there remains, however, a common pathway, a style of thinking, and a coherent working method well understood by those who had the opportunity of following the complete teaching of Paul Nogier. Here are some of the main ideas: auricular somatotopy, the vascular signal, cutaneous photoreception and photoemission, frequencies, the importance of laterality, etc.

The technique I use is similar to that of Pierre Magnin in that I favour photonic projection to diagnose and treat pathologies.

It is these fundamentals of auriculomedicine that we are about to explain in this book. Since 1993, I have tried to simplify and "standardise" the method by using accessible terms, which allows us today to engage in a coherent dialogue with the entire scientific community.

I know that this grooming process has raised and still raises irrational reactions on the part of some of my colleagues, "direct pupils of Paul Nogier". Ignoring the method's future, some have regarded my approach as iconoclastic or even as "murder of the father". Perhaps they will now become more aware of the absolute necessity of working on a synthesis, essential to future generations.

From 1978, when I completed my medical studies, I became the onlooker, the confident, and many a time the collaborator of a man who, despite a considerable entourage, found himself alone, with no opportunity to share his doubts as a researcher. Paul Nogier, naturally optimistic and independent, ploughed on through his own way without worrying about criticism. His many students would not feel in a position to contradict him. But because I was his son, he felt free to engage in informal conversations with me, during which we discussed basic aspects of his method and its development. Together, we had fascinating and exciting discussions.

In 1979, following numerous conversations of which I preciously keep fond memories, Paul Nogier published, at Maisonneuve publishing house, the book *L'Homme dans l'Oreille* (*The Man in the Ear*), of which I was the writer.

It was upon his request that I subsequently started teaching auriculotherapy. Not being able to travel anymore, he asked his foreign correspondents to invite me to speak in his place. I thus visited more than 30 different countries. In 1993, three years before his death, while writing the preface to a book of which I was the author: *Introduction to Auriculomedicine*, Paul Nogier laid on my shoulders the task of opening an objective manner of developing auriculomedicine.

I know it is difficult for a son to carry on his father's work without exposing himself to unflattering comparisons. My aim is not to modify his original work but simply to explain it so as to show its value. Unlike Paul Nogier, I am not myself a researcher, but on the other hand, I am very familiar with his way of thinking, so this gives me a certain ease in interpreting his work. I realised a long time ago that his discoveries had been misunderstood, and I felt it necessary to present them in a more accessible way.

The more recent techniques I am about to explain in the following chapters are based on the same reasoning as that used by Paul Nogier. Hopefully, the students of "The Boss" will forgive me for taking the liberty of presenting my techniques in a manner somewhat different from the initial teaching. They will understand that between what is desirable and what is possible, there is sometimes a rift so deep that it cannot be crossed.

Some years ago, with my friend Anthony de Sousa, we decided to write a book on the RAC. So here it now is. Each of us describes our own practice. Anthony presents a selection of the most basic and outstanding techniques created by Paul Nogier. Apart from attending the Advanced course, he travelled to Lyon every Tuesday for many years to participate in Paul Nogier's research group, thus acquiring valuable training in auriculotherapy and the RAC. Following this, I describe the concepts and techniques I have elaborated during recent years, putting a special emphasis on the importance of the sympathetic system concerning the RAC phenomenon. Thus, the reader will be able to take advantage of a wide range of techniques and choose those best suited to his practice.

Looking back on the experience I have acquired, taking the pulse of all my patients for over 36 years, I sincerely believe that the RAC is an irreplaceable tool. Today, I could not do without it, so great is the importance of the information I receive from it in view of the effective treatment of my patients.

I hope that my colleagues will themselves experience this phenomenon, which in turn will, I am sure, provide tomorrow's medicine with decisive progress. However, it must be understood for what it is.

Pierre Magnin was right in saying: "Auriculomedicine will be scientific, or it will not be".

## CHAPTER 2

# The RAC, General Considerations

**Anthony de Sousa**

## 2.1 WHAT IS THE RAC?

Amongst the numerous medical advances of the 20th century, the discovery of the RAC appears amongst the most surprising. Carried out in the 1960s, at a time when medicine was already strongly influenced by technological and pharmacological progress, the discovery of such a phenomenon could be considered unlikely. Without the aid of any technical means and relying solely on a wide experience of taking the pulse within the field of Chinese acupuncture, Paul Nogier unexpectedly came across a subtle and unprecedented variation in the intensity of the pulse, *as a result of skin stimulation*, a reflex action that was subsequently to entail a vast number of clinical applications, as it were a step back into the Hippocratic spirit of the past (**Figure 2.1**).

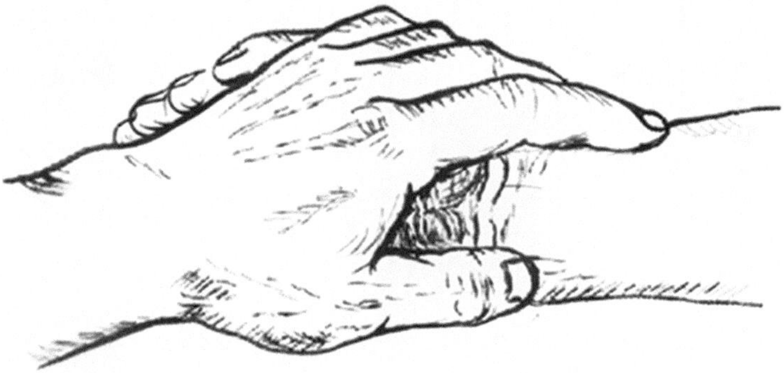

**Figure 2.1** Taking the radial pulse.

The RAC is a neurovegetative reflex, consisting of a temporary variation of the intensity of the arterial resting pulse. Independent of voluntary control, this variation integrates the three fundamental stages of reflex reaction: *stimulation, processing within the central nervous system,* and *response.* Whereas most neurological reflexes are processed within the *cerebrospinal nervous system*, the RAC differs in that it involves the *autonomic neurovegetative system* and the neuro-vegetative nuclei of the midbrain and the posterior hypothalamus [1]. Consequently, the response will not

DOI: 10.1201/9781003753629-2

imply striated muscles in a segmental manner, as would be the case for a cerebrospinal reflex, but rather *smooth muscles* of the entire arterial network, in a ubiquitous manner, regardless of the starting point of stimulation.

Most often, we are dealing with a "***cutaneous-vascular***" type reflex, which can be induced by means of any stimulation of the skin surface, whether mechanical (touch, light pressure), electrical, or thermal. More surprisingly, stimulation can also be carried out *at a distance* (a few centimetres) without direct contact, during a momentary exposure of the skin to a continuous or intermittent white or coloured light source (**Figure 2.2**). It can also consist of an electromagnetic field.

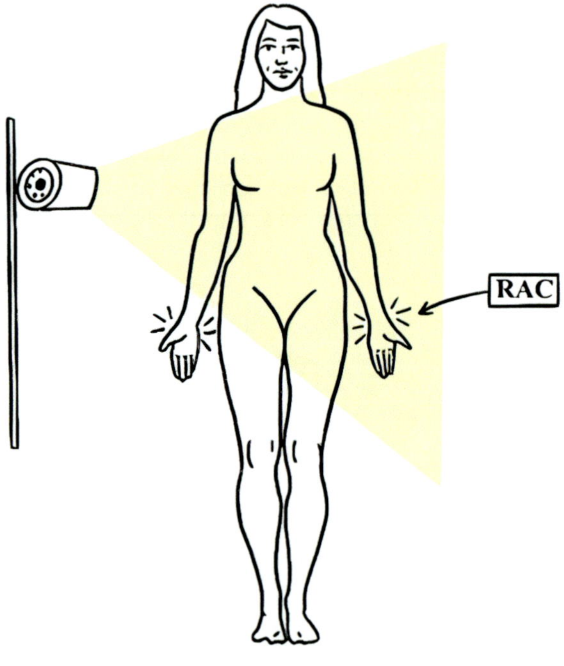


**Figure 2.2** A RAC reaction can be triggered remotely, e.g., by means of a light source.

At the time of its discovery, Paul Nogier was puzzled as to what could be the possible usefulness of such a reflex. Initially, considering the stimulation of reflex action as limited to the skin surface of the ear, he imagined it might serve the purpose of a new method of detecting pathological points on the ear. Later, however, he realized that this reflex was a much more general phenomenon, and that a vascular signal could be obtained not only by stimulating the ear, but in fact, any part of the skin. Considering the type of skin stimulation (e.g., a colour or a light frequency) and the pulse response obtained, the reflex action obtained could be used as a method of *diagnostic measurement*. The arterial reflex then appeared as a very general clinical tool, a new way of *questioning* the organism, hence leading to a genuine *semiology method* based on the arterial reflex.

Moreover, it should be noted that the origin of the stimulation is not necessarily *cutaneous*, i.e., *external*. Because of the sensitivity of our neuro-vegetative system to emotions, a vascular reaction can often be the expression of an emotional reaction [2]. The source of stimulation is then *internal*, and in this case, the reflex could be named "***neuro-vascular***" (as opposed to "*cutaneous-vascular*"). This type of arterial reflex can in many cases be used when treating emotional disorders. During the verbal exchange with the patient, the therapist simultaneously takes the pulse (Section 28.1.1–3).

For the sake of clarity, let us finally specify that the RAC is by no means the same as the pulse used in Chinese traditional medicine. The RAC implies a dynamic aspect, linked to the notions of *reflex* and stimulation, which is not the case regarding the Chinese pulse.

## 2.2 DEFINITION OF THE RAC

We have seen that the RAC appears most often as a *cutaneous-vascular reflex*, the response to which is immediately perceptible by taking the arterial pulse. Paul Nogier (see **Figure 2.5**) compared the resting pulse to a carrier wave, capable of conveying an additional signal, the RAC. In 1979, several years after its discovery, he spoke of it in the following terms: "*The human body reacts to external stimuli by an unconscious vascular response*" [3]. In 2012, this definition was somewhat amplified by Raphaël Nogier: "*The vascular signal is a manually perceptible transient arterial reaction located on distal arteries. This phenomenon exists within any healthy individual and consists in a transient activity of the neuro-vegetative system during adaptation*" [4].

## 2.3 PURPOSE OF THE RAC

This notion of adaptation leads us to the interesting question of the biological significance of the vascular reflex. The ability of the skin interface to transmit all sorts of stimuli from the outside world into the organism is part of a dynamic equilibrium between the organism and its surroundings. According to Paul and Raphaël Nogier [3], any information from the outside world is received by the skin and transmitted to the nerve centres, which in turn analyse the information in order to produce a response that best ensures adaptation and the maintenance of homeostasis via the sympathetic system.

The other aspect of this adaptation system concerns pathology. According to Pierre Magnin [1], "*the neuro-vegetative nervous system has a permanent function of monitoring the state of health of the organism in terms of nervous physiology. The*

*RAC must therefore be considered as a mode of signalling, identifying and locating parasitic or damaged territories or tissues*".

## 2.4 HISTORICAL ASPECTS

### 2.4.1 The Concept of Pulse

History of medicine shows that the concept of pulse took a long time to emerge. At the time of Hippocrates and Aristotle, there was no precise notion of pulse, and the arteries were supposed to contain air! It was Galen, during the 2nd century AD, who first observed that the arteries were filled with blood, and who established a relationship between the heart and the arteries. His views persisted for fifteen centuries until the discovery of blood circulation in the 17th century by the British physician William Harvey (**Figure 2.3**). Harvey asserted that the pulse resulted from cardiac ejection, and this gradually led to the notions of fluid transmission and pulsatile wave during the 18th and 19th centuries.

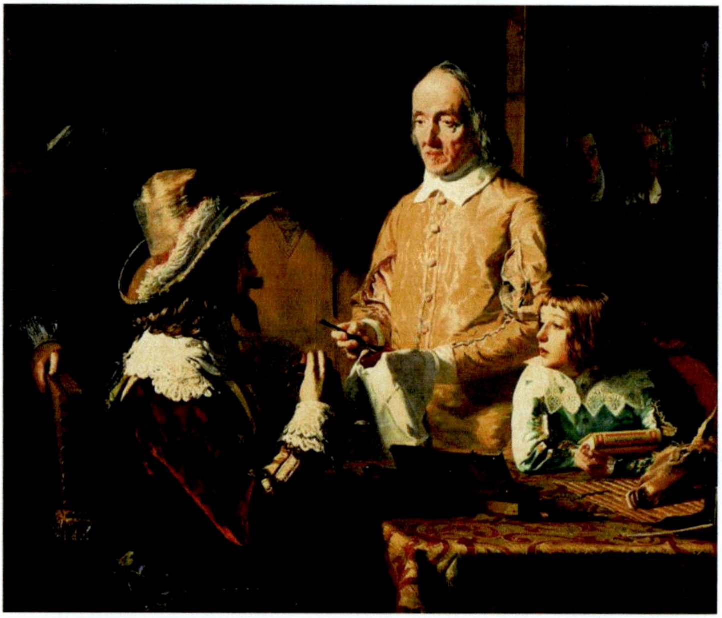

**Figure 2.3** William Harvey explaining his theory of blood circulation to King Charles 1st and his heir. (*Source*: Painting by Robert Hannah. Medical Tribune.)

In 1859, the French physician Etienne-Jules Marey designed a device, the *sphygmograph*, which enabled him to make the first experimental recording of the pulse, thus opening the way to the study of *haemodynamics*.

### 2.4.2 A Precursor, René Leriche

Finally, it was during the troubled context of the Great War of 1914–18, that the notion of *reflex variation of the pulse* first appeared, with René Leriche (1879–1955), a French surgeon famous for his achievements in several fields, particularly vascular surgery, pain surgery, and the sympathetic system [5]. In 1917, at that time, a war surgeon, Leriche, made a remarkable observation on soldiers suffering from arterial lesions: he noticed that the wounded vessel would "beat" whenever he touched the surrounding skin (**Figure 2.4**).

A few years later, in 1943, Leriche published another very similar observation made two years earlier, in his book "*Physiologie pathologique et chirurgie des artères*" [2]. After having operated on a patient suffering from an arterio-venous aneurysm in the left thigh, Leriche observed that while renewing the dressing, the simple fact of touching the surrounding skin produced a characteristic "beat" on the residual aneurysm. Moreover, the patient reported to Leriche that a similar "beat" occurred while he was reading a detective novel, when coming to the more gripping passages.

Noticeably, this example can be said to illustrate by itself both the external *cutaneous-vascular* aspect (stimulation by the skin) and the internal *neuro-vascular* aspect (mental, or emotional stimulus) of the reflex, as described earlier.

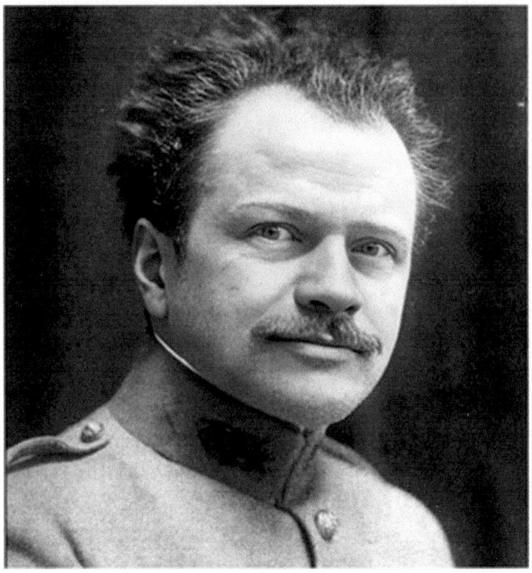

**Figure 2.4** René Leriche, at the time of the Great War. (*Source*: Wikipedia.)

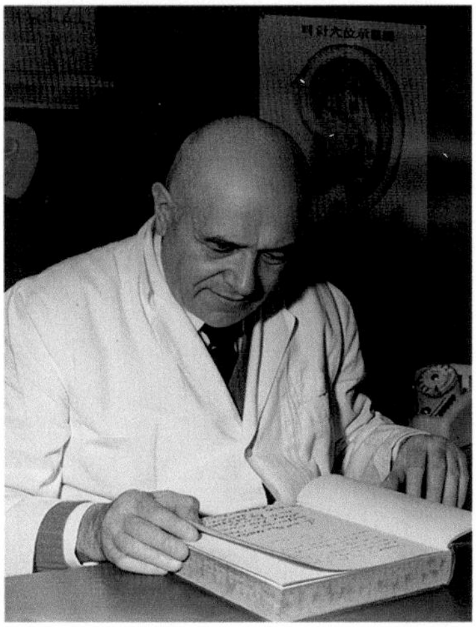

**Figure 2.5** Paul Nogier at the time when he discovered the RAC. (Copyright Raphaël Nogier.)

Despite his wide knowledge regarding the sympathetic system, Leriche is not known to have pursued the study of this phenomenon, considering it merely as a local reflex. Nevertheless, he did make a remarkable comment in relation to his observation, saying that: "*Pathology can reveal phenomena which are thus amplified, and which could not have been observed under normal physiological conditions*". Indeed, it can be said that the arterial reaction, which would later prove so fine and subtle to perceive on a healthy artery, was observed by chance by Leriche, thanks to an *amplification* resulting from the pathological weakening of the arterial wall.

While regrettably Leriche did not live to know about the work of Paul Nogier (**Figure 2.5**) many years later, it must be acknowledged to what point, without knowing it, Leriche turned out to be such a remarkable precursor.

### 2.4.3 Discovery of the RAC

Twenty-three years later, in 1966, the discovery of the RAC on a *normal* artery occurred very unexpectedly. Paul Nogier would later refer to it in the following terms: "*This new discovery, due to very particular circumstances, or should I even say incredible chance, revived my appetite for knowledge*" [3].

This comment suggests a well-known process in science, known as *serendipity*, according to which a researcher is suddenly faced with a new, unforeseen discovery, at a time when he was in the process of exploring something very different. The most characteristic aspect of this notion is the fact that, whereas an unprepared person might well miss the opportunity, by contrast chance will favour an open, flexible, and curious mind, capable of grasping the meaning and significance of the unexpected observation. So indeed, this process might well be said of Paul Nogier, whether referring to his initial findings on auricular mapping in 1951, or to his discovery of the arterial reflex 15 years later.

How did this "second discovery" come about? In Nogier's own words [3]: "In 1966 I had already been working on auriculotherapy for more than 15 years. The time spent on studying it ensured a maximum of precision". Nogier had by then shifted on to a different field. Resuming his knowledge of acupuncture, he had begun to explore the Chinese pulse, in search of a new, intermediary parameter linking yin and yang, and which he called yu [1]. But so doing, he had always kept the habit of examining the ear of all his patients while at the same time taking the radial pulse (**Figure 2.6**).

*"One day", continues Nogier, "while examining a patient, I realized that when I touched his ear, the pulse became totally different and collapsed. I stopped touching the ear, and the pulse became normal again. Once more I stimulated the auricle, and the pulse collapsed. I repeated the experience several times before dismissing the patient. The phenomenon would not fail to repeat itself"* [3].

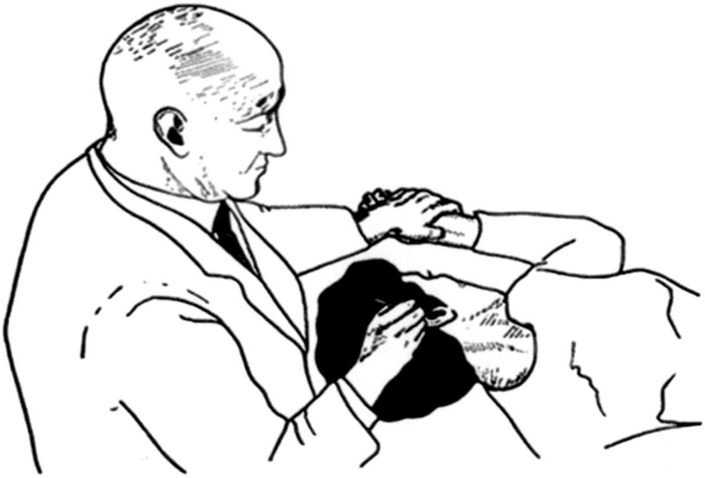

**Figure 2.6** Drawing of Paul Nogier, simultaneously examining the ear and the radial pulse. (Copyright Raphaël Nogier.)

At first, Nogier felt somewhat puzzled by his discovery: "*It was in 1966 that I discovered this reflex, first step into an unexplored territory. But I must confess that [at that time] it did not get me anywhere*". It was only gradually, as mentioned earlier, that Nogier saw it as possibly a new means of detecting pathological points on the ear. Later on, he studied the reactions of the pulse when touching an ear point with different kinds of rods (cork, cold, heat), but eventually considered this process long and tedious in the context of medical examination (Chapter 7). So, understandably, it took Nogier some time to grasp the full potential linked to the vascular reflex he had discovered, thus opening a vast and impressive field of exploration during the following years.

At the time of his discovery, Nogier had no knowledge of Leriche's observations, and the phenomenon remained unheard of within the medical and scientific community. Furthermore, it is noteworthy that without knowing it, his discovery led Nogier to implicitly contradict Leriche's remark, according to which such a phenomenon would remain unnoticed within normal arteries.

## 2.5 NAMING THE ARTERIAL REFLEX, A LONG PROCESS

Naturally, this new phenomenon had to be found a name. After having discovered the reflex in 1966, Paul Nogier had imagined it as being possibly analogous to the oculo-cardiac reflex, hence naming the new phenomenon (in French): Réflexe Auriculo-Cardiaque (Auriculo-Cardiac Reflex), abbreviated **RAC**.

Carrying on with his research, however, Nogier realized that the possibility of eliciting the reflex was in no way limited to the ear but could just as well be triggered by touching the skin on any part of the body. Such an important change required finding a new name, and for this purpose, Nogier took advice from Pierre Magnin, a friend of his and professor of pathophysiology. Magnin devised an English designation: the **Vascular Autonomic Signal**. Abbreviated **VAS**, this new name was thought to be more consistent with the physiology of the reflex, whilst at the same time bearing a more international connotation. At the same time, several other names were suggested, generally with the idea of honouring Paul Nogier's discovery. Amongst others (translated from French): Nogier's vascular signal, or Nogier's arterial reflex, imagined by René Bourdiol, or even Nogier's sign, devised by Frank Bahr. However, none of these designations took over.

In fact, as could be expected, most French-speaking practitioners, long since habituated to using the expression RAC, naturally continued to do so. Besides, it was felt that a French discovery should have a French designation. To that effect, the abbreviation RAC was reintroduced, however, with a different meaning: **Réflexe Autonome Circulatoire**. Eventually, it was decided to standardize both expressions **RAC** and **VAS** as two generalized **acronyms**.

Throughout this book, the arterial reflex will be referred to as **the RAC**.

## 2.6 WHAT TACTILE SENSATIONS CORRESPOND TO A POSITIVE OR NEGATIVE RAC?

Considering that perception of the RAC is a purely subjective sensation, it is important to describe what kinds of tactile impressions are to be expected. Taking the pulse requires concentration for the purpose of carrying out ***a mental comparison*** between two different states of hardness of the arterial pulse.

The observer is to feel a subtle variation in the tension or hardness of the pulse beat following stimulation of the skin, in comparison with the hardness of the pulse during steady state at rest (**Figure 2.7**). This sensation is often compared to what might be felt when applying one's finger on a bicycle tyre when it is being inflated or deflated. When the pulse becomes *harder* with skin stimulation, this is a **positive RAC**. When the pulse becomes *softer,* it is called a **negative RAC**, or a **collapsed pulse** (see **Figure 5.15**). It is interesting to recall here that Paul Nogier described his very first observation of pulse change as a *negative RAC*.

The polarised nature of the vascular response (positive or negative RAC) is somewhat like that of a neurological cerebrospinal reflex, which may appear "enhanced" or "diminished". In practice, experience shows that a *positive RAC* represents the most frequent response to most pathological situations. Whereas a *negative RAC* is more

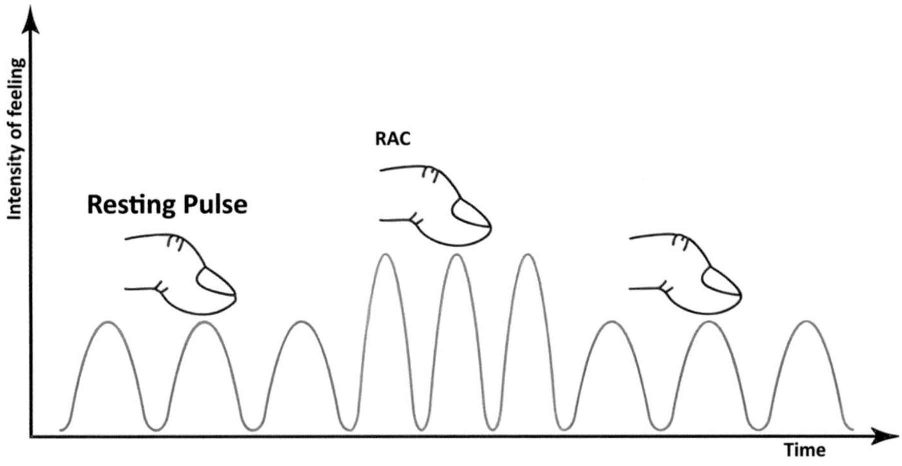


**Figure 2.7** Subjective representation of resting pulse intensity (blue curves) and a positive RAC intensity (red curves). Negative RAC is not represented here.

specifically the expression of loss of vitality. Practically speaking, a negative RAC can be found typically in the following situations, which will be discussed in later chapters:

1. when applying light touch to a *pathological scar* (Section 16.2.1),
2. in case of *food intolerance*, when placing the food test ring on the patient's chest (Section 27.4.4),
3. in the event of *RAC exhaustion*, when repeatedly flashing a light on the patient's chest (Section 10.1.5). However, in this case, the lowering of intensity of the RAC is progressive, at least over 3 cycles or more, whereas in the other two examples, (1) and (2), the collapse of the RAC is immediately perceptible from the very first cycle.

## 2.7 QUANTITATIVE ASPECT OF THE RAC

Whether positive or negative, the vascular reaction also has an important quantitative aspect. This means that for a given measurement, the *number* of RAC reactions produced is not random. The reaction will be maintained over a definite number of cycles. This is important to specify because it determines the intensity or importance of the measured parameter. Examples include: the degree of pathology of a point detected at the ear, the intensity of a person's addiction to tobacco, or the importance of a food hypersensitivity. Once the number is reached, the intensity of the pulse will return to its resting value from one cycle to the next. The threshold for a significant response is generally two to three reactionary pulses, i.e., the first two reactionary pulses are normal, related merely to the skin contact.

This rule of quantification has an exception: the so-called **rebound** reaction: this is a non-quantifiable positive RAC. It only lasts for the time of one, or at most two pulses, but with strong intensity, felt as a sort of blow, before the pulse immediately returns to its resting intensity.

N.B. If one wishes to note the number of cycles obtained, the correct spelling of *RAC* in the plural reads ***RACs***. *VAS*, however, does not change in the plural.

## 2.8 THE RAC IS NOT ESSENTIALLY LINKED TO AURICULOTHERAPY

The circumstances of the discovery of the RAC have created a certain ambiguity in relation to auriculotherapy. True enough, the discovery was carried out by an auriculotherapist, who was working simultaneously on the auricle and the pulse at the time of his observation. And indeed today, auriculotherapy remains an area in which the RAC plays an important part. However, many other techniques using the RAC, such as investigation of food hypersensitivity, drug intolerance, or the diagnosis of somatic pathology, do not necessarily involve the ear. The RAC is a diagnostic tool that can be applied to both general medicine and to auriculotherapy, and as such, basically remains a witness of sympathetic activity.

## BIBLIOGRAPHY

1. Magnin Pierre. *The RAC*, Annales du GLEM 2010-2011: 38
2. Leriche René. *Physiologie pathologique et chirurgie des artères* (Masson) 1943: 113–14
3. Nogier Paul and Raphaël. *L'Homme dans l'Oreille* (Maisonneuve) 1979: 101–102; 106; 114
4. Nogier Raphaël. *L'Alimentation personnalisée* (Sully) 2012: 1067
5. Rouxeville Yves. *The lessons of Professor Leriche*, Annales du Glem 2010–2011: 102
6. Asis Daniel. *Le traitement des traumatismes psycho-émotionnels par auriculothérapie*, 7e symposium international d'auriculothérapie, Lyon 2012
7. Nogier Paul. *From Auriculotherapy to Auriculomedicine* (Maisonneuve) 1981
8. Sinoue Gilbert. *Avicenna or the Road to Ispahan* (Gallimard) 1990: 104–124

CHAPTER 3

# The Neurovegetative System (Autonomic System) Organ Function

**Raphaël Nogier**

As we have seen, the RAC is an expression of the sympathetic system, so it seems important to review the physiology of this system to understand its mechanisms.

## 3.1 BASICS AND DEFINITIONS

Basically, our nervous system can be divided into two parts: on the one hand, a conscious, will-dependent system, and on the other hand, a system that functions automatically, independent of will. The first is called the **cerebrospinal system**, the second the **neurovegetative** or **autonomic nervous system (Table 3.1)**.

**Table 3.1 Differences between the Cerebrospinal and Neurovegetative Nervous Systems**

| | Cerebrospinal nervous system | Autonomic nervous system Neurovegetative system |
|---|---|---|
| | **Relationship with the outside world** | **Controls homeostasis** |
| Mode of function | Voluntary and conscious | Involuntary, unconscious, self-regulated |
| Effector organs | Striated muscle | Smooth muscle, cardiac muscle, probably also striated muscle, glands |
| Type of pathways | Monosynaptic | Bi- or poly-synaptic |
| Neurotransmitters | Acetylcholine | Acetylcholine and Noradrenaline |
| Action | Fast and focused<br>Sensitive and motor | Multiple, diffuse, slower<br>Sensory and motor components |
| Central regulation | CNS, brainstem, anterior horn of medulla | Brainstem, solitary tract, peri-acquaducal grey matter, hypothalamus, amygdala |

1. **The cerebrospinal system** consists of:
   - the encephalon (brain, cerebellum, brainstem) and the spinal cord,
   - the peripheral nervous system, composed of the cranial, motor, and sensory nerves.
2. **The neuro-vegetative (or autonomous nervous system ANS)** innervates all the structures of the body: smooth muscles and striated muscles

DOI: 10.1201/9781003753629-3

(according to recent research), viscera, and the glandular (endocrine) system. It is involved in most metabolisms and ensures homeostasis and adaptation to the environment.

Independent of will, the ANS is made up of two complementary and sometimes antagonistic systems, the sympathetic and the parasympathetic.

Maintaining the stability of the internal environment and adaptation to external stresses is ensured by three major communication systems within the organism:

- Intercellular exchanges are managed locally
- The endocrine system, which operates at the humoral level
- The neurovegetative NVS or autonomous nervous system ANS [1]

The targets of the NVS are multiple:

- Secretory glands
- Smooth muscle
- Striated muscle
- The heart
- Blood vessels
- Bronchi
- The liver and gastrointestinal tract
- The kidney, bladder, large intestine, and rectum
- The genitalia
- The immune system

In other words, the neurovegetative system is omnipresent in the body and is constantly involved in the proper functioning of the organs.

## 3.2 GENERAL ORGANISATION OF THE AUTONOMOUS NERVOUS SYSTEM ANS

The ANS is composed of the sympathetic and parasympathetic systems, both of which work in harmony (**Table 3.2**). Each has its own action on the internal viscera. The two systems are organised in a specific way and work with specific neurotransmitters (**Figure 3.1**).

**Table 3.2 Differences between Parasympathetic and Sympathetic Systems**

| ANS / NVS | Parasympathetic | Sympathetic |
|---|---|---|
| Location of pre-ganglionic neurons | Brainstem sacral part of the spine | From T1 to L3 intermedio-lateralis column |
| Pre-ganglionic neurons | Very long, acetylcholine, Myelinated | Short, acetylcholine, Myelinated |
| Post-ganglionic neuron | Very short, acetylcholine, Non-myelinated | Noradrenaline, Non-myelinated |

*(Continued)*

**Table 3.2 (*Continued*) Differences between Parasympathetic and Sympathetic Systems**

| ANS / NVS | Parasympathetic | Sympathetic |
|---|---|---|
| Nerves | *Cranial nerves*: III, VII, IX, X<br>Sacral parasympathetic from S2 to S4 | Distribution of segments:<br>T1: head<br>T2: neck and upper limbs<br>T3 to T6: thorax<br>T7 to T11: abdomen<br>T12, L1, L2: inferior limbs |
| Activity | Works on the long-term<br>*Active over long periods*: digestion, anabolism | Rapidly active<br>Emergencies<br>Prepares for fight or flight, fright, sexual desire |
| Receptors | Nicotinic (parasymp. ganglia, acetylcholine)<br>*Muscarinic*: target organs, acetylcholine | |
| Local or general action | Local action<br>Possibility of stimulating part of the parasympathetic system | Works according to the all-or-none principle<br>Stimulation of part of the sympathetic system spreads to the whole system |

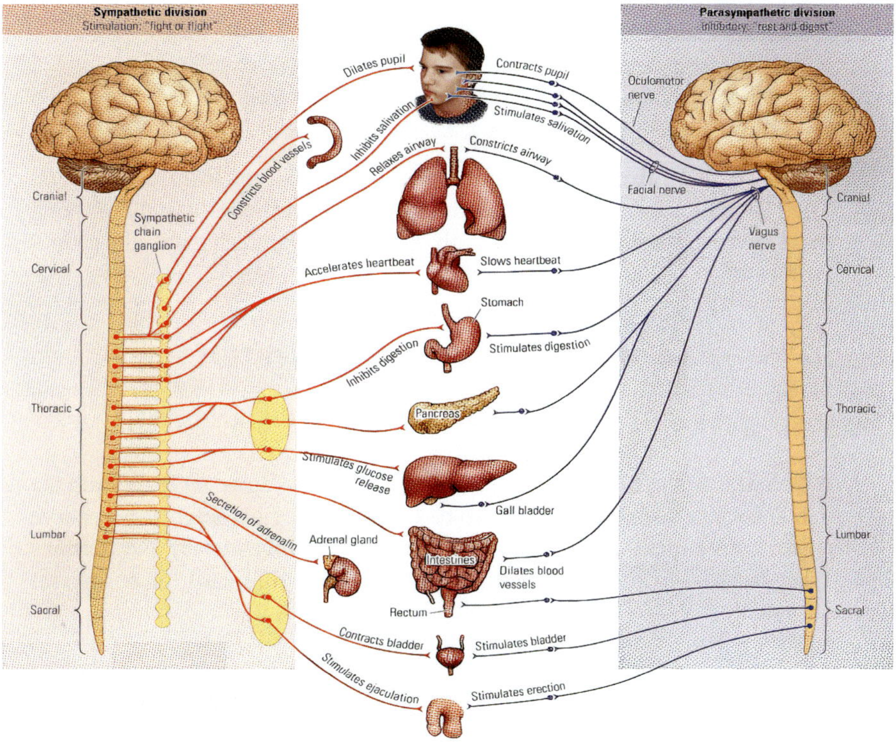


**Figure 3.1** The neuro-vegetative nervous system. (After Kolb, Cerveau et Comportement, 2nd edition 2006, page 105.)

## 3.3 THE SYMPATHETIC SYSTEM

The sympathetic system can be divided into different parts:

1. **Afferent pathways from the viscera and the skin.** These are sensory nerves that lead to the spinal cord at segmental levels from T1 to L2. The fibres end up in the spinal cord via the dorsal root and then relay to neurons located in the pars-intermedio lateralis. This part of the spinal cord is made of white matter.
2. **Sympathetic centres located on the spinal cord from T1 to L2** on a long column called the pars intermedio-lateralis. They give rise to efferent fibres that innervate the viscera.
3. **Efferent pathways consist of axons which emerge from the spinal cord through the anterior root** in the **spinal** nerve and relay in a ganglion (latero-vertebral or pre-vertebral) with a second neuron which will innervate the corresponding viscera. The pre-ganglionic neuron is myelinated; the second post-ganglionic neuron is unmyelinated.

   **The efferent sympathetic pathways are distributed as follows:**

   - T1 segment fibres go to the head
   - T2 segment fibres go to the neck and upper limbs
   - Fibres from segments T3 to T6 go to the thorax
   - Fibres from segments T7 to T11 go to the abdomen
   - Fibres from segments T12, L1, L2 go to the lower limbs
4. **Supra-segmental centres**, which receive information from the viscera. Their function is to control and modulate **sympathetic** activity. Among these centres, we not only find mainly the hypothalamus but also the reticular formation of the brainstem.

## 3.4 THE PARASYMPATHETIC SYSTEM

The parasympathetic system consists of:

1. **Afferents**: About 80% of the afferents travel in the Vagus nerve (X) and the pelvic nerves. Afferents are also to be found in the glossopharyngeal nerve (IX). A great deal of peripheral information is processed by the Solitary Tract Nucleus in the Brainstem, as it were a shunting yard for peripheral information.
2. **The centres**: These are located in the brainstem (cranial parasympathetic) and in the sacral part of the spinal cord (pelvic parasympathetic).
3. **Efferents**: The parasympathetic system has two neurons. The first neuron originates in the bulbar region and leads to a synapse with the second neuron, near or within the organ. Both neurons produce acetylcholine.

### 3.4.1 Interoceptors: Gathering Information

The body is full of sensors at all levels. These sensors send signals to the central nervous system, which processes the information and responds accordingly in a coherent manner to ensure that the internal environment is well-balanced. The sensors measure blood pressure, heart rate, muscle stretch, pH, glycemia, and partial pressure of $O_2$ and $CO_2$. The central nervous system will be alerted by the slightest abnormality and will generate a response.

### 3.4.2 Processing of Information by the Central Nervous System

The parts of the central nervous system involved are not only mainly the hypothalamus but also the tractus solitarius, the locus coeruleus, the hippocampus, and the amygdala.

The response may be either sympathetic or/and parasympathetic. It can be of four different types:

- **On/Off type**: (blood vessels of the skin which are innervated solely by the sympathetic).
- **Reciprocal type**: double innervation, one opposed to the other: e.g. mydriasis, miosis.
- **Synergistic type**: both innervations work in the same direction: e.g. salivary glands: parasympathetic > aqueous secretion; sympathetic > viscous secretion.
- **Cooperative type**: action in the same direction, and complementary: e.g. parasympathetic > erection; sympathetic > ejaculation.

A ***parasympathetic response*** will be localised. The parasympathetic system can indeed activate its different functions independently of each other (for example, only urination).

A ***sympathetic response*** is global. This means that all sympathetic functions will be activated at the same time but to different degrees. The sympathetic system can modulate its activation according to the levels of innervation (weak, moderate, or strong, basically) but the **sympathetic response is global** (Agnès Jacquin Piques). This can be explained by the close relationship existing between the pre-synaptic sympathetic ganglions. True enough, some small segments can be activated separately, but much more classically, sympathetic activity takes place throughout the whole organism when the circumstances motivate activation (Vander, Traité de Physiologie, 5th edition, page 204).

This network-type organisation of the sympathetic system explains the RAC. Stimulating one part of the sympathetic system, the skin, for example, is enough to alert the whole system and trigger a vascular reaction.

### 3.4.3 Under Physiological Conditions

The parasympathetic system is dominant during periods of rest and digestion, whereas the sympathetic system is dominant in periods of stress and activity (**Table 3.3**).

**Table 3.3 Different Actions of the Parasympathetic and Sympathetic Systems on Target Organs**

| Target organs | Parasympathetic rest and digestion | Sympathetic fight or flight |
|---|---|---|
| Heart rate | Reduced | Increased |
| Lungs, bronchi | Constriction | Dilation |
| Liver, glycogen | No effect | Glycogen utilisation Increase in blood glucose |
| Stomach | Increases HCl secretion | Decreases HCl secretion |
| Intestine | Increases mobility | Reduces mobility |
| Bladder | Promotes urination | Inhibits urination |
| Rectum | Promotes defecation | Inhibits defecation |
| Eye | Contracts the iris | Dilates the iris |
| Genitalia | Stimulates erection | Stimulates ejaculation |

In the event of stress or pathology, the autonomous nervous system will adapt its responses to the existing situation.

## 3.5 UNDER PATHOLOGICAL CONDITIONS

In the event of anoxia, inflammation, tissue suffering or of a lesion anywhere in the body, interoceptors will alert the CNS, which in turn will elicit a response in the neuro-vegetative system. Since it represents aggression, the response will be essentially sympathetic. It is a global response in which the immune system, placed under tension, will elaborate specific responses. This results in a whole series of reactions intended to circumscribe and eliminate the inflammation or lesion.

## 3.6 THE RAC AND THE AUTONOMOUS NERVOUS SYSTEM

The arterial reflex RAC, described by Paul Nogier, can be considered as an epiphenomenon of a physiological sympathetic reaction, which takes place during **adaptation** to a change in the environment or during stress (**Figure 3.2**). It is also present in case of aggression or pathology. In this case, it witnesses a **defence** process in which the sympathetic system takes part. In this case, the RAC takes on a different aspect, and represents a valuable signal that allows us to appreciate the global activity of the NVS. Until now, classical semiology had not yet described many clinical means of evaluating the activity of the sympathetic system.

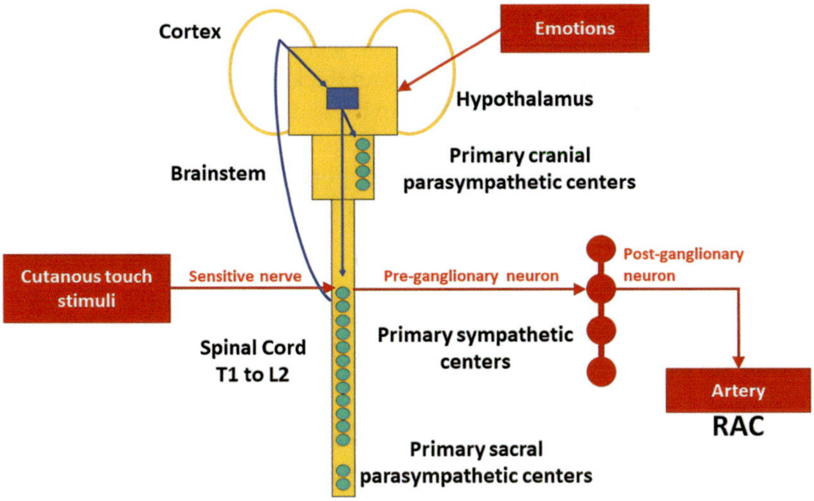


**Figure 3.2** Schematic representation of skin, sympathetic and parasympathetic systems, emotions, and RAC.

By using this vascular signal, it will be possible to establish diagnoses, all of which will focus on the neurovegetative aspect of the disease. We will primarily use the skin as an interface to assess ANS responses. While taking the radial pulse to feel the RAC reactions, we will stimulate the skin surface, which, as we have seen, is innervated only by sympathetic fibres. These skin stimulations will enable us to measure **two kinds of reactions** and, hence, make the difference between physiological and pathological reactions.

In the first place, the **general physiological reaction** of the sympathetic system. To investigate this aspect, we will stimulate very large areas of the skin. This is *the white light test*, (Chapter 9) consisting of a flash of light, for example, over the entire chest and abdomen (the stimulation must indeed be sufficiently wide and powerful to elicit a response, because in a healthy individual, a *narrow* light beam will not produce a RAC, whereas a *wide* beam will elicit a general RAC response, which may be altered in case of pathology.

Secondly, the **local reactions in search of pathology**. In this case, by contrast, we will stimulate only a very localised part of the skin, either by touch or with light. Normally, as we have seen, this type of stimulation by means of a narrow light beam does not trigger a RAC reaction, unless the skin surface that is exposed to the light beam is already subjected to stimulation by an underlying pathological viscera. The skin acts as a functional mirror of the viscera. Areas corresponding to the underlying viscera can be outlined on the skin. Even if the viscera is only mildly impaired by some functional problem, that will be sufficient for the corresponding skin portion to become painful, a phenomenon that

Dr Henri Jarricot of Lyon had highlighted with the description of *reflex dermalgia* (**Figure 21.3**). We know today that when a viscera is sick, there are sympathetic repercussions on the skin, leading to pain and thickening on palpation of the skin (palpation-roll method). This is due to the existence of viscero-cutaneous reflexes. If, for example, we examine a patient suffering from an inflamed sigmoid colon, the simple fact of mildly stimulating the skin portion that corresponds to the sigmoid colon will lead to a RAC reaction. This is due to convergence phenomena on the spinal cord segments.

Stimulation of a portion of skin already under tension because of some underlying pathology is what will trigger a RAC reaction.

## BIBLIOGRAPHY

1. Bonneau D. "*La peau, du diagnostic à la thérapeutique*", FEMMO Congress, Mulhouse 2003
2. Magnin Pierre, VIDAL Pascal. *Photonic medicine*, 2013
3. Nogier Raphaël. *History of auriculotherapy.* In Le livre Blanc de l'auriculothérapie. Coordinator Yves Rouxeville. Sauramps Médical 2020
4. Sauleau P., Jacquin-Piques A. *Vegetative nervous system.* Course in neurophysiology Aphysionado. https://sites.google.com/site/aphysionado/
5. Revillard. *Immunology* 2nd edition De Boeck Université 1995
6. Vander, Sherman, Luciano: *Human Physiology.* 5th edition. Pages 203 to 207, Maloine 2009

CHAPTER 4

# Practical Aspects of Taking the RAC

**Anthony de Sousa**

This chapter is primarily intended to provide a starting point for those wishing to train [1] in techniques using the vascular response. Taking the RAC is an act of subtle and fine perception, so it must be based on well-structured conditions.

## 4.1 DIFFERENT POSITIONS FOR PATIENT AND EXAMINER

We have seen previously that skin stimulation in view of eliciting a vascular reaction (RAC) can be performed on any part of the ear or body (soma). In practice, this will require some flexibility in choosing the most suitable position for examining the patient.

### 4.1.1 Classical Position for the Practice of RAC-Assisted Auriculotherapy

The examiner, if right-handed, positions himself in line behind the recumbent patient's head (**Figure 4.1**) to be able to take the patient's left radial pulse with his left hand. This leaves the right hand free to handle instruments, take measurements, and treat the auricles. This position also gives access to the head and is practical for working with test rings or frequency generators on the chest, arms, and head. A left-handed examiner can, of course, easily work in the inverse position, taking the right radial pulse with his right hand.

### 4.1.2 Taking the Pulse on the Patient's Opposite Wrist

This positioning (**Figure 4.2**) can be of use in various types of situations. For instance, the examiner may occasionally find it difficult or even impossible to feel the left radial pulse due to some individual anatomical variation, e.g. when the radial artery is located too deep under the skin surface, particularly in overweight patients. More seldom, the artery may follow an unusual anatomical pathway on the lateral or even the dorsal side of the wrist, which will turn out to be less stable and tend to roll under the effect of palpation. Moreover, the pressure wave travelling at high speed inside the artery may lead to a lateral escape phenomenon also called buckling (see **Figure 4.14**) [1], which in turn will distort perception of the vascular signal. Naturally, the patient's left wrist may also be temporarily inaccessible due to a cast or the local presence of allodynia (when touch is perceived as painful), for example.

DOI: 10.1201/9781003753629-4

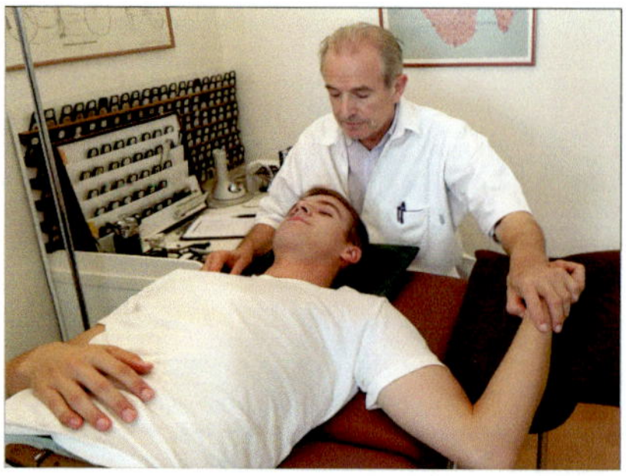

**Figure 4.1** Classical position for examination of the ear using the pulse. (From Ref. [2].)

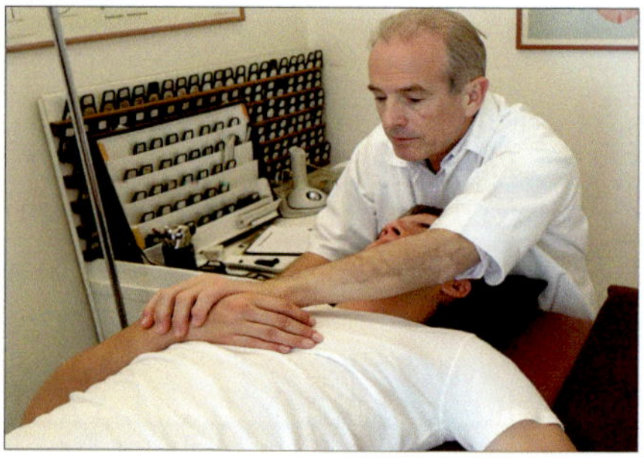

**Figure 4.2** Pulse measurement on the opposite wrist.

All these situations can be a minor drawback, but on the whole should not prevent a good quality examination.

The following positions are applicable both in the context of an auriculotherapy [3] examination and as a diagnostic tool for general medicine.

### 4.1.3 Examination of the Soma, Face-to-Face Position

Taking the pulse face-to-face is mainly used for dental examination or in case of a sinus pathology, for example. In **Figure 4.3**, the examiner takes the patient's right pulse with his left hand while scanning a colour filter over the sinus region with his right hand.

### 4.1.4 Examination of the Anterior Wall of Chest and Abdomen, with Patient Supine

In this position, the examiner stands on the patient's side, takes the (left or right) radial pulse with his left hand (**Figure 4.4**), while scanning an instrument (e.g. a

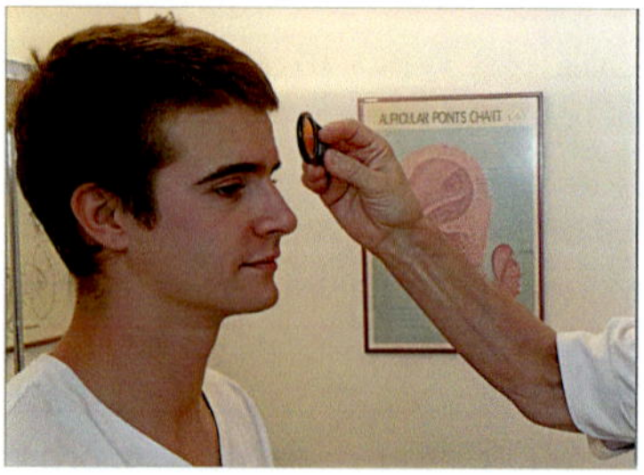

**Figure 4.3** Taking the pulse face-to-face.

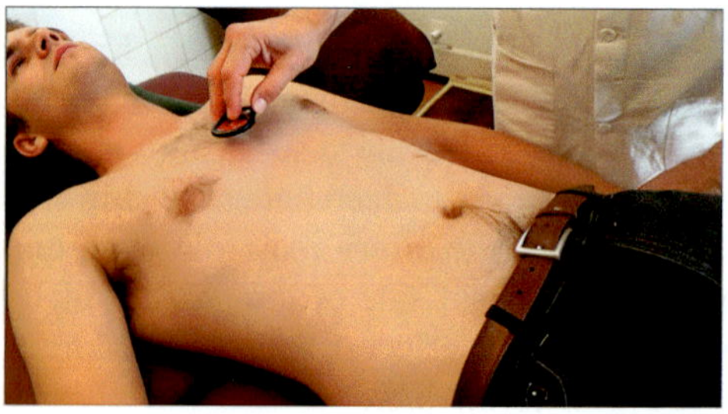

**Figure 4.4** Scanning an instrument over the anterior wall of chest and abdomen. (From Ref. [4].)

colour filter or lamp) with his right hand over the anterior wall of chest or abdomen (at one or two cm distance). A RAC reaction may appear when the filter reaches a part of skin under that lies an impaired organ. This is due to convergence onto a particular level of the spinal cord, between the reactive part of the skin and the underlying impaired organ (see Chapter 3).

### 4.1.5 Examination of Back and Spine, with Patient Standing

This positioning, patient standing, gives access mainly to the spine and the lungs.

Similarly to the preceding example, the examiner takes the patient's left radial pulse with his left hand while scanning an appropriate instrument (e.g. a colour filter) along the spine or over the lungs with his right hand. A RAC reaction will indicate, for example, the level of an osteopathic block on the spine (**Figure 4.5**).

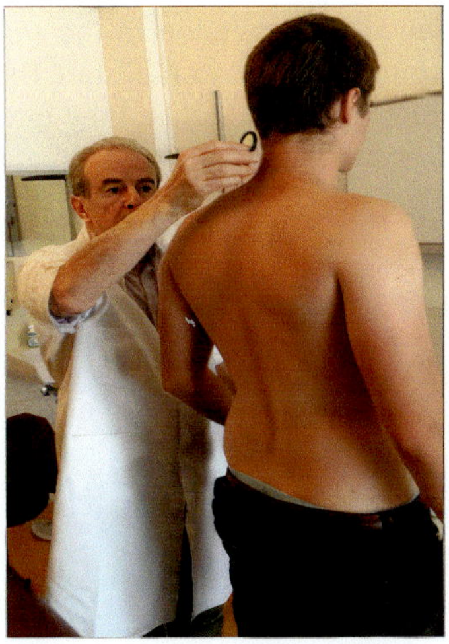

**Figure 4.5** Scanning a colour filter over the spine.

## 4.2 AT WHICH ARTERIAL SITE IS THE RAC BEST PERCEIVED?

In theory, the RAC is a ubiquitous reflex occurring on all parts of the arterial system, but [5] most clearly on distal muscular arteries. The problem consists of finding the best access to the artery. Just as for the classical pulse at rest, the most favourable site for perception of a RAC reaction is the ***radial artery*** on the anterior aspect of the wrist, at a level corresponding to *the slope of the styloid process of the radius,* situated between *apex* and *base* (**Figure 4.6**).

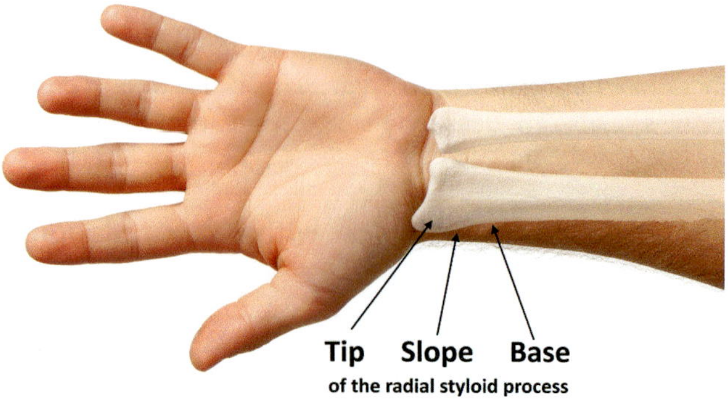


**Figure 4.6** The slope of the styloid process of the radius, between its apex and base, on the anterior aspect of the wrist.

These three parts of the styloid process are easy to feel by palpation. Locating these bone markers is a starting point for locating *the radial artery*, which can normally be felt *slightly inwards* in relation to the slope of the styloid process (**Figure 4.7**). For didactic purposes and to facilitate the learning process of taking the RAC, beginners are encouraged, once they have located the bony structures and the artery, to then mark these anatomical features on the skin, as shown in **Figure 4.7**.

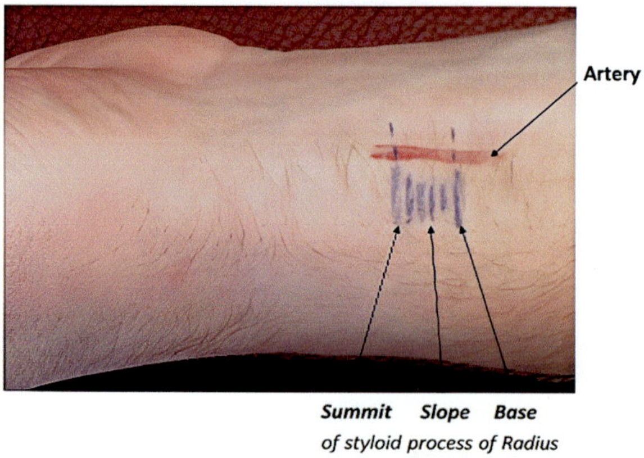


**Figure 4.7** Marking of the skin projection of styloid process slope and the artery.

The radial artery at wrist level has clearly shown to provide the best access to both the resting pulse and the RAC, because at this particular anatomical site, the artery runs directly under a thin surface of skin, and at the same time rests close to the flat surface of the styloid process slope (**Figure 4.8**), thereby providing both good access and stability of perception.

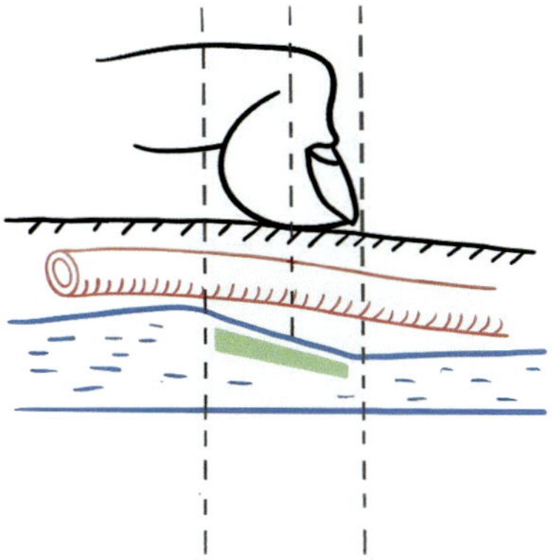


**Figure 4.8** Longitudinal section showing the passage of the artery between the slope of the styloid process (green) and the skin.

### 4.2.1 Other Possible Sites for Taking the RAC

Nevertheless, anatomy is subject to individual variation, and it is not exceptional to come across situations where access to the radial artery is difficult or even impossible. A good alternative may then be to try on the **ulnar (cubital) artery**, which is often well perceived as it passes through the ulnar aspect of the anterior wrist.

On a more experimental basis, it is possible to have access to and feel a RAC on many other muscular arteries, such as the superficial temporal artery, the facial artery, or even *the femoral or the pedal artery.* As for taking the pulse at the *common carotid* artery, it is more difficult because, paradoxically, the pulsatile amplitude of this large elastic vessel is disproportionate and tends to drown the subtlety of the vascular response RAC. Additionally, this area lacks a stabilising underlying bony plane.

### 4.2.2 Which Finger Should Be Used to Take the Pulse?

Theoretically, tactile perception of the pulse, whether at rest or during a RAC, can be considered from the point of view of *transduction of information* between *the patient's artery* (which bears the pressure variations), and the *skin captors sensitive to pressure variations, located in the examiner's finger pads* [2]. One of the factors on which the quality of this *transduction* depends is the density of skin captors within the finger pads. And it is generally admitted that this density is at its highest at the fingertips under the nails.

On the practical level, and considering these factors, experience has shown that there are two most efficient ways of taking the pulse: either with the *thumb alone* or with *both index and middle finger (medius).*

**Taking the pulse with the thumb** has always been taught and practised by Paul Nogier [3] and is now the most widely used technique. With the examiner's left thumb, flexed completely, the part of skin pad just below the nail is placed in line with the patient's forearm (**Figure 4.9**). It rests lightly onto the *inner* part of the blue area (projection of the *slope* of the styloid process), in such a way as to straddle the axis of the artery, and with the nail placed at the proximal limit of the blue hatched area (i.e. at level with the *base* of the styloid process), as represented on **Figure 4.10**. This description may appear somewhat complicated at first. However, a good perception of the pulse depends on a precise positioning of the fingers over the artery, and with habit, takes merely a few seconds.

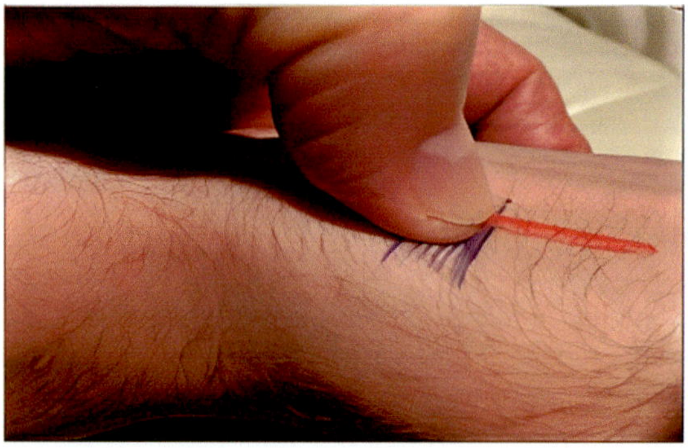

**Figure 4.9** Contact position of the flexed thumb on the skin surface corresponding to the slope of the styloid process.

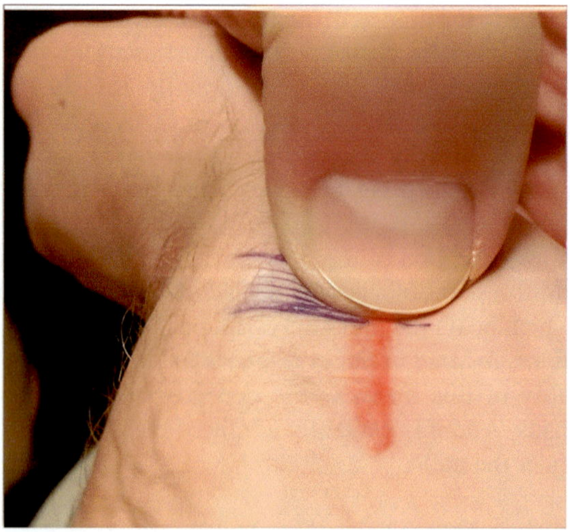

**Figure 4.10** The thumb straddles the axis of the radial artery passage, towards the inner part of the blue area.

To ensure stability of the thumb over the artery, it is important to avoid space between the patient's and the examiner's palm (**Figures 4.11** and **4.12**). Both palms should be in contact. This can also be done by extending the patient's wrist downwards [4]. According to Paul Nogier, *this manual "grip" must be gentle, flexible, and above all, avoid stiffness. It should, however, give the patient an impression of firmness* [3].

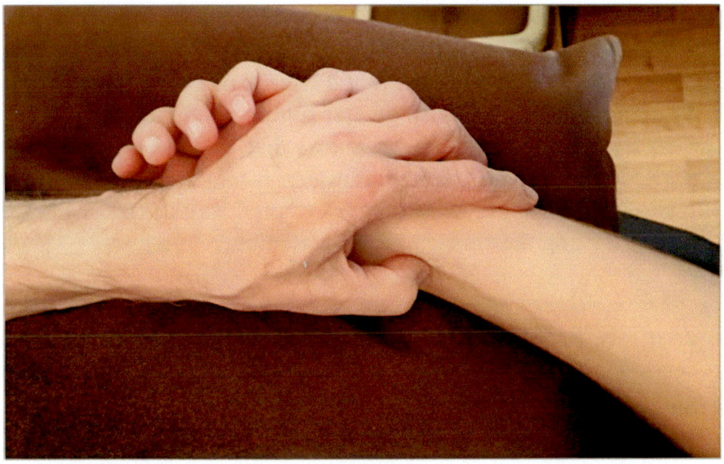

**Figure 4.11** Taking the pulse with the thumb flexed.

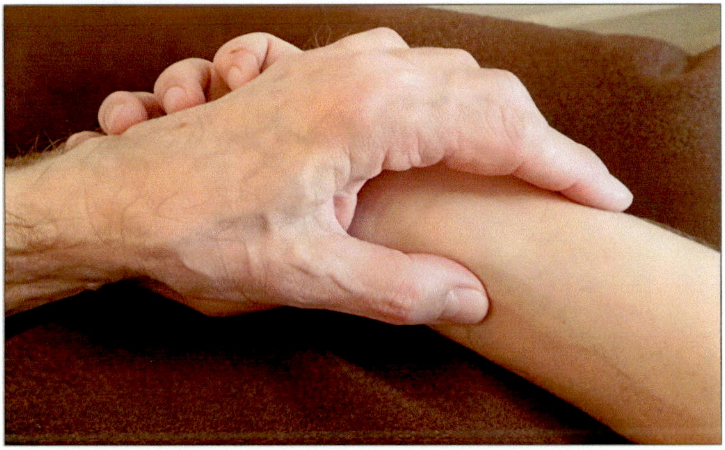

**Figure 4.12** Taking the pulse with an extended thumb ("flat thumb").

Finally, **flexion of the thumb** (**Figure 4.11**) is considered preferable. However, some practitioners perceive the pulse better with the thumb in a flat position (**Figure 4.12**) or **semi-flexed**.

**Taking the pulse with two fingers: index and middle finger (medius)** was initially used by some physicians in the early days of the RAC, before the thumb technique became more widespread. Although less used nowadays by practitioners of signal medicine, in our opinion, the two-finger technique (which is the classic technique used by internists and cardiologists) offers a valid and efficient alternative for good quality perception of the RAC.

Indeed, it appears likely that perception of the arterial reflex through the skin captors of two separate fingers may generate a greater summation of afferences reaching the sensory cortex. By and large, experience shows that, depending on the patient and the anatomical configuration of the radial artery, it may be either the thumb technique or the two-finger technique that proves to produce the clearest perception of the RAC, thereby leaving the choice to each practitioner.

In practice, *the examiner's index and middle finger* are placed (**Figure 4.13**) on the same wrist location as with the thumb technique, i.e. over the slope of the styloid process of the radius. But in this case, the examiner's hand will be placed in a perpendicular or oblique direction in relation to the axis of the radial artery, and the patient's forearm must be placed in a position of slight pronation (internal rotation). With this technique, it is no longer possible to establish contact between the palms.

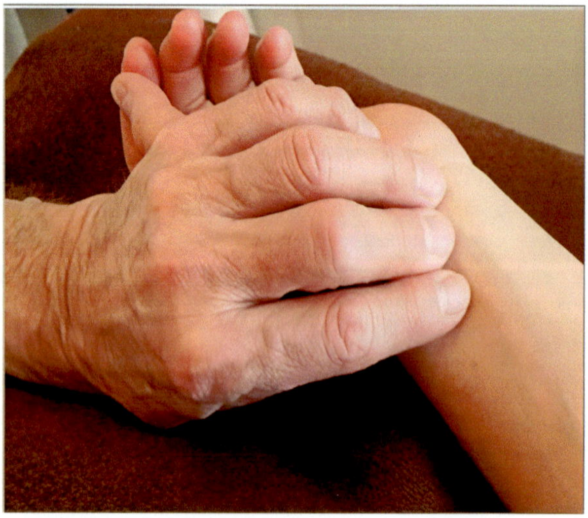

**Figure 4.13** Taking the pulse with the index and middle fingers.

### 4.2.3 A Precaution: Verticality of Contact over the Artery

Whichever method is chosen for taking the pulse, it is important to ensure that the examiner's finger(s) are placed as *vertically* as possible over the artery, on its *medial flank* (**Figure 4.14**). The idea is to avoid taking the pulse *obliquely on the lateral flanks*, that is to say, at an angle of more than a few degrees from verticality [1, 5]. This is because an oblique finger position over the artery tends to displace it sideways, a tendency enhanced by the mechanical effect caused by the repeated passage of each pulse wave (see Chapter 6). Such *lateral escape* of the artery, sometimes called *buckling,* can distort RAC responses, even to the extent of inverting a positive and a negative RAC.

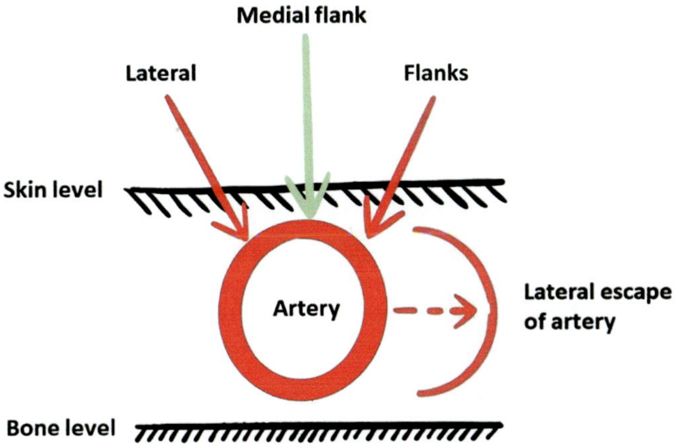


**Figure 4.14** Lateral escape of the artery (buckling), due to oblique finger pressure.

### 4.2.4 Pulse Amplification

Experimentally, a significant amplification of both the resting pulse and the RAC can be done by obliterating the radial artery by means of mechanical compression applied to the distal side of the styloid process of the radius, i.e. slightly downstream from the site at which the pulse is felt. This obliteration can be performed by placing a clamp (**Figure 4.15**) or by an aid compressing the artery with a finger. This has the effect [3] of short-circuiting the downstream layout of anastomoses and arteriolar network, which normally dampen the reflection of the wave. Therefore, this arterial clamp device creates a more sharply defined wall for reflection of the pulse wave, which, hence, is considerably amplified (see Chapter 5).

In practice, this simple device can be helpful when the pulse turns out to be too tenuous and can also facilitate RAC perception for beginners. However, it is not designed for routine use.

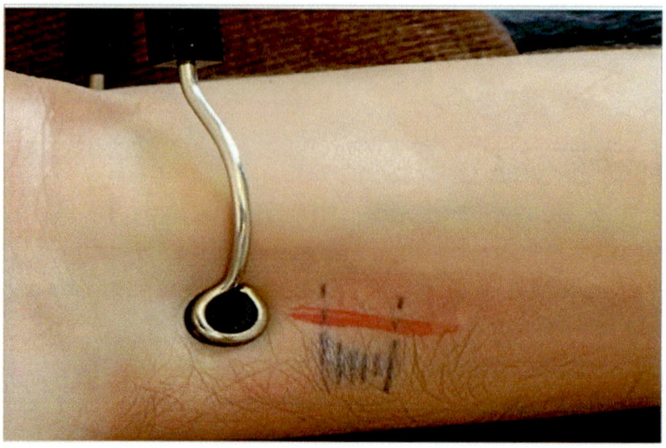

**Figure 4.15** Pulse amplification by compression of the radial artery with a clamp placed distally to where the pulse is felt.

## REFERENCES


1. Marignan Michel. *The VAS or Nogier pulse*, Physical, physiological and biomechanical vasculaire bases. Published in: [5]
2. Guyton Arthur. *Textbook of medical physiology* (Saunders), 8th edition 1991, 496 12
3. Nogier Paul. *From Auriculotherapy to Auriculomedicine* (Maisonneuve) 1981, 75–79
4. Nogier Raphaël. *Introduction pratique à l'auriculomédecine* (Haug) 1993, 20–25
5. Nogier Paul. *The perception of the pulse signal*. Revue Auriculomédecine 28.23, 1982

CHAPTER 5

# Physiological Aspects of the RAC

**Anthony de Sousa**

## 5.1 INTRODUCTION

Our knowledge of the arterial reflex does not originate from any experimental discovery. As we have seen, it was a clinical finding resulting from a random observation based on a tactile sensation. To better understand the dynamic mechanisms underlying this reflex, and before we discuss the experimental aspects, we will begin by considering a tentative model of the RAC in terms of the existing classical physiological descriptions of the arterial resting pulse.

## 5.2 PRESSURE WAVE AND BLOOD FLOW

The heart generates two distinct effects with each cardiac contraction (systole). While launching a volume of blood of approximately 60 millilitres, known as the stroke volume, the heart simultaneously propels a pressure wave into the arterial system.

These must be seen as two separate entities. In the radial artery at the wrist level, the blood volume travels slowly, about 0.9 metres per second. Whereas, by contrast, the pressure wave travels approximately ten times faster, i.e. 9 metres per second (equivalent to a speed of over 30 km per hour). To illustrate this difference in velocity, and all things considered, the pressure wave could be compared to a miniature tsunami travelling at a very high speed within a much slower liquid medium. In the arterial system, the rhythmical passage of the pressure wave is essentially responsible for the tactile sensation of the pulse. Displacement of the actual blood volume plays only a very small part, if any at all [1].

## 5.3 INCIDENT AND REFLECTED WAVES

The pressure wave generated by the heart, also called the incident wave, will travel through the aorta, the large elastic trunks, and the muscular arteries before finally dispersing into the peripheral arterioles (of the hand, in the case of the radial artery) (**Figure 5.1**).

The *arteriolar resistance* caused by this complex network made up of innumerable anastomoses and connections, will gradually result in a decrease in the power of the *incident wave*, to the point of virtually generating a "*wall*", against which the

DOI: 10.1201/9781003753629-5

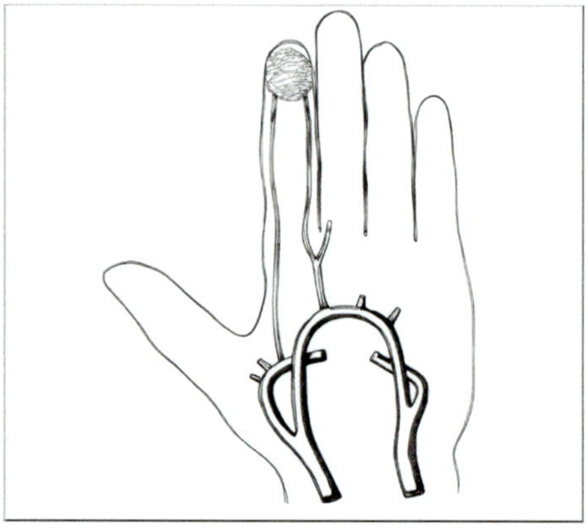

**Figure 5.1** Schematic representation of the muscular arteries and the peripheral arteriolar network of the hand. (Copyright Raphaël Nogier.)

incident wave will eventually *reflect* and then travel back up in the direction of the heart, forming a *reflected, or retrograde wave*. The reflection of the incident wave against the peripheral wall will finally lead to a *crossover* and *summation* of the incident and reflected waves (**Figure 5.2**).

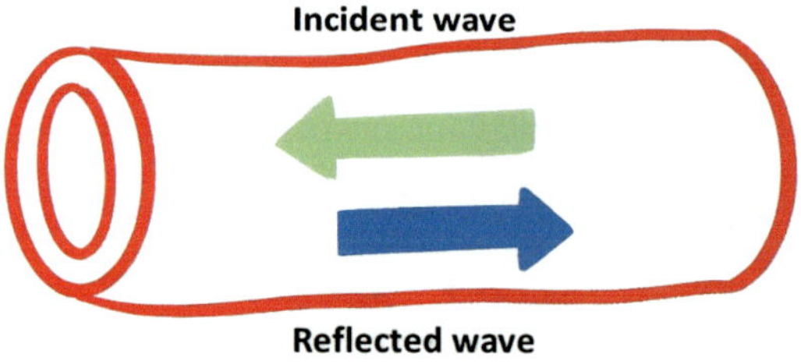


**Figure 5.2** Crossover of incident and reflected waves.

Given the high velocity of the pressure wave, the incident wave will be inversed and produce the reflected wave *before the systole is completed* [2]. Consequently, what we feel when taking the pulse is, in fact, a *summation of both the incident and the reflected waves*.

N.B. It should be added that the drop in power of the incident wave caused by the arteriolar network can, a contrario, explain the mechanism of pulse amplification, which has been described in **Figure 4.15**. This is a situation where the arteriolar network is short-circuited by a clamp placed on the muscular artery at wrist level, suddenly obliterating the vessel and creating an artificial wall resembling the conditions of a terminal artery. As a result, the incident pressure wave, instead of being gradually slowed down by the arteriolar network, maintains its full power when hitting the clamped artery. This results in an increase, up to four to six times, in the amplitude of the resting pulse and the RAC.

## 5.4 A HISTORICAL ASPECT, THE STANDING WAVE HYPOTHESIS

In fluid dynamics, the intersection of two waves travelling in opposite directions may, under certain conditions, produce a standing wave. This can be observed within elementary systems, such as a bowl filled with water, in the middle of which a small pebble is dropped or is subjected to vibrations. Waves are formed, which can be observed to move centrifugally (incident waves) and then reflect onto the walls of the bowl and turn back (reflected waves). When the incident waves meet the reflected waves, they both become stationary, no longer moving in either direction (**Figure 5.3**).

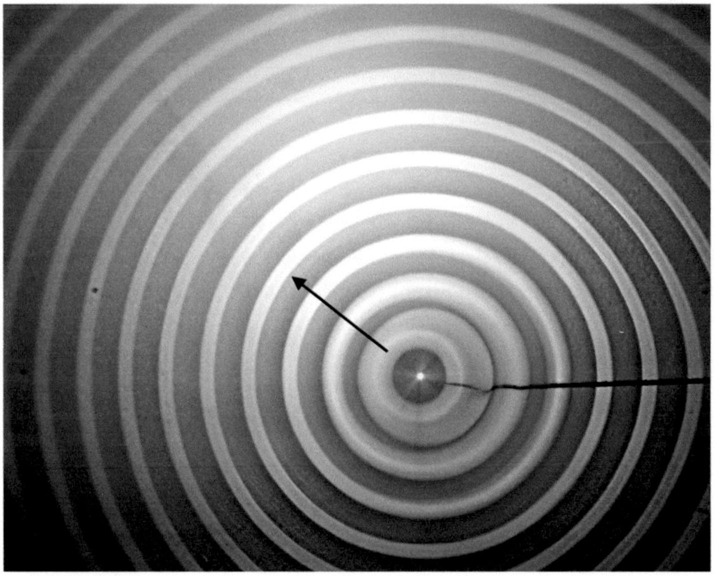

**Figure 5.3** Formation of standing waves in a bowl of water.

In 1967, in search of a haemodynamic explanation of the arterial reflex he had discovered, Paul Nogier approached Raymond Comolet, a physicist specialising in fluid mechanics, to study an analogue model of the pulse. This resulted in a device called the *Comolet tank* (**Figure 5.4**), somewhat like what we have just described: a simple system consisting of an elongated tube filled with water, covered on one side with a rubber membrane, and connected to a pump at one end, and a tap at the other. The device was specifically designed to produce standing waves, which were visible through the rubber membrane (the shape of which was determined by a standing wave under the rubber membrane) and the sensation felt by a finger placed on the artery.

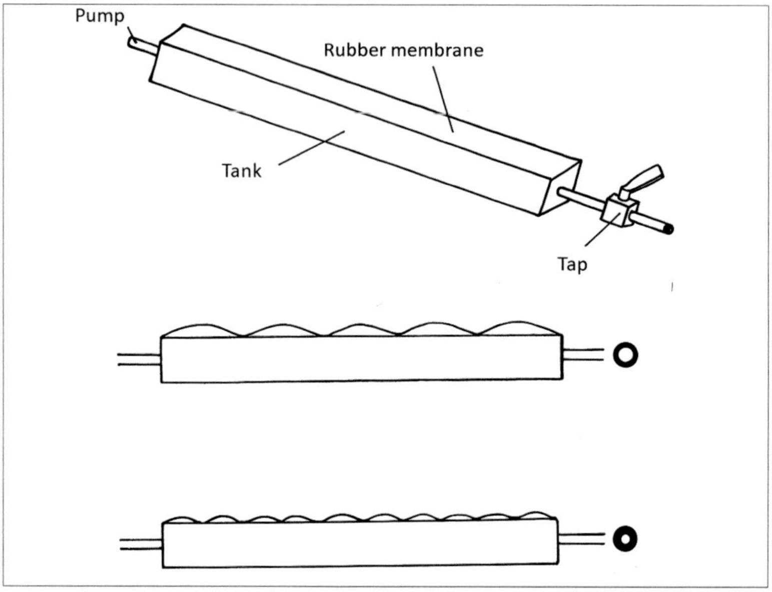


**Figure 5.4** The Comolet tank, an analogue model of the pulse. (Copyright René Bourdiol.)

The analogy implied that the arterial pulse at rest was, in fact, a standing wave and that the RAC would consist of a slight displacement of this standing wave, distally for a positive RAC or proximally for a negative RAC (**Figure 5.5**). These effects would be caused by a variation of the arteriolar "wall", due to an autonomic sympathetic discharge.

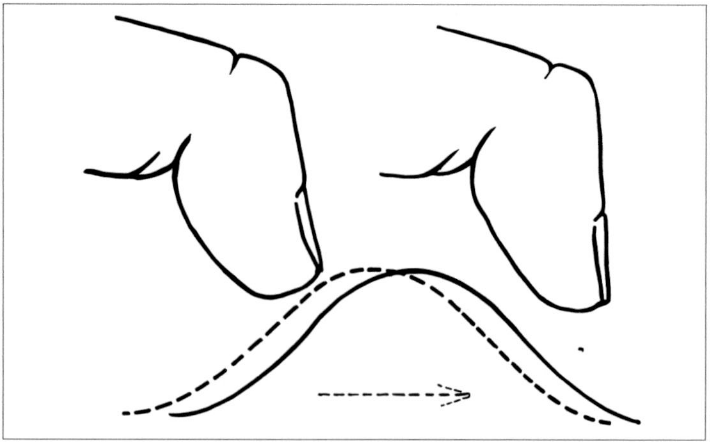

**Figure 5.5** Displacement of a standing wave. (Copyright Raphaël Nogier.)

Historically speaking, the standing wave theory has provided an interesting hypothesis for understanding the physiology of the RAC and, as such, has prevailed for many years in publications and the teaching of signal medicine throughout many countries. However, the theory has neither been confirmed nor pursued, theoretically or experimentally, suggesting that it is, in fact, an oversimplification.

It so appears that the problem deserves reconsideration. As we have seen, the formation of individual standing waves is possible within an elementary system such as a bowl of water subjected to vibration and, as such, is easy to implement. By contrast, the arterial network can obviously not be considered an elementary system. To emphasise this, three separate aspects can be considered [3]:

1. The calculated wavelength of the arterial pressure wave (which depends on the velocity of the wave and the duration of systolic ejection) can be shown to be theoretically long enough to exceed even the length of the upper limb and so would have no resemblance with a simple wave, as represented for example in **Figure 5.5**.
2. The intersection of an incident and a reflected wave does not necessarily imply the formation of a well-individualised standing wave. In fact, a standing wave represents a special case, requiring the distance between the summit of the standing wave and the reflection wall to be a multiple of half its wavelength (**Figure 5.6**).

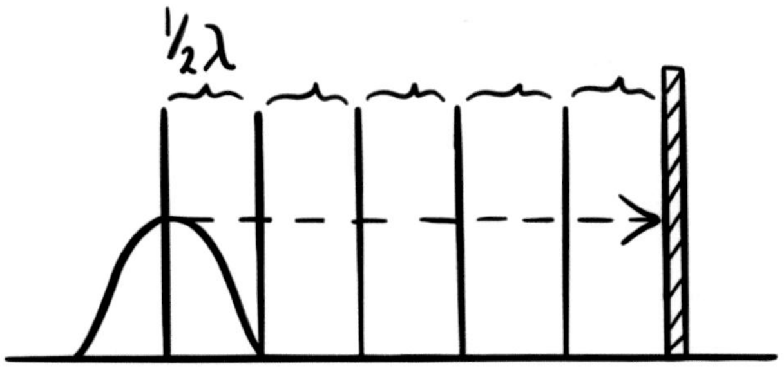


**Figure 5.6** The distance from the summit of a standing wave to the reflection wall should be a multiple of half its wavelength.

3. Anatomically, the reflecting "wall" formed by the arteriolar network is clearly much more complex than the wall of a simple bowl. This entails that the system formed by the muscular arteries and the arterioles does by no means meet the hemodynamic conditions for the formation of individual standing waves. Only one vessel could possibly be capable of doing so: the abdominal aorta (8), a very large vessel in which the velocity of the pressure wave is considerably slower and the wavelength

shorter. Furthermore, in this case, the reflection of the wave is not due to a dampening arteriolar network, but to the branching of the right and left common iliac arteries, which could indeed materialize the conditions of a mechanical "wall" (**Figure 5.7**). However, the aorta cannot exactly be said to offer very suitable access for taking the pulse!

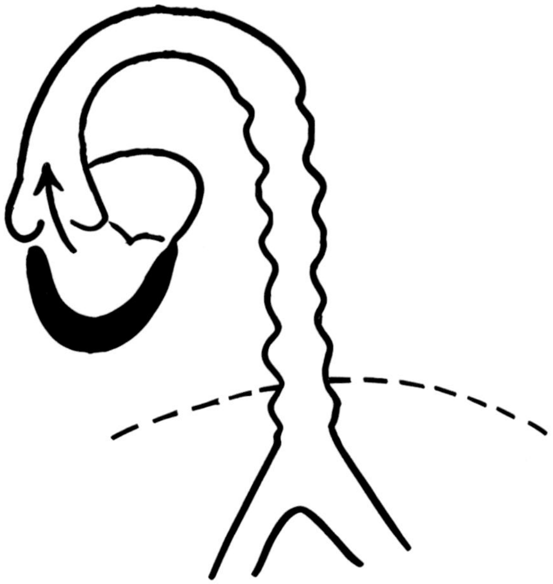

**Figure 5.7** Possible formation of standing waves in the aorta.

## 5.5 FINDING A SUITABLE REFERENCE SYSTEM

At this point, it is important to introduce the notion of a *pressure curve,* bearing in mind that a *pressure wave* and a *pressure curve* are two distinct representations of the same phenomenon. As such, they both define a different *reference system,* and the problem of understanding the pulse and the RAC may well lie in selecting the suitable reference system.

Indeed, the fact is that the complexity of the arterial system makes it inappropriate, if not impossible, to measure the pressure wave directly as such; in other words, by using a reference system that considers the spatial dimension of the wave using a graphical reference where the x-axis represents length (**Figure 5.8**). Yet this was precisely the case in the standing wave theory.

By contrast, ***time*** appears as an adequate and measurable parameter and can *replace length on the x-axis.* The pulse is thus no longer referred to as a *wave*

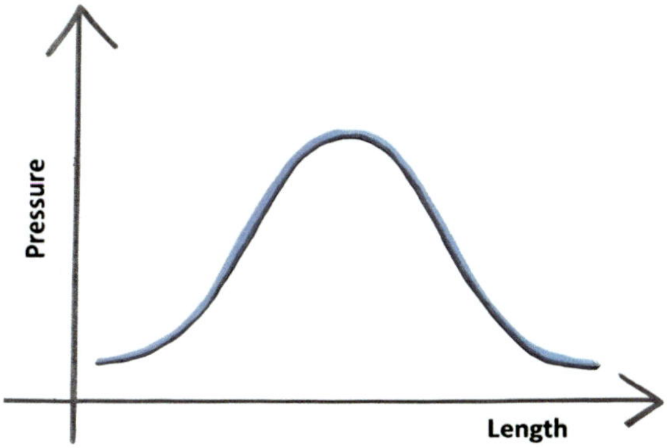


**Figure 5.8** The pressure wave, represented on a graph with length on the x-axis.

but rather as a *curve*. And indeed, in the field of haemodynamics, physiologists have long since described the pressure wave indirectly as a *curve* representing *the pressure variation at a given point on the artery, per unit of time, due to the passage of the pressure wave. Graphically,* the x-axis represents ***time*** instead of *length* (**Figure 5.9**).

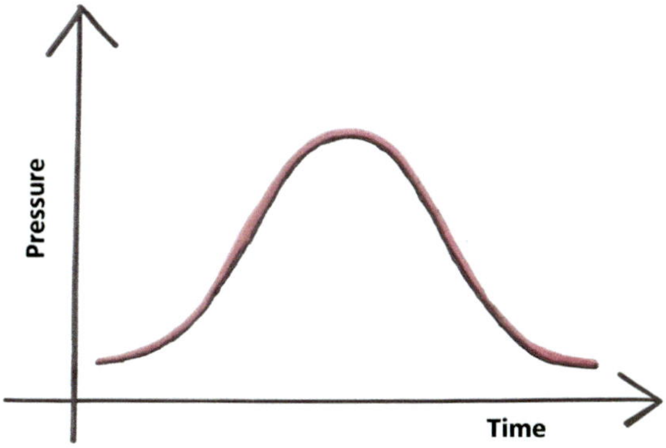


**Figure 5.9** The pressure curve varies through time and is represented on a graph with time on the x-axis.

It appears interesting that in 1978, Paul Nogier, after having described the pulse for many years as a standing wave, probably became implicitly aware of the issue of *reference*, speaking of "*variation in the shape of the pulse*" [4]. Similarly, during a course given in Paris in 1980, he mentioned "*that the standing wave was perhaps not the only mechanism implied to explain the arterial reflex" and that "the shape of the curve could be implied*" [5]. See also [6].

## 5.6 GENERAL ASPECT OF THE PRESSURE CURVE

Although the pressure curve profile varies progressively along a gradient between the aorta and the peripheral muscular arteries [1, 2], the general aspect of the curve [2, 7] is shown schematically in **Figure 5.10**.

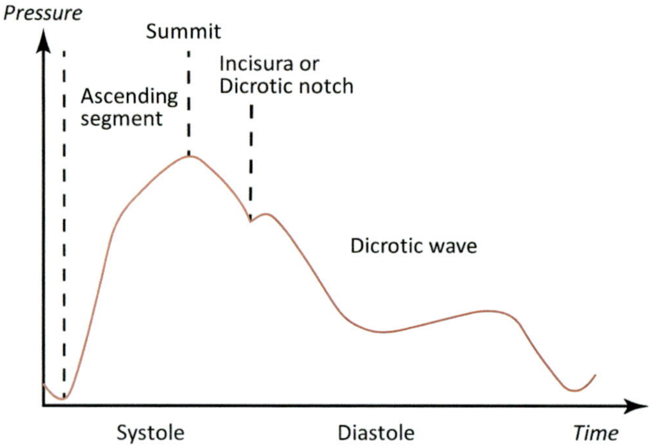


**Figure 5.10** Schematic aspect of the pulse curve.

The cardiac cycle starts off with the ***systole***, consisting of the initial rapidly ascending segment, up to the summit, after which the ***diastole*** begins with the descent. The first part of the descent ends abruptly at the *incisura*, resulting from the closure of the aortic valve, and is followed by the remaining part of the descent, including the second, less abrupt peak called the *dicrotic wave*.

As shown in **Figure 5.11**, it is important to bear in mind that the pulse curve is, in fact, a *compound curve* representing, as described above, the *summation* between the curve generated by the *incident wave* and the curve resulting from the *reflected wave*. Incidentally, it should be added that the systolic, ascending part of the pulse curve mostly represents the *incident wave*, whereas the reflected wave mainly determines the diastolic part of the curve.

## 5.7 PERCEPTION OF THE PULSE

As mentioned earlier (Chapter 4), our sensory ability to perceive the pulse depends on *transduction of information* between the artery, which bears the pressure curve variations, and the skin captors located in the examiner's fingertip pads [8]. In this respect, two types of receptors are involved, both of which are said to be "rapidly

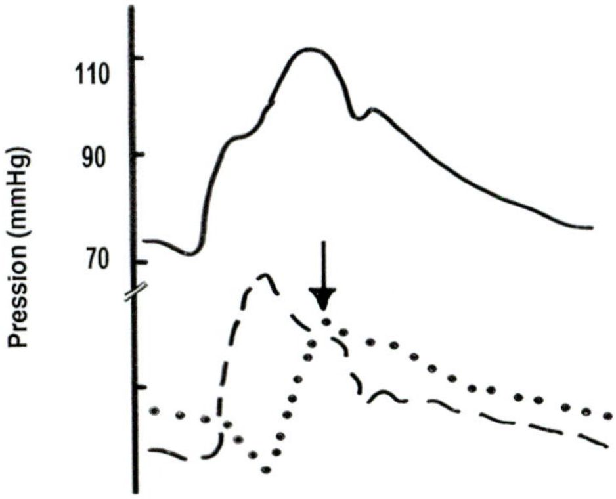


**Figure 5.11** The upper pulse curve results from the summation between the incident wave (segmented curve) and the reflected wave (dotted curve). (Copyright Roland Asmar [1].)

adapting": *Meissner's corpuscles*, which react to the *speed of* pressure increase, and the *Pacini corpuscles*, which are sensitive to the *acceleration* of pressure increase (**Figure 5.12**).

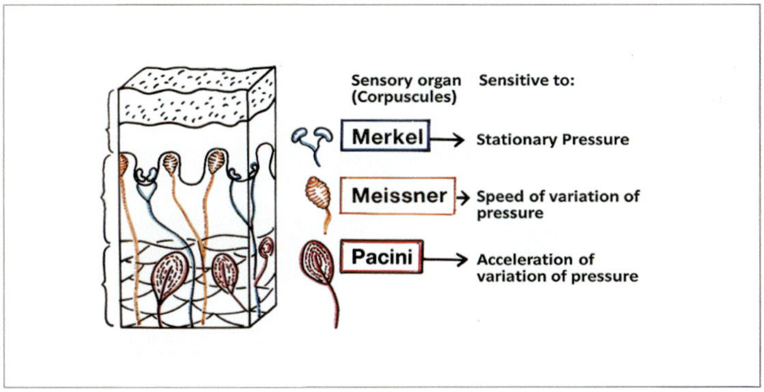


**Figure 5.12** The rapidly adapting skin captors involved in the perception of a sudden pressure change: the Meissner and Pacini corpuscles.

However, presumably because these captors specifically respond much more to a rapid *increase* than to a *decrease* in pressure, experience shows that we distinctly perceive the initial *ascending* systolic segment of the curve up to the summit (**Figure 5.13**). In contrast, our tactile perception of the diastolic *decreasing* part of the curve is very imprecise or even non-existent. By contrast, an instrumental recording of the curve would uniformly register the entire curve.

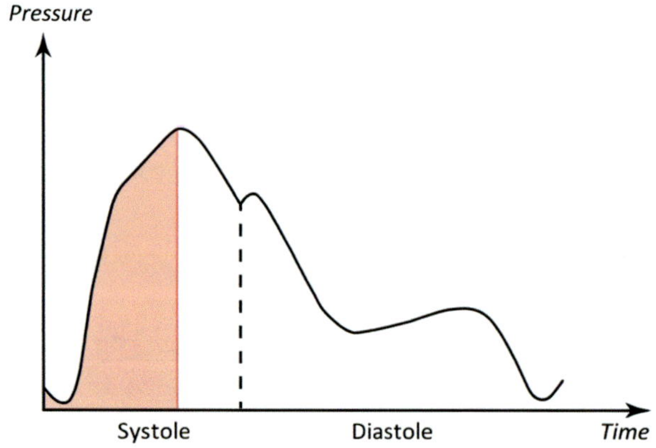


**Figure 5.13** Our rapidly adapting skin captors allow us to perceive the first rapidly ascending part of the pressure curve (segment coloured in red) but not the following descending part of the curve.

## 5.8 HOW CAN WE EXPECT THE PULSE CURVE TO VARY DURING A RAC?

At this stage, partly by deduction and partly based on experimental data described in Chapter 6, we can endeavour to anticipate the variations that the pressure curve will probably undergo under the effect of a RAC reaction (**Figure 5.14**). Given that the RAC results from an adaptative process of the *autonomous sympathetic system*,

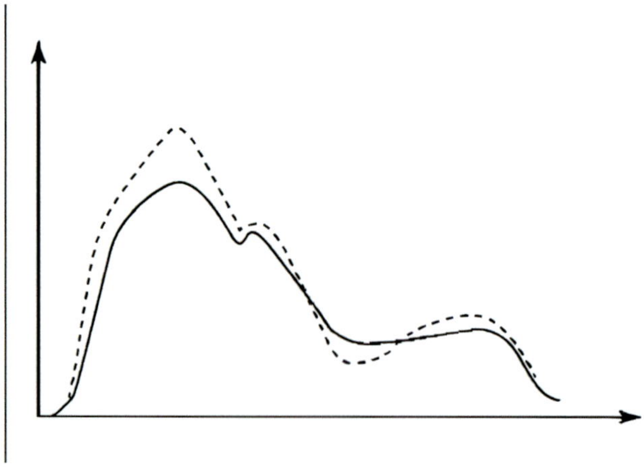

**Figure 5.14** Schematic representation of the probable variations in pressure curve profile under the effect of a sympathetic discharge.

let us first recall the main effects of a sympathetic discharge on the cardiovascular system as a whole [2]:

- An increase in stroke volume.
- An increase in the speed of contraction and shortening of myocardial fibres.
- Vasoconstriction of the muscular arteries and variation of their compliance.
- An increase in peripheral arteriolar resistance.

This now enables us to anticipate (**Figure 5.14**) the impact of a sympathetic discharge on the pressure curve profile.

The main variation will be *an increase in the slope and amplitude of the initial ascending (systolic) segment.* This variation is supported by experimental evidence (**Figure 6.9**).

Secondly, there will probably also be changes in the profile of the diastolic part of the curve, but these are more difficult to predict, and the experimental evidence is tenuous (**Figure 6.2**). However, at least for the manual perception of the pulse, this can be considered less important since the diastolic part of the curve is probably not perceived (see above: **Figure 5.13**).

## 5.9 TACTILE PERCEPTION OF THE RAC

By and large, manual perception of the RAC can be considered to result from *variation in slope and amplitude of the initial ascending part of the curve* (**Figure 5.15**)

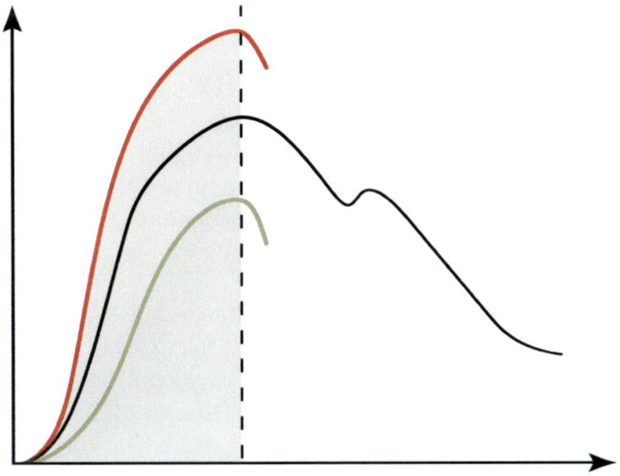

**Figure 5.15** The tactile sensation of a positive or a negative RAC result from an increase (red curve) or a decrease (green curve) in the slope and amplitude of the initial systolic segment. The black curve represents the *steady state of* the pulse at rest. The changes in the shape of the curve result in a variation of the area *surface* underneath the curve.

because of a sympathetic discharge and finally perceived by the examiner as a "harder" positive RAC (red curve) or "softer" negative (green curve).

Variations in the profile of the pulse curve will be discussed again in relation to the experimental aspects described in the next chapter. It will be interesting to note that **Figure 6.9** confirms the variation of the *slope* of the initial ascending segment, which in turn leads to a change in the *surface of the area* between the ascending segment of the curve and the horizontal x-axis (**Figure 5.15**, grey area). The change of surface area is also an expression of the RAC, because it produces an increase in the *energy* developed and, therefore, in the "kinetic" impact of the pressure wave when it hits against the pulp of the examiner's finger, leading to the characteristic impression of a stronger pulse.

## 5.10 DISCUSSION

Perception of the RAC can be made easier by having a clear mental representation of the theoretical aspects. In our description, we have referred to the classical physiological descriptions of the pulse to offer a model of the possible variations of the pressure curve. However, these descriptions are by no means exhaustive, and the mechanism of RAC perception may consist not only of the activity of peripheral skin captors. It may well involve additional factors that are more complex, such as micro-vibrations of the arterial wall due to vasoconstriction or the integration of various associative regions of the central nervous system, implying sensory impressions and interpretations. Discussion of the experimental data of the RAC in the following chapter will provide us with more information about these aspects.

## BIBLIOGRAPHY


1. Asmar Roland. *Arterial stiffness and pulse wave velocity* (Elsevier Paris) 1999: 17–19
2. Selkurt Ewald. *Physiology* (Little, Brown) 2nd edition 1966: 333–341
3. de Sousa Anthony. *Reflections on the hemodynamic theory of RAC*. Annals of the First International Symposium of Auriculotherapy and Auriculomedicine, GLEM Lyon 1994
4. Nogier Paul. *Connaissance pratique du RAC*, Revue Auriculomédecine 1978: 13–35
5. Nogier Paul. *Cours d'auriculomédecine* (GLEM Lyon) 1980
6. Nogier Paul. *From Auriculotherapy to Auriculomedicine* (Maisonneuve) 1981: 69–74
7. Bray John. *Lecture notes on human physiology* (Blackwell) 2nd edition 1993: 423–428
8. Guyton Arthur. *Textbook of medical physiology* (Saunders) 8th edition 1991: 496

# CHAPTER 6

# Experimental Aspects

**Michel Marignan and Anthony de Sousa**

## 6.1 EARLY TRIALS

The first attempts to record and objectify the arterial reflex go back to the late seventies and is summarised below.

**Bernard Bricot (Marseille, 1978)** undertook one of the very first trials by recording the *flow of blood* using an echo-Doppler device (**Figure 6.1**). A RAC reaction was obtained by stimulating the skin of the ear with a punctual pressure of approximately 70 grams/mm$^2$. This initiates what will be referred to later as the 4/4 rhythmic response of the *middle layer* (Chapter 16).

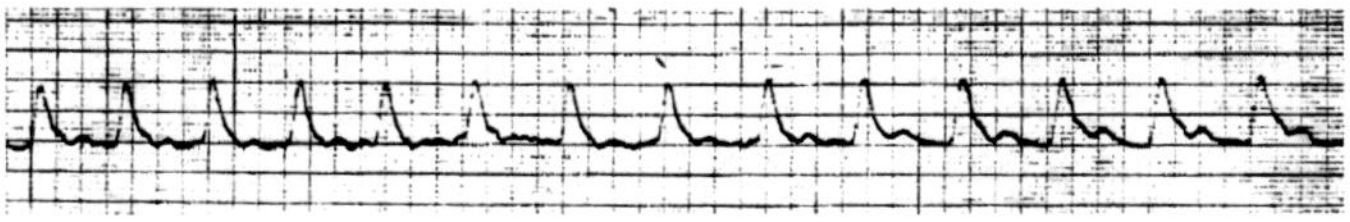

**Reference plot. Pulse at rest. No stimulation**

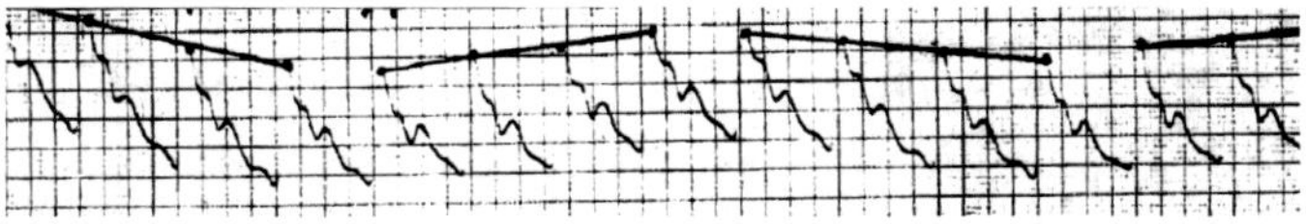

**Plot after stimulation by specific skin pressure of 70 gr/mm2: 4/4 rhythm of the middle layer? (see Chapter 16).**

**Figure 6.1** Pulse recording by echo-Doppler. (*Source*: Review Auriculomedecine n°12.)

It is doubtful that this type of recording could be considered representative of the arterial pulse because, as we have seen (Chapter 5), variations in blood flow play, at most, a very minor role as far as the manual perception of the pulse is concerned. In addition, it is surprising that the shapes of the curves do not vary. As for the rhythmic variation of the baseline, it most probably reflects blood flow oscillations due to the negative intra-thoracic pressures induced by the respiratory movements of the chest.

DOI: 10.1201/9781003753629-6

Nevertheless, a second series of echo-Doppler recordings [1] took place shortly afterwards by **Henry, Magnin** *et al.*, but the results were not considered statistically significant.

In 1980, **Paul Nogier** undertook a different type of recording of the RAC, using a *piezoelectric sensor*, capable of measuring the deformation of the arterial wall under the effect of the passage of the pressure wave, while stimulating the skin by touch on the forearm (**Figure 6.2**) [2].

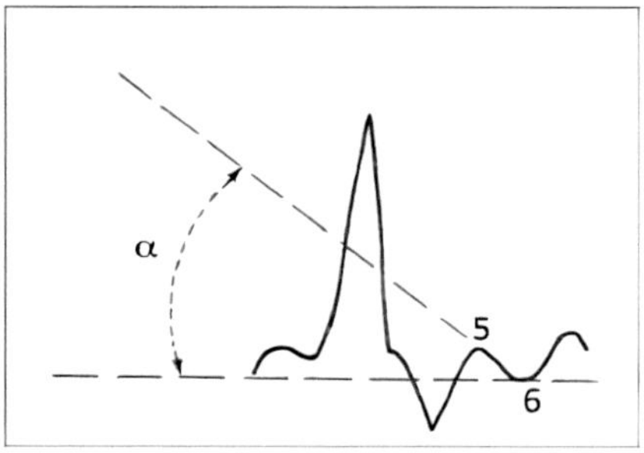


**Figure 6.2** Under the effect of a RAC obtained by touching the skin of the forearm, Paul Nogier observed, on the second part of the curve, a variation of the angle formed by the descending segment 5–6 of the dicrotic wave. (*Source*: Review Auriculomedicine.)

No change in the shape of the curve was observed on the first systolic, rapidly ascending segment, although this part of the curve is, in fact, what is perceived manually (**Figure 5.13**). However, on the second part of the curve (dicrotic wave), Nogier measured a slight variation in the angle formed by the descending segment of the dicrotic wave (segments 5–6) and the horizontal line. This is consistent with the fact that the variations in the shape of the curve under the effect of a RAC concern the entire curve. But paradoxically, what is perceived by manual palpation of the pulse and what can be recorded instrumentally does not concern the same parts of the curve, probably due to a difference in the sensitivity of skin captors on one side and artificial captors on the other.

The same year, Paul Nogier continued his research and published a study in collaboration with two signal-processing engineers, **M. Chiollaz and J. Larcher** [3]. Again, recording the radial pulse with a *piezoelectric sensor* and stimulating the skin by applying light touch on the forearm, the experiment, this time, consisted of recording the spectral density energy curve on several healthy patients, defined as the frequency composition of the signal obtained and the energetic participation of each frequency.

In comparison with **Figure 6.3** showing a recording obtained at rest, i.e. the absence of stimulation, the spectral density curve shown in **Figure 6.4** resulting from skin stimulation clearly indicates a rise in the 4–8 Hertz range.

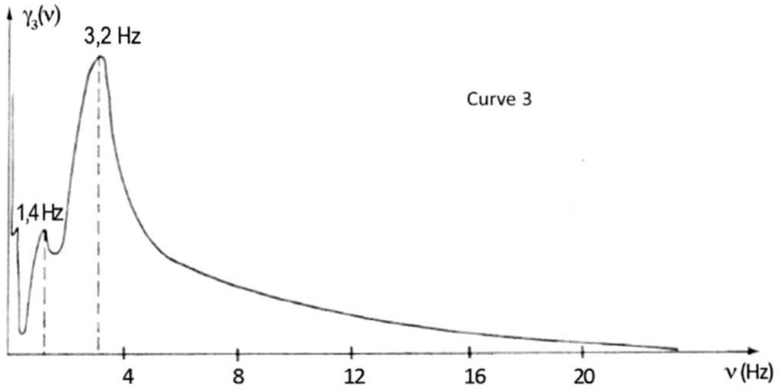


**Figure 6.3** Curve representing the spectral density of the pulse at rest. (*Source*: Review Auriculomédecine no 20.)

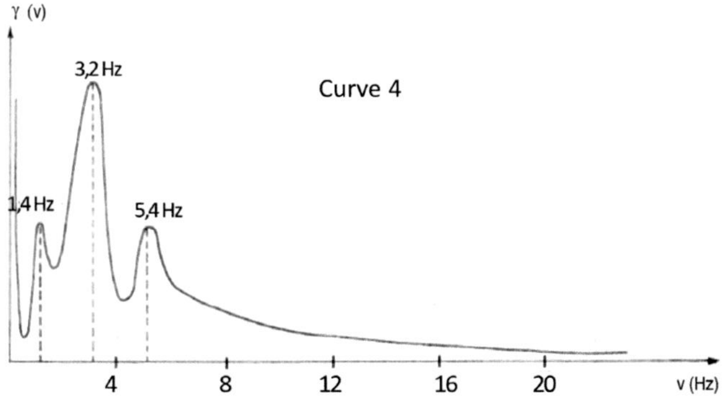


**Figure 6.4** Spectral density curve obtained under the effect of skin stimulation. (*Source*: Review Auriculomédecine no 20.)

## 6.2 MICHEL MARIGNAN'S RESEARCH

During the 1990s, Dr Michel Marignan of Marseille, at the time a scientific attaché at the CNRS (National Centre for Scientific Research) in France, aimed to achieve more convincing results using new equipment and concept These results, obtained thanks to cooperation between Marignan, the GLEM (Lyon Group for Medical Research), the Métravib RDS Company, and the AVENTI research group of the Marseille-Luminy Faculty of Sciences, have proved to be the most significant to this day. Extracts have been published at international congresses.

Marignan chose to use a pressure sensor made of PVDF (polarized vinylidene fluoride), capable of detecting very small variations in pressure without disturbing the pulse (thickness approximately 2 microns) (**Figure 6.5**).

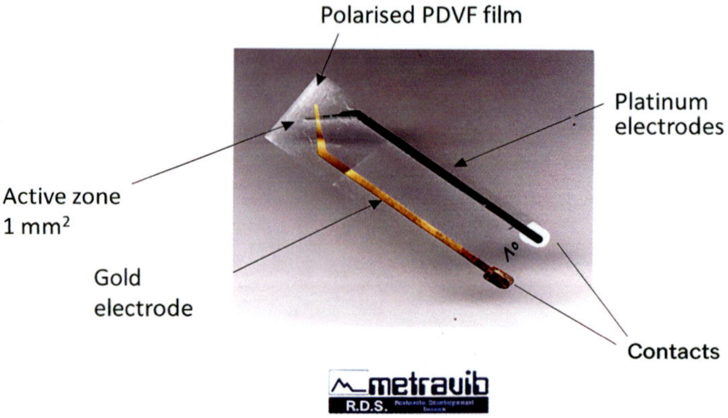


**Figure 6.5** Polarised PVDF micrometric sensor. (Copyright Michel Marignan.)

This high-performance sensor allows the pressure variations exerted by the radial artery on an examiner's finger to be collected without disturbing contact of the finger, as it can be placed between the latter and the artery.

The conditioning electronics (charge amplifiers) make it possible to collect the pressure curve as accurately as possible (**Figure 6.6**).

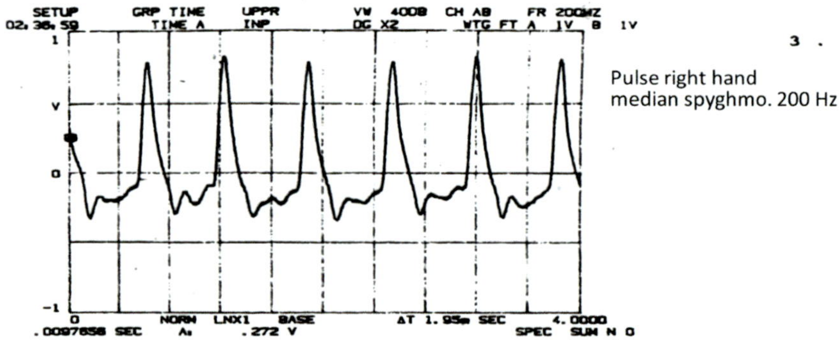


**Figure 6.6** Pulse curve collected by the sensor. (Copyright Michel Marignan.)

Considerably surprising was that these curves were in phase opposition (**Figure 6.7**), according to whether the sensor was oriented towards the artery's radial or ulnar side (or flank). This confirms a clinical observation of Paul Nogier, who recommended a median vertical pulse measurement between these two flanks to avoid errors in perception (**Figure 4.14**).

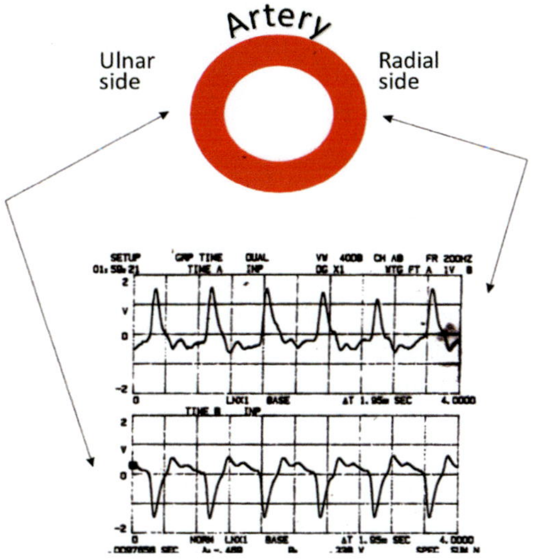


**Figure 6.7** The pressure curves are in phase opposition between the radial and ulnar flanks of the radial artery, in this case, using two sensors simultaneously. (Copyright Michel Marignan.)

This led the team to the conclusion that in its free portion along the radial styloid process, the artery does not undergo systolic load in a so-called *respiratory mode* (swelling of the artery in all directions) but rather in a *flexion mode* (displacement and elongation of the artery), also known as buckling (**Figure 6.8**).

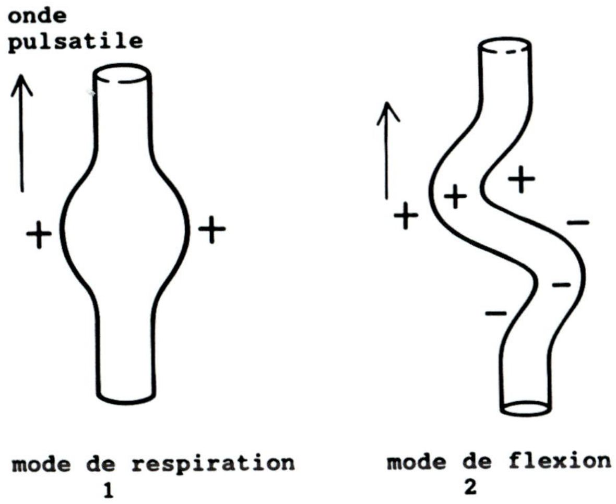


**Figure 6.8** Buckling of the radial artery. (Copyright Michel Marignan.)

This phenomenon has been modelled mathematically and validated by the Institute of Fluid Mechanics in Marseille, France. Indeed, buckling can only occur with frequencies close to the cardiac frequencies and with arterial diameter of the order of the radial artery (**Figure 6.8**). However, this is not directly related to the RAC phenomenon.

To "see" the RAC, the system was connected to a curve analyser in a single-blind experiment.

The effect on the radial pressure curve of white light stimulation (cold, i.e., without local heating) on a subject's arm, tested several times in one day, shows a constant and very significant modification of the **rising phase** of the curve (**Figure 6.9**).

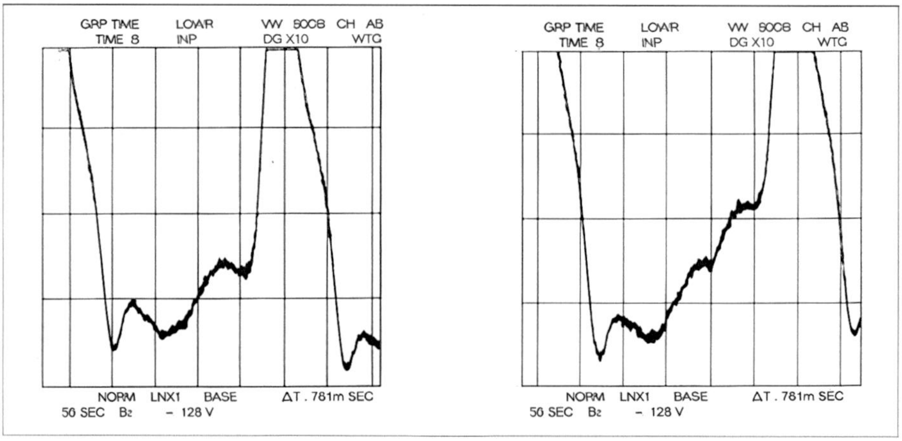


**Figure 6.9** A significant change in the initial rising phase of the curve. Left curve: at rest. Right curve: after white light stimulation of the arm. (Copyright Michel Marignan.)

Such a variation is potentially likely to be felt by an examiner's finger. Because the amount of energy developed during this upward phase of the curve, which can be calculated as the *area* (or integral) between the curve and the time axis (x-axis), is significantly greater (**Figure 5.15**).

This was the subject of a limited-edition research report in June 1991 entitled:

**CHANGES IN PULSATILE WAVEFORMS IN THE RADIAL ARTERY FOLLOWING EPIDERMIC STIMULI**

**By Michel MARIGNAN, MD - Paul AUBERT, MD - Reynald SEZNEC, PhD - CASTELLS, Eng.**

In science, inter-individual reproducibility is a major criterion for validating a physiological phenomenon. In this case, it could not be done, as most of the scientists in the project did not have the opportunity to test the response on a population of individuals.

Furthermore, pulse curves vary considerably from one individual to another, so visual recognition of a change in the curve is perhaps not the best method.

Therefore, a new concept considered that the RAC might be identified not so much by shape changes in the pressure curve but rather by a different "style" of curve. The classic example is that one can easily distinguish by ear between jazz music and a Mozart symphony, whilst it would clearly be more difficult to differentiate them visually on a graphical representation of their sound curves.

Such considerations led the team to turn to other advanced (pulse) signal processing techniques from the artificial intelligence and signal processing field using chaotic learning methods with artificial neural networks. So doing, the team joined up with a new partner, the research company Aventi, Faculty of Science at Luminy, France (**Figure 6.10**).

**Figure 6.10** The logo of the Avanti Research company.

## 6.3 REPORT ON RAC SIGNAL DETECTION BY ARTIFICIAL NEURAL NETWORKS DECEMBER 1997

A full report of this work was published in December 1997. Here is an excerpt from its introduction:

> *An extremely powerful detection technique in advanced signal processing consists of obtaining a modelization of the signal, based on its short-term prediction based on its past achievements. By subtracting, at any moment, the predicted value from the*

> *observed value, it is possible to detect with great detail any change in the signal's dynamics in frequency or amplitude or any external event that would transiently be added to the basic signal.*
>
> *This technique has been successfully used in radar detection, using artificial neural networks to obtain an optimal non-linear modelling of radar signals.*

Without going into excessive technical detail, the experiment can be described as follows:

> Digital pulse samples were collected by Dr Chantal Vulliez, with the previously described equipment, from 10 individuals. During the recording of each of these samples, stimulations by light, known to trigger a RAC reaction, were randomly applied to the skin. At the same time, a physician trained to feel the RAC noted the (subjective) moments of the onset and disappearance of the arterial signal.

The periods without stimulation, when stimulation began and ended, and the perception of RAC's beginning and ending times were all noted with precision.

The samples were submitted to Aventi for analysis, each with the periods of stimulation and those during which the physician had detected a RAC.

The question put forward to the Aventi research group was: "Can you identify *a difference in pulse style* between periods *with* and periods *without* manual identification of a RAC?"

The technique described in the report consists, for each individual, of using the learning capabilities of an artificial neural network organised as a "two-layer perceptron", working according to Takens's theorem (concerning non-linear, so-called chaotic, dynamic systems).

For each subject, the network first "learnt" the *style* of the pulse on the recording during the period without neither stimulation nor manual detection of the RAC (neutral period).

What the network had learnt was fixed and was then used to predict and plot the following part of the pulse curve. The result was remarkable: over periods when the RAC was supposedly absent, the prediction of the neural network was fantastically accurate, with the predicted curve (red) overlapping the recorded curves (green) precisely (**Figure 6.11**).

By contrast, during periods when a manually perceived RAC *had* been reported, the network lost the quality of its prediction and made errors.

This can be represented in several ways, the most convenient being calculating the error's square at every instant (**Figure 6.12**).

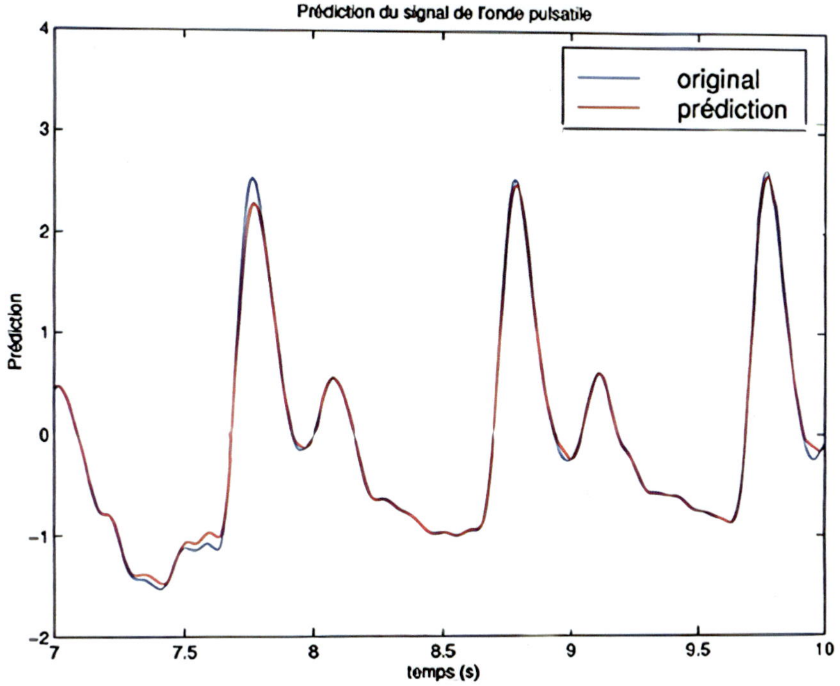


**Figure 6.11** A neural network, after learning, can predict the course in time of a pulse curve based on its past achievements. (Copyright Michel Marignan.)

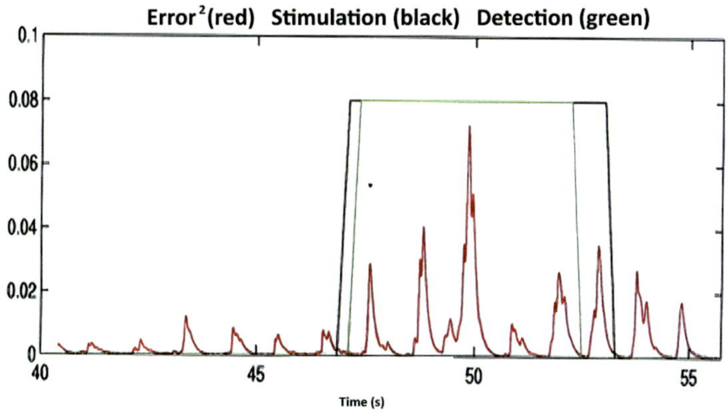


**Figure 6.12** Error in network prediction when a RAC had been manually detected—red: prediction error; black: stimulation; green: manual detection. (Copyright Michel Marignan.)

The red curve represents the prediction error (and not the recorded curve), whereas the black rectangle frames the stimulation, and the green rectangle frames the examiner's manual detection of an RAC.

### 6.3.1 The Full Conclusion of the Report

*The method for RAC detection used in this study shows encouraging results. The network has demonstrated excellent performance in learning and generalization. These results are better than those obtained with a linear or simple network that would predict future values based on preceding values.*

*The results obtained strongly encourage us to carry on with this method of study and research. Remarks which could lead to an improvement in RAC detection include the following:*

1. *The signal has an ample baseline that cannot be simply subtracted from the signal. The baseline can be explained by the fact that the sensor is placed under the examiner's finger and, therefore, records simultaneously the patient's and the examiner's pulse wave signals, but also the variations in pressure of the examiner's finger on the patient's wrist. The multiple acquisition of these various items makes any type of processing that isolates the patient's pulse wave signal alone extremely complex and uncertain. The best solution would be to make the signal acquisition without positioning the examiner's thumb on the sensor, which would be the only reliable way to obtain a signal that is not disturbed by the signals generated by the examiner.*
2. *The identification model used in the study assumes that the signal remains stationary for at least several seconds. However, the signals obtained, which have the appearance of a non-linear periodic signal, show a fluctuation in frequency (the peaks of the spectral density of power are wide) and amplitude throughout the recording. Oscillation of the signal in frequency and amplitude is clearly shown by spectrograms of different portions of the analysed signal, which show an oscillation of the signal at a frequency slower than that of the pulse wave. This permanent oscillation could be linked to the patient's respiratory dynamics.*
3. *These phenomena cannot be reproduced with theoretical identification models with constant control parameters like the one we used for this study. The solution would be to consider these phenomena at the level of the identification model. Preliminary results obtained from theoretical non-linear dynamic models with oscillating control parameters have indeed shown that it is possible, under these conditions, to generate signals, the characteristics of which are identical to those of the pulsatile wave signals. This oscillating control parameter, which appears to be generated by the patient's respiration, could be integrated into the*

*model using a respiration commonly available measurement sensor to acquire the respiration signal.*

4. *Calculating the attractor's reconstruction timeframe and the network's learning process must be redone before each stimulation. This is due to the signal's instationarity (translator's note: term meaning instability through time), which does not allow learning of a global model with constant control parameters. One solution would be to implement an adaptive network, the learning of which would evolve continuously throughout the signal. An alternative solution to this problem could be the choice of the identification model, which should include, as mentioned earlier, control parameters varying through time. Their absence from the model might, at least in part, explain the lack of stability of the signal through time (which would then only be a consequence of the dynamics of the model). Including them could allow for global learning of the network.*
5. *Considering these improvements in signal acquisition and the neural identification model, we are confident that it will be possible to perform fine detection of the RAC signal by identifying and predicting the dynamics of the pulse wave signal.*

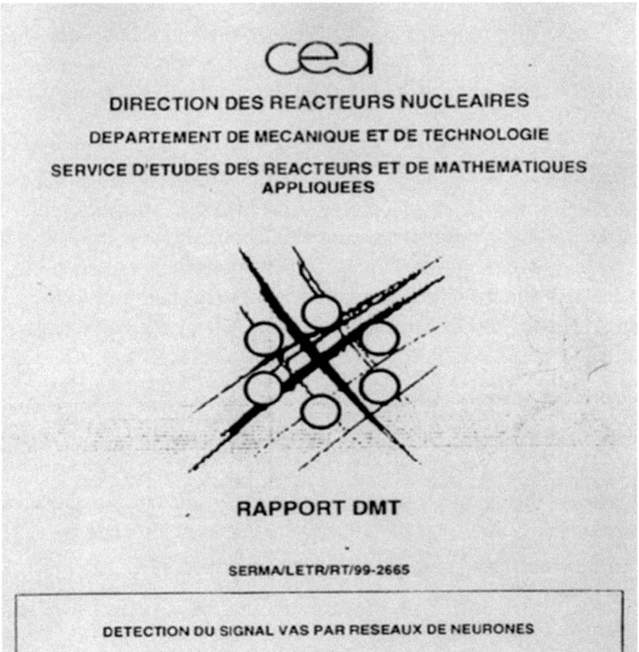

DIRECTION DES REACTEURS NUCLEAIRES

DEPARTEMENT DE MECANIQUE ET DE TECHNOLOGIE

SERVICE D'ETUDES DES REACTEURS ET DE MATHEMATIQUES APPLIQUEES

RAPPORT DMT

SERMA/LETR/RT/99-2665

DETECTION DU SIGNAL VAS PAR RESEAUX DE NEURONES

**Figure 6.13** The "counter-expertise" report from CEA.

It is apparent from this report that the vascular autonomic signal RAC has been identified by this method.

Unfortunately, our research team was later disbanded because its members eventually scattered around the globe. The Metravib team now works for the military, and the Aventi team has moved to Canada.

It should be noted that for additional validation, this report was subjected to a "counter-expertise" by a team of mathematicians from the CEA in Cadarache (research centre in Southern France) in 1999. The report confirms the scientific validity of the Aventi study and provides solutions, some of which are difficult to implement, for the follow-up concerning this research (**Figure 6.13**).

In the future, the final scientific validation of the RAC and the possibility of producing a reliable instrument capable of measuring RAC lies in the continuation of this expertise and the mobilisation of technical and human resources within a new research team.

## BIBLIOGRAPHY


1. Henry J.C. Henry E., Cardot J.C., Bazin R., Magnin P. Methodological approach for the detection of V.A.S., Revue Auriculomédecine 18, 1980, 11
2. Nogier P. A new approach to V.A.S., Revue Auriculomédecine, 19, 1980, 29, and 20, 1980, 29
3. Chiollaz and Larcher. Study of the V.A.S. by spectral analysis, Revue Auriculomédecine 20, 1980, 31
4. Bricot B. Recording of the RAC, Revue Auriculomédecine 12, 1978, 7
5. Marignan M, Sesnec B. Changes in pulsatile waveforms in the radial artery following epidermic stimuli, Institut de Mécanique des Fluides de Marseille, June 1991
6. Marignan M. "V.A.S., Vascular Autonomic Signal" or Nogier pulse - Physical, physiological and vascular bio-mechanical bases. Published in the book "Introduction Pratique à l'Auriculomédecine", Raphaël Nogier (Ed. Haug), 1993.
7. Marignan M. Overview of current basic research in auriculotherapy and acupuncture medicine. Presented and published at the XVI Czech and Slovak International Congress of Acupuncture - BRNO - October 1996 - Czech Republic.
8. Nogier P. La rançon d'une découverte, Revue Auriculomédecine, 11, 1978, 5
9. Nogier P. Le R.A.C. ou le V.A.S., Revue Auriculomédecine, 12, 1978, 9
10. Nogier P. Connaissance pratique du R.A.C., Revue Auriculomédecine, 13, 1978, 35
11. Nogier R.V.A.S., Stimulations lumineuses cutanées sur le lapin. Leur influence sur le taux d'amines vasopressives plasmatiques, Revue Auriculomédecine, 25, 1981, 31
12. Nogier P. The perception of the pulse signal, Revue Auriculomédecine, 28, 1982, 23

CHAPTER 7

# Paul Nogier's Five Main Stages of Research on the Use of the RAC

**Raphaël Nogier**

Many of our colleagues are not aware of how Paul Nogier progressed in his understanding of the RAC. So, it appears important to describe the main steps he took before reaching the method we know today.

Let us bear in mind the fact that the RAC was initially considered by Paul Nogier as a means of improving auriculotherapy, and he first used it as such.

His progression can be roughly divided into five stages.

## 7.1 THE FIVE STAGES

### 7.1.1 First Stage: Study of the RAC by Mechanical and Physical Stimulation of Ear Points

To understand Paul Nogier's approach, we must not forget that he practised acupuncture and, as such, was influenced by the theory of Yin and Yang. To treat the ear points, he used needles made of different metals: gold, silver, and steel. And faced with the difficulty of knowing on what grounds one could choose the right metal, it did not take him long to realize that the RAC might well help solve this problem. To this effect, he studied the reactions of the pulse when stimulating the point with touch, heat, and cold.

Empirically, he elaborated a relatively simple procedure. First, he located the auricular point with an electric detector, after which he studied the point with the pulse. He applied pressure to the point with a very thin piece of cork (TN: presumably to obtain a neutral reference), then stimulated the point with a cold instrument, and finally with a hot instrument, while at the same time observing the reactions on the radial artery. He used glass rods previously put into contact with ice or hot water for cold and hot stimulation. Depending on the nature of the stimulation, he obtained a positive RAC+ or negative RAC−, enabling him to choose a gold, silver, or steel needle. Here is a protocol published in 1969 in his book *Traité d'auriculothérapie* (**Table 7.1**).

This process was abandoned many years ago because gold and silver needles are no longer used for hygiene reasons. Today, we use only disposable steel needles. In those days, however, this research on the ear points undoubtedly enabled Paul Nogier

DOI: 10.1201/9781003753629-7

**Table 7.1 Choice of Needle Metal According to Vascular Reactions**

| Examination | | | Treatment | |
|---|---|---|---|---|
| **Cork** | **Warm** | **Cold** | **Needles** | **Current** |
| + | + | − | Silver | Negative |
| + | − | + | Gold | Positive |
| − | − | + | Silver | Negative |
| − | + | − | Gold | Positive |
| − | + | + | Steel | Positive negative |
| + | − | − | Steel | Positive negative |

to familiarise himself with manual perception of the RAC, which, at that time, was a new procedure that he probably had not yet mastered perfectly.

### 7.1.2 Stage 2: Study of the RAC by Photonic Stimulation of Ear Points

The second step certainly influenced the following stages of Paul Nogier's research, when he became aware of the fact that it was possible to trigger a vascular response by stimulating certain auricular points not by way of a mechanical process, but with a simple beam of punctual white light (**Figure 7.1**). It was then no longer necessary to *touch* the point but merely to *illuminate* it, to initiate an autonomic circulatory response (RAC). **When illuminated, only points of diminished REC (cutaneous electrical resistance) will cause a RAC, whereas stimulation of other types of points will not induce any response.**

In other words, if one wants to detect auricular points correlated with a functional pathology, one can simply explore a subject's ear by manually scanning a punctual light above its surface to locate points that trigger a RAC.

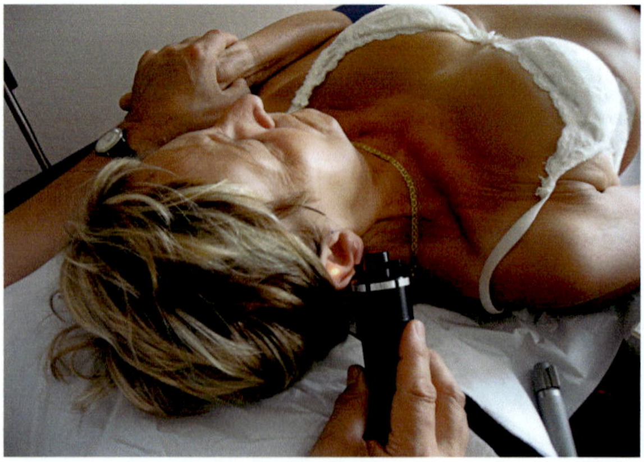

**Figure 7.1** Illumination of pathological ear points triggers a RAC response.

This discovery eventually led auriculotherapy along the path of what is sometimes referred to as "energetics", with all that this may imply, whether positive or negative. This was a major step. Until then, it was easy to understand that mechanically stimulating an ear point could trigger a neurovegetative reaction. Indeed, touch, pressure, cold, and heat all stimulate the cerebrospinal system, which has a well-known relationship with the neurovegetative system. With photonic stimulation, however, it becomes difficult to understand how a neuro-vegetative response can be obtained without stimulation of mechanical receptors within the skin. Why and how would the mere illumination of an auricular point or area of skin create a vascular response? We must suppose the existence of photosensitive cells capable of having a direct or indirect effect on the neurovegetative system, consistent with the fact that an immediate vascular response is obtained following stimulation by light.

Surprisingly, a RAC will only be triggered if the auricular point exposed to light is related to a pathological state and has an electrical activity that can be identified by *a lesser REC* (cutaneous electrical resistance).

It should be remembered that points of lesser REC are histologically related to active *neuro-vascular complexes (CNV)*, which appear to be involved in levels of thermoregulation of the organism.

Exposing a point of diminished electrical resistance to light always induces a vascular response, except if there is *a state of RAC exhaustion* (Chapter 10). The reaction can be more or less important, implying two, five, ten, or more vascular responses (RAC). It is always important to count the number of RACs when exposing the point to light, for assessing the importance of the pathology it represents.

### 7.1.3 Stage 3: Study of the RAC by Stimulating Areas of the Ear

This is the stage that explains the discovery of stimulations by means of *frequencies* used all over the world today.

In the case of a healthy subject, lighting an ear point with a narrow beam does not produce a RAC. But if the light beam is widened, then a RAC may appear (**Figure 7.2**). This fact enabled Paul Nogier to define homogeneous *zones* or *areas* of the ear. At first, six areas were found, and later, seven. These areas, also called territories or *zones, named A, B, C, D, E, F, G*, were then studied with intermittent light (*frequencies*), thus enabling Paul Nogier to isolate the well-known *seven fundamental frequencies*. These frequencies, known today as *the "Nogier frequencies"*, have specific properties used in auricular therapy but also in general medicine. An eighth frequency was described by the author of this chapter in 2006: the L frequency (Chapters 8 and 21).

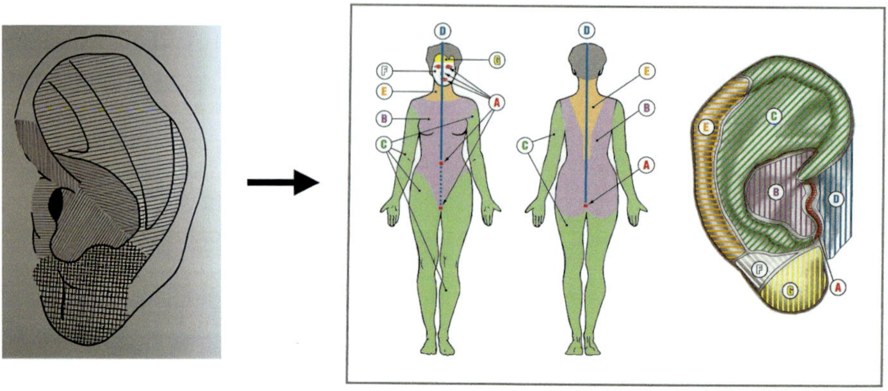


**Figure 7.2** The lighting of ear zones led Paul Nogier to define seven areas.

### 7.1.4 Stage 4: Study of the RAC by Coupled Stimulation of Ear and Periphery

This stage allowed Paul Nogier to study the RAC during simultaneous stimulation of the periphery and the ear. The periphery is defined as all the body areas except the ear and the central nervous system.

We have seen that, in a healthy person, exposing an ear point with a narrow beam of light does not trigger a RAC.

Let us now take the example of a healthy subject artificially exposed to blue light on the right knee. Suppose a RAC is triggered when the auricular point representing the knee is illuminated with blue light bearing the same wavelength. Moreover, the RAC no longer appears as soon as you stop exposing the right knee to blue light. This reaction is called *coupled stimulation*. In this case, we have used the example of blue light, but the phenomenon can be seen with many different types of stimulation. If the right knee of a healthy person is exposed to yellow light, the corresponding auricular point will induce a RAC reaction if illuminated with a yellow beam.

This phenomenon is interesting for several reasons.

It can be used to study localisations on the ear by illuminating some part of the skin with coloured light and then searching for an ear point reacting to the same colour. For example, this procedure can be used in pathologies such as neuropathies of the lower limbs. This consists of exposing the lower limbs to a coloured light and then searching the ear for the point (or points) that appear to react to the same colour. For this, one can use the Italian Microlight device, which allows us to simultaneously expose a region of the body and search for auricular points with the same colour.

This phenomenon also makes it possible to study the transfers of information between the periphery and the ear (Chapter 17). The mechanism we described appears to be physiological and disappears in certain pathologies such as cancer.

### 7.1.5 Stage 5: Triggering RAC without Using the Ear

This stage is probably of interest to a wide medical audience because it involves using the vascular reaction outside the field of auriculotherapy. It is indeed possible to trigger a RAC:

By inducing emotions within the patient. It is with this technique that diagnoses can be made following psycho-emotional traumas or during interpersonal conflicts (Chapter 28). While taking the patient's pulse, the physician will have the patient recall items about their life, activities, and environment. When the patient evokes a painful or traumatic event, the pulse will react. The diagnosis will then entail, in a second phase, the introduction of a treatment, most of the time auriculotherapy.

- By stimulating the skin at a distance from the ear (**Figure 7.3**). This can be done by:
  - white light
  - coloured light
  - pulsed light
  - polarized light
  - colour filters
  - test rings containing biological or chemical substances

This stage opens up auriculotherapy to a broader method in which it is possible to study a patient's reactions by taking their pulse. This is what we call ***signal medicine***.

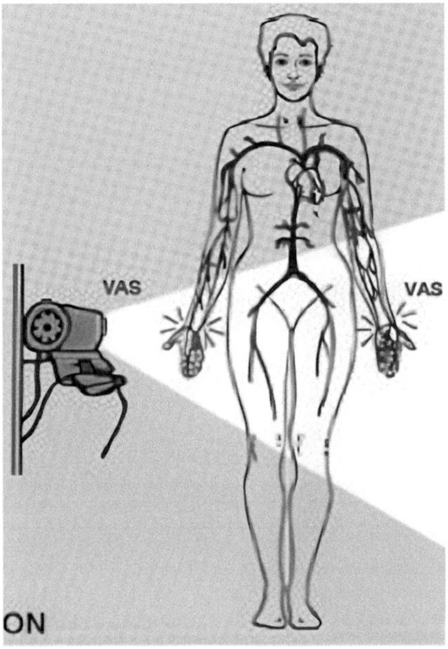


**Figure 7.3** Exposing the skin to light triggers a RAC. (Copyright © Dr. Raphaël Nogier.)

## BIBLIOGRAPHY

1. Bourdiol René. *L'auriculo-somatologie.* Maisonneuve Éditeur. 1981
2. Nogier Paul. *Le traité d'auriculothérapie.* Éditions Maisonneuve. 1969
3. Nogier Paul. *Practical introduction to auriculotherapy.* Maisonneuve. 1977
4. Nogier Paul in collaboration with Raphaël Nogier. *The man in the ear.* Éditions Maisonneuve. 1979
5. Nogier Raphaël. *Comment Paul Nogier a-t-il établi les cartes auriculaires?* Acupuncture and Moxibustion Jan–Mar 2016.

CHAPTER 8

# Use of Colour Filters Photoemission Photoreception Areas Frequencies

Raphaël Nogier

Before describing these topics, we would like the reader to remember the importance of what follows. In auriculotherapy, among other instruments, we use test rings and filters, some of which evaluate photoemission and others photoreception.

In his practice, Paul Nogier used colour filters. These round Kodak Wratten filters (see Chapter 12) have a diameter of 35 mm, i.e. a small surface, which he approached towards the ear or placed on the skin. He had noticed that the RAC reactions varied according to the patient's pathology when approaching these filters towards the ear.

In addition to filters, he also projected coloured light onto ear points using lamps (Chapters 12 and 18).

This implies two different techniques: the first is using colour filters to measure the body's photoemissions; the second is using lamps to activate the body's capacity for photoreception.

Paul Nogier wrote: "*The effects obtained by projecting colours onto the ear are very different from those obtained by approaching, touching or withdrawing filters from the ears. Whereas with filters we measure the energetic emissions from the auricle; by projecting coloured lights, we study receptive areas*" [1].

## 8.1 PHOTOEMISSION

As mentioned above, Paul Nogier evaluated RAC reactions while approaching or placing colour filters on the skin. He even observed that this phenomenon was also active in complete darkness, a fact that formally excluded a classic type of stimulation with light. He realized that what he was measuring using this technique of approaching filters was photonic emission from the organism.

These findings were confirmed by the experiments of Dr John Ackerman, an American neuropsychiatrist who devoted a passionate interest in the clinical use of RAC.

DOI: 10.1201/9781003753629-8

In 2005 and 2006, Ackerman conducted experiments on the emission of body bio-photons when approaching a Wratten Kodak red 25 colour filter. This paper earned him the GLEM (Lyon Group for Medical Studies) Prize in 2006.

The experiments took place in Neuss, Germany, in a biophysics laboratory equipped with instruments designed for counting photons emitted by the organism in complete darkness. The emission of bio-photons is indeed not limited to small organisms but can also be observed in humans. The wavelength of these emissions corresponds to oxygen and lipid radical peroxidation processes (**Figure 8.1**).

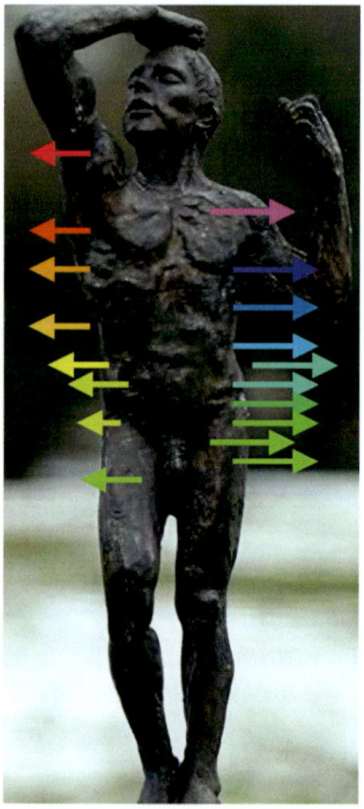

**Figure 8.1** The skin emits bio-photons.

The experiment consisted of placing a red Kodak Wratten no. 25 filter at 7 cm from the palm of a subject's left hand for 200 seconds and measuring the photonic emission on the back of the hand and on the forehead before and after placing the filter at 7 cm from the palm. The results suggest that approaching a filter has a systemic action because it entails an increased emission of bio-photons, not only from the hand itself but also simultaneously from the forehead.

The most logical explanation for this phenomenon would be that the filter partly reflects bio-photons emitted by the skin of the hand and will, therefore, return to stimulate the skin. This would explain why in signal medicine, a red filter does not have the same effect as a blue or green filter because the reflected photons differ. By definition, a filter lets a certain number of photons through while absorbing some and reflecting others. This seems to us the most likely hypothesis.

In signal medicine, the study of photoemission using the RAC will allow us to assess the severity of a disease. For this, we use seven colour filters. Each filter has a letter and a number. The letter corresponds to the territory described on the body, and the number to the Wratten Kodak classification:

- Orange A21
- Red B25
- Yellow C3 or yellow C4
- Red D24
- Blue E44
- Violet F98
- Magenta G30

It is important to understand that these filters bear a correspondence with the territories on the body and not with the so-called Nogier frequencies. They are mainly used to study the photoemission of an area. For example, if a patient comes to us suffering from abdominal pain, we can evaluate photoemission of the abdomen with the B25 filter since the abdomen is part of the B territory. While taking the patient's pulse, we slowly scan the B25 filter at about 2 cm over the abdomen to locate RAC reactions. If a pathological area exists, the pulse will become harder over this area, and we will observe a RAC+. The degree of photoemission and the importance of the pathology will be proportionate to the number of RAC reactions. The maximum is 9 RAC. Above 5 RAC, the pathology can be serious.

Along the same lines, if we were to study a pathology of the limbs, we would use the C3 or C4 filter. If we were to examine the neck, we would use filter E, etc.

## 8.2 PHOTORECEPTION

Paul Nogier began working on the concept of cutaneous photoreception at the end of the 1960s, without giving it a precise name at the time. It was mainly during the eighties, following experiments carried out at the INSA (National Institute for Applied Sciences, France) with Professor Roger Santini, that this concept was studied at length. At first, it was erroneously called skin photo-*perception*. Erroneously because the word "perception" implies sensoriality, which is not the case here.

Initially, the experiments at INSA were intended to prove the existence of the RAC by biological instead of mechanical measurements. Indeed, since its discovery in

1966, no recording of the RAC had been convincing, despite numerous trials. It was, therefore, decided to proceed in a different way and to see if stimulation of the skin could lead to a variation of the circulating catecholamines (adrenaline, noradrenaline, dopamine), which are natural vasopressive substances of the organism and, therefore, capable of modifying the arterial tone. It was assumed that if stimulation of the skin by light could lead to disturbances in circulating catecholamines, this would bring indirect evidence of the existence of RAC.

The research was conducted on rabbits. Each rabbit was placed in a box with a rounded hole a few centimetres in diameter on one side, allowing it to keep its head out. It was, therefore, possible to expose the rabbits to light inside the box without involving the eyes. They were "blind" rabbits, so to speak. They had not been shaved, and their coats were normal.

Three lots were studied:

- A control lot
- A lot exposed to continuous white light for 1 minute
- A lot exposed to discontinuous white light (9 cycles/second) for 2 minutes

The rabbits received the same number of photons, whether exposed to continuous or discontinuous light.

Blood samples were taken: 1 minute before exposure to light, then at 5 seconds, 30 seconds, 1 minute, 5 minutes, and 10 minutes after exposure.

The results were very clear. Compared to the control, the rabbits exposed to discontinuous light had increased blood levels of catecholamines, which was not the case for the rabbits exposed to continuous light.

In other words, a "blind" rabbit can biologically recognize the difference between continuous and discontinuous light, projected onto its coat. The rabbit, therefore, has a special ability to discriminate between photonic stimuli of different qualities on its coat. This implies the presence of photoreceptors within the skin, which is unsurprising given that photoreception is a faculty found in many single-cell beings.

Using the same procedure, the influence of light on sugar and acetylcholinesterase blood levels was also studied.

The experiments on rabbits were then continued at Professor Kahn's laboratory in Neuilly, France. This time, the aim was to study the influence of coloured light on pain in a vigilant rabbit. A rabbit was prepared by inserting an electrode into the thalamus to produce nervous influxes induced by infra-somaesthetic electrical stimulation of one of its legs. The animal was then placed in a box with a hole at one end to keep its head out and avoid seeing what was happening inside the box, where a system was installed to expose the rabbit to different coloured lights.

The experiment consisted of stimulating a rabbit's hind leg and, using the electrode located in the thalamus, collecting data for a so-called "pain curve". The aim was to observe whether this curve was altered due to the rabbit's coat being exposed to different coloured lights. What we obtained confirmed our hopes, as indeed the pain curve was found to be altered by the photonic atmosphere in the box. The curve decreased when the rabbit's coat was exposed to blue light, whereas the curve increased significantly with yellow or red light. This experiment suggests that the colour of light projected onto the rabbit's coat alters the transmission of nociceptive information and, thereby, also chemical neuromediation.

### 8.2.1 Why Does Skin Photoreception Exist?

That is the question we have been trying to answer since 1985. It appears the skin could act as a vast receptor of electromagnetic information (**Figure 8.2**).

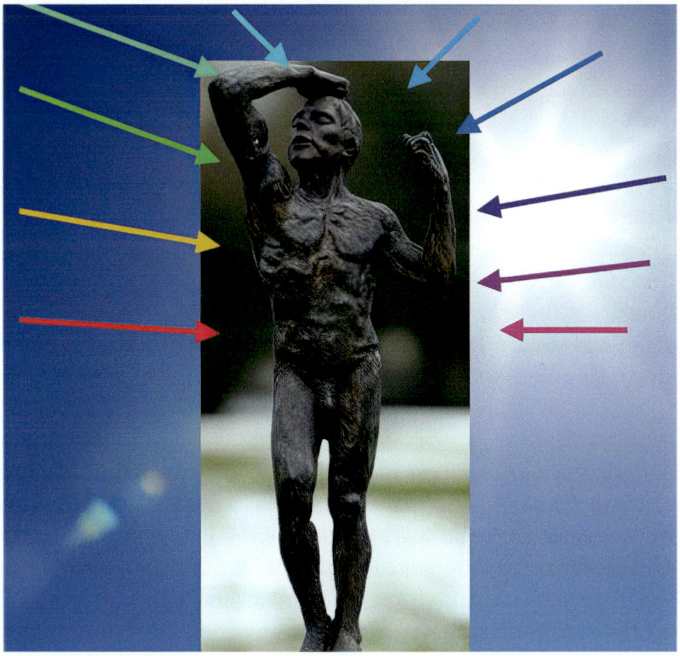

**Figure 8.2** The skin surface acts like a photoreceptor.

It has been known for a long time that many single-cell beings have a more or less developed photosensitivity. Phototactism is a known and well-studied property in certain bacteria and larvae. Everyone has in mind the experiments carried out with a Petri dish, covered on half its surface by a mask, and where a difference in microbial presence can be observed on the side exposed to light, compared to the dark side. Some single cells are attracted to light. This is positive Phototactism. Others turn away from it, which is known as negative phototactism.

In Humans, certain cells are photosensitive. We are all familiar with visual perception due to the properties of retinal cells. The eye contains photosensitive captors and is designed much like a photographic camera. Its function is to receive and transform electromagnetic vibrations produced by light into nerve impulses, which in turn are transmitted through the optic pathways to the visual areas of the cortex. The retina contains photoreceptive cells containing pigments that are decomposed by light absorption, giving rise to a receptor potential through depolarisation. Cones contain rhodopsin, and rods contain iodopsin. Vision is a property observed in a great number of animal species: insects, birds, and mammals. The question arises as to whether any other cells in the body could be photosensitive. And how exactly does light act upon the organism?

Benoit's experiments on ducks are demonstrative, showing that their fertility is increased by 15% by switching from 6 hours of light per day to 15 hours per day. Benoit observed that only red and orange lights stimulate the gonads, whereas other colours have no effect. This phenomenon can be explained by stimulation of the hypothalamus via the eyes.

Disclos studied the development of Anura frogs. When subjected to a regular photoperiod, they require 244 to 260 days to become adults. By exposing the tadpoles to light 24 hours a day, the maturation time will then be reduced to 130 days. Disclos wanted to find out whether the eyes were involved in this process, and surgically destroyed the eyes of the tadpoles, exposed to light 24 hours a day. There again, the maturation time was reduced to 130 days. The eyes are therefore not involved in the process, and it is possible to consider the existence of deep receptors, the action of which is favoured by the transparency of the teguments.

It seems likely that photoreception is involved in the regulation of chemical neuromediation. If we give credit to Darwin's thesis, we cannot imagine that there is no adaptation to electromagnetic waves within living beings. Biologically speaking, adaptation can be defined as the adjustment of an organism to its environment. For example, it will help the organism become consistent with the surrounding air or water and bring it to "get the most" out of its environment through lungs or gills. Functional and structural modifications of the organism itself will follow. This principle of adaptation, which cannot be questioned, gives us a glimpse of the possibilities of cutaneous photoreception.

As it is, we are permanently absorbed within an electromagnetic "soup" made of various waves that come to us from the stars and mainly from the sun. How could we imagine that terrestrial organisms would not have made use of this soup to develop? These waves range from very short to long waves, including visible waves ranging from 400 nm to 780 nm. Why would various organisms not have used these waves in various ways in their development?

The skin surface appears to act like a huge electromagnetic wave sensor, rather like a parabolic antenna. In our view, these waves will influence certain functions but also regulate and repair them by stimulating chemical neuromediation.

We believe that stimulation of a neuromediator via the skin can only be conceived within a precise range of wavelengths and that a given wavelength projected onto the skin will stimulate the production of a specific chemical neuromediator. Red light does not have the same effect as green or blue light.

The skin surface is not uniform, and certain areas or territories will be receptive to given wavelengths, while other areas will receive other wavelengths. As far as photoreception is concerned, the skin resembles a kind of patchwork.

## 8.3 THE SEVEN AREAS (TERRITORIES) OF THE BODY AND THE EAR

Using the RAC, Paul Nogier described seven different territories of photoreception on the body. At first, however, he had begun by defining seven territories on the ear, showing that in a healthy individual, a vascular reaction (RAC) could be triggered by exposing the ear to light. The area had to be sufficiently large because a narrow beam of light on the ear would not normally produce a RAC.

The seven territories (or areas) **on the ear** were named by letters (**Figure 8.3**. See also Section 21.3.1):

- **Territory A**: the subtragal region, overlooking the external acoustic meatus
- **Territory B**: the concha
- **Territory C**: the anthelix and the anterior part of the helix
- **Territory D**: the external part of the tragus
- **Territory E**: the posterior part and the tail of the helix
- **Territory F**: the posterior part of the lobule
- **Territory G**: the anterior part of the lobule, just behind the cheek

In the second stage, Paul Nogier, working with the pulse, wanted to know if these auricular territories had specific properties regarding *pulsed* light stimulation as opposed to *continuous* light. He, therefore, acquired a light-emitting device capable of projecting a *punctual* pulsed light that could range from 1 to 10,000 Hz. At that point, he found out that each different territory reacted to stimulation by a specific pulsed frequency (**Table 8.1**).

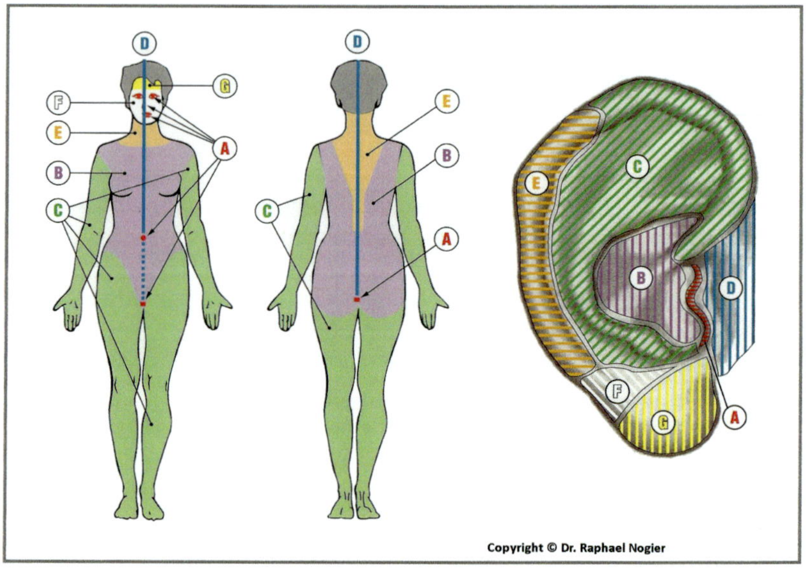


**Figure 8.3** Paul Nogier described seven territories on the ear and the body.

**Table 8.1 Ear Territories and the Frequencies to Which They Respond**

| Ear territory | Responds at (Hz) |
|---|---|
| A | 2.28 |
| B | 4.56 |
| C | 9.12 |
| D | 18.24 |
| E | 36.5 |
| F | 73 |
| G | 146 |

In the third stage, Paul Nogier was able to determine that the frequencies to which the areas of the body respond are the same as those to which the areas of the ear react, provided the pulsed light frequencies were applied to specific territories or zones.

So Nogier could now define seven zones on the body (**Figure 8.3**). These territories (or zones) on the body are distributed as follows:

| | |
|---|---|
| Body zone **A**: | *Orifices*: eyes, nostrils, mouth, navel, urinary meatus, vagina, anus |
| Body zone **B**: | Anterior part of the trunk between the bi-clavicular line and the insertion of the deltoids at its upper limit and the inguinal folds at its lower limit |

| | |
|---|---|
| Body zone **C**: | Upper and lower limbs |
| Body zone **D**: | Median sagittal line 4 cm wide, starting from the pubis, goes up along the Linea alba of the abdomen, the sternum, and the bridge of the nose, up to the apex of the skull, and goes down on the back, passing by the spinal processes of the vertebrae, ending at the anus |
| Body zone **E:** | Essentially the neck and scalp |
| Body zone **F:** | Face |
| Body zone **G:** | Forehead and alar part (wings) of the nose |

## 8.4 WHAT DO THE NOGIER FREQUENCIES CORRESPOND TO?

It is important to bear in mind that Paul Nogier was, above all, an experimentalist, keen to undertake research in a great many fields. He did not immediately grasp the implications of his discovery on frequencies, and it took him some time to understand their medical interest. Each frequency has its own biological properties. The A-frequency (2.28 Hz), for example, does not have the same properties as the B-frequency (4.56 Hz) or the G-frequency (146 Hz). The skin, divided into seven territories, constantly receives electromagnetic frequencies of different wavelengths. Every territory specializes in the reception of a particular frequency, and each wavelength will, in turn, stimulate a specific body function.

## 8.5 REMINDER ON LIGHT

To understand the concept of photoreception, it is helpful to sum up the nature of light. Light corresponds to the electromagnetic waves visible to the human eye, i.e. wavelengths from 380 nm (violet) to 780 nm (red). Light comes from matter. Without matter, there is no light. Matter is made up of atoms, which contain a nucleus (protons and neutrons) around which one or several electrons rotate. The nucleus has a positive electric charge and the electron a negative charge.

Electrons gravitate around the nucleus on orbital layers called Bohr orbits, after the physicist who discovered them. The energy of each electron depends on the orbit in which it rotates. The further away the orbit is from the nucleus, the greater the energy of the electron. Under certain circumstances, an electron can change orbit, jumping down to a lower layer. By this, the electron will lose a quantum of energy released as a photon, a speck of light. The colour or wavelength of the light is determined by the amount of energy released. This means that light (with a few exceptions) simply originates from an electron changing orbit (**Figure 8.4**). It will have only one frequency and is therefore called monochromatic.

An electric light bulb is based on this principle. To create artificial light, a tungsten wire is connected to an electric current. This agitates the electrons contained in the tungsten, thus making them jump up and down from one layer to another, producing photons.

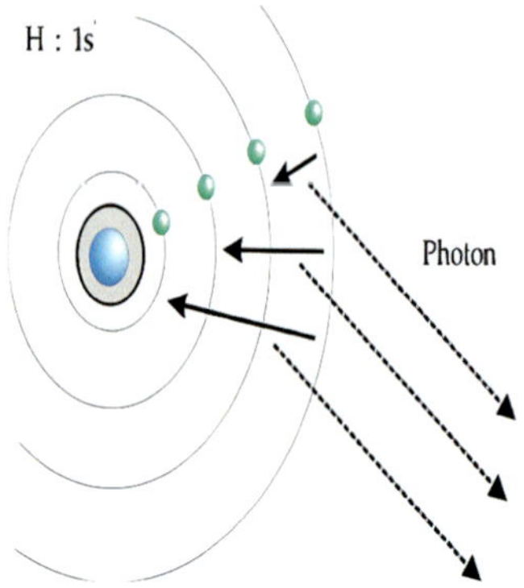


**Figure 8.4** A photon originates from the loss of energy of an electron due to a change of orbit.

Due to the properties of our eye receptors, equal amounts of red, green, and blue light are perceived as (metameric) white light in humans. Also, continuous whole spectrum light, composed of an equal amount of photons of all colours in the visual spectrum, is perceived as white, e.g. the light emitted by the sun or from a halogen light bulb. When light contains photons of more than one wavelength or colour, we call it polychromatic.

## 8.6 FREQUENCY GENERATORS

Paul Nogier worked with various intermittent (pulsed) light generators (Chapter 12) that function like stroboscopes, thus pulsing with a specific pulsation frequency—not to be confused with the colour frequency or wavelength of the light, corresponding to the energy of the photons. In auricular therapy, it is customary to reserve the term frequency to mean pulsation frequency and to use wavelength or colour to denote the energy level of the photon.

The device he used the most was the GIR 30 (Sedatelec), which emits close to a monochromatic red light, and if the nozzle is changed, it can instead emit infrared wavelengths. He also used gallium arsenide infrared lasers (904 nm). Today, we hold the view that when the instrument is too powerful, which is the case with lasers, it tends to be less effective in auriculotherapy than devices with weaker power. The more powerful the stimulation, the lesser the therapeutic response. Conversely, the therapeutic response will be optimal if we use a weaker stimulation.

In our current practice today, we use an Italian instrument, the GL+ (Micropad), which also emits red or infrared (**Figure 8.5**). It has the advantage of being designed for both right- and left-handed practitioners and being able to produce 150 different pulsation frequencies. It is the only instrument offering a choice between the "historical" first-generation frequencies and the second-generation frequencies used in various generators (see **Table 8.2**).

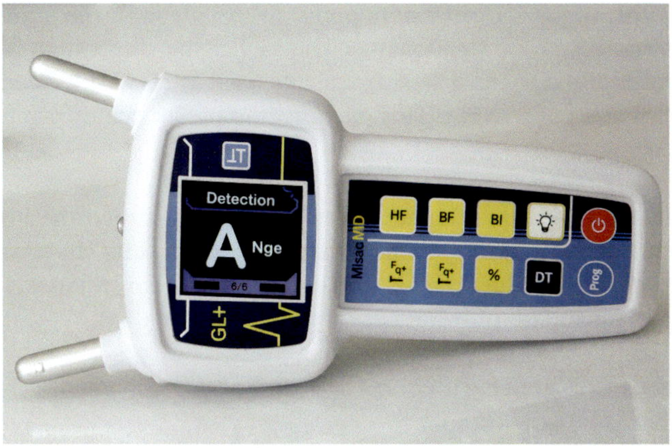


**Figure 8.5** The Micropad GL+ generator can produce 150 different frequencies.

**Table 8.2 First- and Second-Generation Frequencies**

| Name of the frequencies | Historical frequencies in Hz First-generation frequency | Second-generation frequency used in frequency generators |
|---|---|---|
| U | 11.4 | |
| A | 2.28 | 292 |
| B | 4.56 | 584 |
| C | 9.12 | 1168 |
| D | 18.24 | 2336 |
| E | 36.5 | 4672 |
| F | 73 | 9334 |
| G | 146 | 18,688 |
| L | 276 | |

As we can see, there is a geometric progression in the sequence of Nogier frequencies, each of which doubles the previous one: 2.28; 4.56; 9.12; 18.24; 36.5; 73; 146 Hz. These frequencies were described between 1970 and 1978. It turns out that if we continue this progression, a curious phenomenon appears. If we multiply the G-frequency, 146 Hz, by 2, we obtain 292 Hz, a frequency that seems to have the same properties as the A-frequency. Therefore, several A-frequencies would exist: 2.28 Hz and 292 Hz. If we continue multiplying by 2, we obtain a frequency of 584, which has the same properties as the B frequency, and so on. We could compare this phenomenon to an endless spiral (**Table 8.2**).

The frequencies that follow the historical frequencies are called second-generation frequencies.

Manufacturers of frequency generators prefer to use second-generation frequencies to increase the power of the light beams. The higher the stimulation frequency, the greater the power of the beam. The A frequency used at 2.28 Hz has less power than the A frequency used at 292 Hz. This explains the preference of manufacturers for higher frequencies.

The Micropad GL+ allows the practitioner to choose between the historical first-generation frequencies and the second-generation frequencies. In specific pathologies, it seems preferable to use the historical frequencies: for instance, in the case of Parkinson's disease and fibromyalgia.

Two other frequencies are also used.

- The U frequency of 1.14 Hz, described by Paul Nogier, is half the A-frequency (2.28 Hz) and can be used to replace any other frequency (hence the name U for "universal"). It is widely used by medical instrument manufacturers for the electrical stimulation of auricular points.
- The L frequency of 276 Hz, described by Raphaël Nogier in 2006, stimulates laterality functions (see Chapter 26).

## 8.7 BIOLOGICAL PROPERTIES OF FREQUENCIES

Each frequency has its own biological properties.

**A-frequency** is the frequency of cell stimulation. If we expose a cell to frequency A, we stimulate the work processes of this cell. Our colleague and friend, Dr Chantal Vulliez from Lyon, has studied the effect of this frequency on the behaviour of fibroblasts, which are known to produce collagen.

**B-frequency** stimulates all functions related to multicellularity:

- Cohesion between cells
- Coherence in the work of cells
- Intercellular exchanges, nutrition function, digestive system, intestinal absorption
- Respiration
- **Intercellular recognition**: immune system
- **Endocrine system**: thyroid
- Venous system

**C-frequency** stimulates all functions related to motricity:

- Dopaminergic function
- Striated muscle contraction

- Smooth muscle contraction
  - Intestinal peristalsis
  - Bile flush
  - Arterial vasomotricity
  - Cardiac muscle function
  - Contraction of tonic-phasic paravertebral muscles

**D-frequency** stimulates functions related to symmetry in the organism. All animals have a symmetry function resulting in the development of two identical hemi-bodies mirrored on a symmetry axis.

**E-frequency** stimulates the most elementary neurological function: the reflex loop consisting of a motor neuron, a sensory neuron, and a neuron for association.

**F-frequency** stimulates subcortical functions, those related to preservation of the organism and its reproduction, mainly sensations and feelings: hunger, thirst, pain, sensation of heat or cold, thermoregulation, fear, attraction, repulsion, endocrine control.

**G-frequency** stimulates cortical functions: cognition and interpretation.

**L-frequency** stimulates laterality, i.e. the functional asymmetry of the two cerebral hemispheres (**Table 8.3**).

**Table 8.3 Biological Properties of the Nogier Frequencies**

| Frequency | Biological properties |
|---|---|
| A | Stimulates cell work |
| B | Stimulates functions related to pluricellularity: coherence, cohesion, recognition, digestive and respiratory system |
| C | Stimulates motor function (muscles) |
| D | Stimulates symmetry and locomotion |
| E | Stimulates medullary function (reflex loop) |
| F | Stimulates sub-cortical functions: sensations, feelings, endocrine control |
| G | Stimulates cortical functions, cognition, sociability |
| L | Stimulates laterality, asymmetry: learning, decision-making, skills, memory |

## 8.8 INTERPRETATION OF THE FREQUENCY SYSTEM

The French poet Paul Valery is known to have said: *"What is deepest in man is his skin".*

The skin is not just a barrier between the outside and the inside of the body. It is an active interface between what is happening inside and what is going on outside.

The skin reflects our metabolism, emotions, thoughts, and way of life. Neurodermatitis such as prurigo and sometimes eczema is a reminder that stress, for example, can generate skin diseases. This phenomenon has been known for a long time. History reminds us of Queen Marie-Antoinette's or Thomas More's hair turning white very quickly, in a few days, shortly before their execution. These phenomena can be explained because the skin and nervous system are intimately linked, both deriving from the same embryological sheet: the ectoblast.

Although we are aware of the effects of the nervous system on the skin, on the other hand, we do not know the precise details of how the skin influences the nervous system. Of course, we are familiar with the fact that the skin involves perception of temperature, pressure, and pain, all of which are conscious sensations. However, classical physiology lacks knowledge concerning the role the skin plays unconsciously in regulating different functions of the organism.

Thanks to the RAC, we have been able to study the effects of various stimulations on the skin. Today, we believe the skin behaves like a vast receptor of information constantly receiving electromagnetic waves. These waves stimulate, regulate, and repair various functions of the body. The skin is a photoreceptor divided into different territories, each of which reacts to a certain category of waves.

Paul Nogier mainly studied the influence of *pulsed* light on the skin. However, he also studied the influence of *coloured* light, but for cost reasons, he had to use polychromatic filters instead of a single monochromatic colour. So, it was difficult to define precisely which wavelengths induced an RAC. However, he found a correspondence in reaction between Nogier's pulsation frequencies and the wavelengths of light. Projecting coloured light onto the skin or projecting intermittent light would, in fact, have the same effect.

Certain wavelengths of light would have the same effects as A-Frequency, others the same effects as B-Frequency, etc. However, to establish a parallel between the wavelengths of light and the Nogier frequencies, we come up against a technical problem. Ideally, we would work with a combination of numerous monochromatic filters. Their cost, however, was not affordable. With today's LED having very narrow "close to monochromatic" wavelength bands, it might have turned out differently.

So, most research and experiments have focussed on filtered light, and to tap into this knowledge, we are compelled to use polychromatic light. Our mentor, Professor Pierre Magnin, has studied at length the effects of coloured light while taking the pulse of his patients. Without really defining a parallel between Nogier frequencies and wavelengths, he has, however, clearly defined the properties of each coloured light, which entails the possibility of establishing a clinical correspondence.

To understand the frequency system, we must consider Man from a historical standpoint, as indeed the skin seems to be a witness of evolution and more precisely of our evolution.

It is estimated that the earth is 4.5 billion years old. In its early days, the earth contained only minerals, water, and gases and was exposed to electromagnetic waves coming from the stars, especially the sun. It is somewhat difficult to imagine our planet without life, which probably began following the appearance of amino acids. This was a decisive condition for the development of proteins, yet it remains mysterious. It is likely that these elements were brought to Earth by comets. This is called panspermia. In any event, life did not appear suddenly to give rise to what we know today. There was a slow and gradual evolution. It all started with the appearance of single-cell beings and ended with man.

### 8.8.1 Single-Cell Stage: A-Frequencies

Life probably appeared on earth about 3.8 billion years ago in the form of cells that are thought to have colonised the surface of the globe over several hundred thousand years. These first cells were probably rudimentary. They had a hydrophilic membrane on one side and a hydrophobic membrane on the other. To develop, they needed energy, which they drew from the surrounding electromagnetic waves, the sole resources available to them.

Today, we know that intracellular elements are sensitive to certain wavelengths of light and not to others. Some wavelengths facilitate chemical reactions; others inhibit them. For example, cytochrome b, essential for cell respiration, is selectively inhibited by 530 nm, whereas 633 nm at the same power has no effect (Rounds and Johnson). This can be explained by the absorption of light by biological structures. Cells, living in a heterogeneous and complex electromagnetic soup, made use of the waves they needed to be able to develop, and it is likely that different wavelengths of light were selected by the cells. For the sake of convention, let us name 'A-frequencies' all the electromagnetic waves that promote cellular work by inhibiting or facilitating certain chemical reactions.

### 8.8.2 Multi cellular Stage: B-Frequencies

One of the characteristics of evolution is a progressive increase in the complexity of structures, not a simplification. Following the cellular stage, which lasted for several hundred million years, multicellular structures appeared, acquiring new properties essential for survival. Again, the preservation of life appears as an inherent property of life itself.

Evolution towards multicellular beings involved specific requirements. For a living being made of several cells to survive, it is necessary that:

- All the cells of the structure are joined and aggregate with one another,
- There are exchanges regarding nutrition and information between all the cells,
- All the cells work in coherence: multicellular metabolism,
- Each of them can differentiate a self-cell from a non-self-cell.

In a multicell structure, each cell must imperatively serve the structure to which it belongs, much like the "hive effect" where each bee fulfils a role in the overall functioning of the hive. Multicellularity will require the emergence of anatomical and functional structures to ensure intercellular cohesion, coherence, intercellular exchanges, metabolism, and recognition. Anatomically, this multicellularity represents the digestive tract, the respiratory system, the digestive appendices, the immune system, the venous system, and the primitive endocrine system in humans.

For the sake of clarity, let us extend the meaning of the term "multicellularity" to a set of functions that are essential to the maintenance of a multicellular structure.

Let us, by convention, call "B-frequencies" all the electromagnetic waves which, by facilitating or inhibiting chemical reactions, have had a positive effect on the development and functioning of multicellular beings: cohesion, coherence, exchange, metabolism, and recognition.

### 8.8.3 Emergence of Muscle Cells: C-Frequencies

When a multicellular organism grows, it is essential that it is capable of transporting nutrients to all parts of the parenchyma. This requires the existence of pathways (arteries) with an ejection system (pump, peristalsis). In humans, if the heart stops for a few minutes, the system does not survive. We believe that within evolution, the first muscle cells found their purpose in satisfying the need to actively transport food, nutrients, gases, and waste. Let us call "C-frequencies" all the electromagnetic waves that contribute to the emergence and functioning of motor cells.

### 8.8.4 Emergence of Symmetry: D-Frequencies

Symmetry is mysterious. All animals are built around an axis of symmetry, on either side of which there are two identical hemi-bodies. Symmetry does not spare the central nervous system since all developed animals have a brain composed of two parts linked together by commissures. This configuration is undoubtedly linked to locomotion, which almost defines the Animal Kingdom, although some animals do not have locomotion. The sponge, for example, is part of the Animal Kingdom but does not possess the faculty of locomotion and generally does not have elements of symmetry.

For a living being to move, it must acquire at least two functions: a motor function and a symmetry function. Indeed, locomotion cannot be conceived without perfect symmetry. This is a major difference between the animal and plant kingdoms, where symmetry is not an absolute rule. Trees have an asymmetrical development that depends mainly on sunshine and wind. In humans, regardless of the environment, development is symmetrical with respect to an axis because there is an intrinsic function of symmetrisation. Let us call "D-frequencies" all the frequencies that have contributed to stimulating the function of symmetry.

### 8.8.5 Instinctive and Reflex Brain: E-Frequencies

The archencephalon refers to the development level of fish and amphibians. The reflex loop, which is made up of a sensory neuron, a motor neuron, and an interneuron, is the simplest and shortest known nervous circuit allowing motricity to be triggered from a stimulus either mechanical (patellar reflex), by light (pupillary reflex), or by sound (stapedius reflex). The reflex responds to the law of all or nothing and is carried out without the participation of consciousness. In evolution, this reflex loop probably constitutes the first outline of the nervous system. It participates in defence mechanisms and in the maintenance of homeostasis. Let us call "E-frequencies" all the electromagnetic waves that have participated in the emergence and functioning of the reflex loop as well as of the neurovegetative system.

### 8.8.6 Impulsive and Automatic Brain: F-Frequencies

The palencephalon is the stage of development of reptiles and birds. The sub-cortex comprises different nuclei that play an important part in managing sensations, behaviour, and any automatic activity. Let us call "F-frequencies" all the electromagnetic waves that have participated in the development and functioning of the subcortex. In humans, anatomical structures corresponding to the F-frequencies are mainly represented by the limbic system: thalamus, hypothalamus, neurohypophysis, striatum, pallidum, hippocampus, and amygdala.

### 8.8.7 Rational Brain: G-Frequencies

The neoencephalon is the cerebral cortex, which is mainly developed in primates and especially in man. The neoencephalon controls the palencephalon. Let us call "G-frequencies" all electromagnetic waves that have participated in the emergence and functioning of the neocortex.

### 8.8.8 The Functional Asymmetry of the Cerebral Hemispheres: L-Frequencies

While all animals are built on a symmetrical pattern that has induced the existence of two identical, mirrored hemi-bodies, man is not entirely subject to this rule since every human being also expresses laterality. Man is gradually moving away from symmetry. Ninety-six percent of humans are right-handed and prefer using one hemi-body to the other, which is not the case with animals, even superior species such as monkeys. This motor preference is linked to a functional asymmetry of the cerebral hemispheres. In humans, the left hemisphere is functionally different from the right hemisphere. In 2006, the author of this chapter discovered a new frequency (L-Frequency) that stimulates the functional asymmetry of the cerebral hemispheres.

## 8.9 SUMMARY OF PHOTORECEPTION AND PHOTOEMISSION

See **Table 8.4**.

**Table 8.4 Summary of Photoreception and Photoemission**

| | Photoreception | Photoemission |
|---|---|---|
| **Physiology** | • The skin is a photoreceptor<br>• There are 8 photoreceptive areas Each area responds to a specific frequency<br>• There are 8 fundamental frequencies: A, B, C, D, E, F, G, L<br><br>Normally, any projection of white light onto a sufficiently large area of the skin will result in a 3-pulse RAC<br><br>Photoreception is used to stimulate, regulate, and repair certain functions | • The skin emits bio-photons<br>• Eight photoemission areas:<br>• Area A: orange 21<br>• Area B: red 25<br>• Area C: yellow 3<br>• Area D: red 24<br>• Area E: blue 44<br>• Area F: violet 98<br>• Area G: magenta 32<br>• Area L: green 58 |
| **Pathology** | • Photoreception gaps in the photogram<br>• Parasite frequencies<br>• Frequency signature of a lesion<br>• Frequency signature of an auricular point | Photoemission increases with pathology |
| **Diagnosis** | • White light test<br>• Photogram<br>• Projection of frequencies on the body or the ear using frequency generators<br>• Projection of coloured lights on the body or ear points<br>• Laterality frequencies<br>• RAFT (Radial Artery Food Test)<br>• With the white rod, we detect receptor points | • Study of the RAC by approaching coloured filters at a distance of 1 or 2 cm from the skin. Study by approaching a coloured filter towards the ear<br>• Double contact technique. This gives us information on the impaired territory. E.g., filter B25 corresponds to territory B<br>• With the black rod, we look for emitting points |
| **Treatment** | • Treatment with the same frequencies as the signature<br>• The lesion or auricular point will be treated for as long as there is a RAC response | When a lesion is identified on the soma by photoemission, the frequency signature must be determined with a frequency generator. Then, the auricular point corresponding to these frequencies must be found |
| **Comments** | The study of RAC responses to frequency projection will give us information on the nature and quality of the pathology | The study of photoemission will give us information on the severity of the pathology<br><br>Each filter must be used on its own territory |

## BIBLIOGRAPHY

1. Nogier Paul. *From auriculotherapy to auriculomedicine.* Éditions Maisonneuve. 1981
2. Akerman John. *Human biophoton emission and VAS.* GLEM Annals 2006–2007
3. Bourdiol René. *Elements of auriculotherapy.* Éditions Maisonneuve. 1981
4. Bourdiol René. *L'auriculo-somatologie.* Maisonneuve éditeur 1981
5. Magnin Pierre, VIDAL Pascal. *Photonic medicine* 2013
6. Nogier Paul. "*L'auriculothérapie*". Lyon-Méditerranée Médical Tome VII n° 14 September 1971
7. NOGIER Paul in collaboration with NOGIER Raphaël: *L'homme dans l'oreille.* Éditions Maisonneuve. 1979
8. Nogier Paul. *Le traité d'auriculothérapie.* Éditions Maisonneuve. 1969
9. Nogier R. *Auriculotherapy.* Thieme 2007
10. Nogier R. *Health through the ear.* Editions Mango 2018
11. Rouxeville Yves. *The keys to auriculotherapy.* Satas 2015
12. Rouxeville Yves. *Panorama of auriculotherapy and auriculomedicine.* Springer 2000

CHAPTER 9

# The White Light Test

**Raphaël Nogier**

## 9.1 INTRODUCTION

When examining our patients, the very first thing to do is to measure the efficiency of the neuro-vegetative system when faced with a stimulus. This is a prerequisite. To do this, we will stimulate the skin in a global and non-specific manner while observing the reaction of the radial artery pulse. It should be kept in mind that the skin is innervated almost entirely by the sympathetic system, which is also the case with the radial artery. Stimulating the skin will, for a few seconds, stimulate sympathetic activity, thus triggering transient RAC reactions. The skin can be stimulated in different ways, but we have opted for exposure to light because it is simple and easily reproducible. The response obtained through the RAC will give an idea of the subject's ability to react to any stimulus and thus anticipate her or his capacity to react to a more important aggression such as a virus, bacteria, fungi, an accidental or surgical wound, a cancerous cell, or merely frustration. Indeed, if the patient proves unable to adapt to a simple stimulus, how could we expect this patient to face a genuine aggression requiring adaptation and defence on the part of the organism?

So, among the many techniques available for triggering RACs, *the white light test* is one of the simplest. All that is needed is a light bulb of approximately 75 watts, placed at about 60 cm from the patient, to light up a wide area on the front wall of the chest. The patient (shirtless, if possible) lies supine on the examination couch, eyes open. The room should be comfortably heated, quiet, and dimly lit. The patient must not be under stress.

The examiner, positioned behind the patient's head, feels the patient's left radial pulse with his left thumb (**Figure 9.1**). To allow the patient to get used to the examiner's

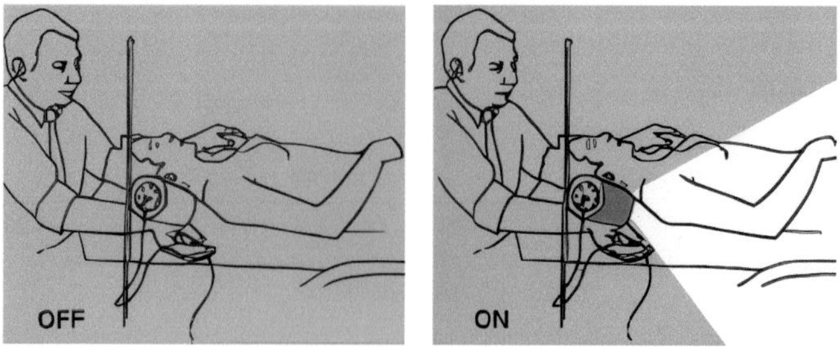


**Figure 9.1** Triggering a RAC by exposing the chest to white light.


DOI: 10.1201/9781003753629-9

presence, the latter should remain in this position for at least ten seconds before beginning the test. The pressure on the radial artery should be neither too strong nor too light. Strong enough to feel the arterial beats but not to the point of blocking the artery (**Figures 4.1** and **9.1**).

The test involves exposing the patient to a flash of white light by directing a wide beam onto the chest (**Figure 9.1**). Under normal physiological conditions, this will immediately trigger a RAC+ response.

## 9.2 THE REACTIVITY INDEX (RI): MEASURING THE SYMPATHETIC RESPONSE: ADAPTATION

Exposing the chest to a flash of white light normally triggers 3 RAC responses (**Figure 9.2**), known as a *reactivity index (RI)* of 3. The index is precious information because it will allow us to appreciate the proper functioning of the neuro-vegetative system and its capacity to correctly ensure the balance of the internal environment as well as defend the organism in the event of aggression.

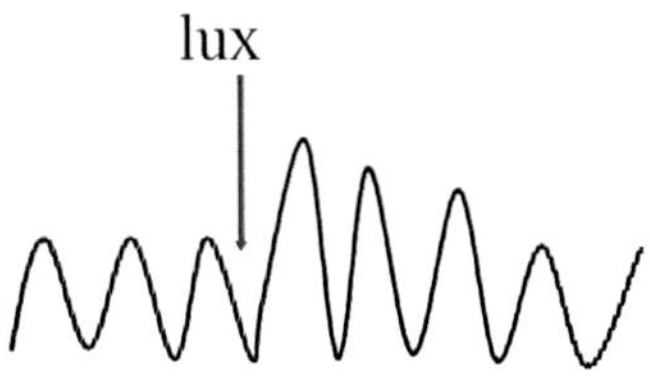


**Figure 9.2** Curve symbolising the examiner's sensation after a flash of light. Three RACs are triggered immediately after the light has been turned on ("lux").

Claude Bernard (1813–1878) was the scientist who discovered the importance of the stability of the internal environment, without which life could not exist. Following environmental aggressions, the organism will generate a series of responses, aiming to maintain the physiological balance. These responses involve the neuro-vegetative system and are essentially non-conscious. The balance of the internal environment is ensured mainly by the sympathetic nervous system, together with the ***adrenal medulla gland***, which releases adrenaline. Due to the action of sense organs (touch, hearing, sight, smell, taste), the central nervous system will be aware of changes in the external environment and of possible threats. At the same time, reacting to internal sensors called interoceptors, the CNS will be informed of changes in the internal environment. An appropriate response is then initiated by the neuro-vegetative system, mainly through the hypothalamus.

Hans Selye (1946) has pointed out that harmful agents, regardless of their nature and in a non-specific manner, will induce a characteristic pathological state, known as ***the general adaptation syndrome***, in which Selye describes ***three stages***:

1. ***A rapid alarm reaction***.
2. If the agent's action persists, a ***stage of resistance or struggle*** follows with an increase in the secretion of the adrenal cortex gland controlled by the anterior pituitary gland and identified in 1949 (Hench *et al.*) as cortisol in humans.
3. If the aggression continues, a ***stage of exhaustion*** follows.

In signal medicine, we evaluate the sympathetic response by counting the number of RAC+ pulses that follow white light stimulation until the pulse returns to its steady state while the subject is still exposed to the lamp. This number is called the reactivity index. A **reactivity index (RI) of 3** indicates a normal response.

If the index is greater or smaller than three, this indicates an adaptation disorder.

### 9.2.1 RAC Reactions to Aggression

When faced with aggression, the RAC reactions will be modified. The aggression may be an infectious agent (influenza, for example), a traumatic event, or an intense fear. If the aggression is brutal, we will observe *three successive phases*: ***prostration***, ***struggle***, and ***exhaustion*** (**Figure 9.3**).

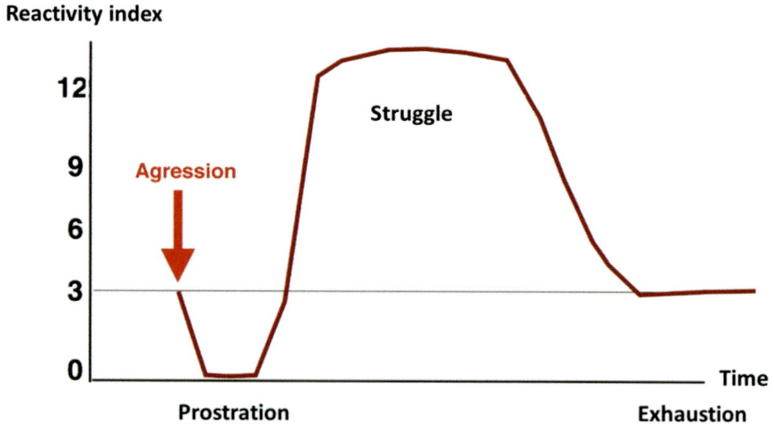


**Figure 9.3** Reactivity index following aggression. The three stages.

#### *9.2.1.1 Prostration Phase*

It lasts for a few minutes. During this phase, there is no RAC when the subject is exposed to white light. The reactivity index is equal to zero. In standard practice, this phase is rarely observed unless the physician happens to be with a patient immediately after intense stress. This phase probably corresponds to an adrenal response.

#### 9.2.1.2 *Struggle Phase*

This phase begins a few minutes after the aggression and immediately follows the prostration phase. It can last for several hours, several days, or several weeks. The organism enters a phase of struggle, which results in hyperreactivity of the neurovegetative system, with a reactivity index that can reach 10, 12, and even 15 in some cases. We are faced with a disproportionate response that can no doubt be explained by the adrenergic discharges. This phase is important to diagnose because the physician can act, using auriculotherapy, and work on auricular points representing cortisol, thus avoiding the third phase, exhaustion.

#### 9.2.1.3 *Exhaustion Phase*

If the aggression continues, the NVS can no longer fulfil its role because it is "overwhelmed". We then observe a phase of RAC exhaustion, which can be demonstrated by repeated flashes of light onto the skin. After several flashes, the RAC reaction disappears (Chapter 10).

As we can see, the reactivity index enables us to assess the body's capacity to adapt. A patient comes to us with fatigue that has been present for many months. Measuring his reactivity index will lead us to a diagnosis. If the RI is 10, we know that the patient is in a phase of struggle and that his sympathetic system cannot ensure a coherent response to any kind of stress. In this case, we must search for some contemporary disruptive element such as a scar, a dental focus, a viral disease, or a stressful element. If the RI is normal, we will orient ourselves towards pathology without a disruptive element: for example, a laterality disorder (Chapter 26).

## 9.3 SPECIAL CASES WITH ABOLITION OF THE RAC

In various cases, exposing the patient to light does not produce a RAC, i.e. the RAC is suppressed. Such cases could be:

- Beta-blocker treatments
- Wearing a thick metal necklace
- Wearing insoles with electromagnetic stimulation under the feet
- Various cancers
- Compression of the stellar ganglion

### 9.3.1 Beta-Blocker Treatments

Beta-blockers induce suppression of the RAC when prescribed at high doses and can be an obstacle to examination using the pulse. Being unable to refer to the vascular reflex is unfortunate; for example, when treating migraines, a typical situation where the RAC is especially useful for dietary tests.

If the migraines are very disabling, one may possibly consider reducing the dose of beta-blockers, with the aim of restoring the vascular response. **Except** if the beta-blocker has been prescribed for cardiac reasons, in which case, the beta-blocker must imperatively be maintained.

### 9.3.2 Wearing a Thick Metal Necklace

Another frequent example of abolition of the RAC is when the patient wears a necklace made of thick metal links. To observe this, the chain must be closed. Even a slightly open chain or bearing a nylon link will not suppress the RAC. This phenomenon is difficult to explain, especially as it is not systematic. One can imagine that large metallic chains inhibit certain reactions, such as photoreception. One thing is sure: people with no RAC because of a necklace are prone to develop functional pathologies such as fatigue, headache, etc. The RAC immediately reappears if the chain is removed, and the associated disorders rapidly recover.

I recall the case of a hairdresser who came to see me for intense fatigue, which had begun seven years earlier, following the birth of her daughter. The white light test showed a reactivity index equal to zero, and she was wearing a thick, flashy gold chain. When asked about this necklace, she said that she had received it from her husband for the birth of their daughter. After removing the necklace, the reactivity index immediately returned to normal. In this case, the treatment was simple, consisting of no longer wearing the chain.

I have come across this phenomenon hundreds of times with necklaces. But only once have I observed it in the case of a patient wearing a gold wristwatch. I saw this patient regularly every month for the follow-up of prostate cancer. His RAC responses were always perfect. One day, I was surprised to find that the RAC failed to respond, with a reactivity index of zero. Normally, he never wore a watch, but on this occasion, he had decided to wear one that his wife had given him. Having had an accident on his left wrist, he wore it on his right side. As soon as he removed his watch at my request, the RAC reappeared, and the white light test returned to normal.

### 9.3.3 Wearing Electromagnetic Insoles

Certain insoles labelled "postural reprogramming insoles" are designed to create an electromagnetic field to stimulate receptors under the feet, thereby regulating the tone of the paravertebral muscle chains. These insoles are liable to suppress the RAC. When taking the patient's history, it is, therefore, necessary to enquire whether they wear insoles and what type. If so, it is important to examine the patient with the shoes on and wearing the insoles to see if they influence the RAC.

### 9.3.4 Various Cancers

I have always been surprised to observe that the white light test was not impaired in the case of certain cancers. I have often had the opportunity to examine women with very advanced breast cancer. The RAC reactions were not abolished. The same is true for prostate cancer. However, it is not the case for lung cancer, in which the white light test is altered.

My patients often ask whether I can detect the presence of cancer using the pulse. The answer is no. However, if you know a patient well and have examined her or him on numerous occasions, a sudden and unexplained change in the white light test should make you think of the possibility of cancer.

## 9.4 THE SPECIAL CASE OF FIRST RIB SYNDROME

On performing a white light test, it may happen that no RAC reaction is perceptible on the left radial pulse. If so, checking whether the RAC is present on the right radial pulse is necessary. If it turns out to be maintained on the right, this often indicates compression of the stellate ganglion by the head of the first rib on the left side. This leads to what we call the *first rib syndrome*. Apart from the fact that the situation will interfere with a pulse examination, it is important to know that compression of the stellate ganglion will always have a clinical effect. One should, therefore, handle this problem before treating any other pathology with auriculotherapy. The first rib syndrome, although described several decades ago, is not widely known throughout the medical community. It consists of a group of symptoms and signs all due to compression of the stellar ganglion, resulting in abnormal stimulation of the sympathetic system. The first rib syndrome is considered an obstacle to auricular therapy.

### 9.4.1 Anatomy, a Brief Recall

Anatomically, the stellate ganglion, also known as the cervico-thoracic ganglion, is part of the latero-vertebral sympathetic chain. It is naturally vulnerable because of its location just above the head of the first rib. The anterior part of the first rib is attached to the manubrium sterni, whereas its posterior extremity is inserted on the first thoracic vertebra, forming the costo-vertebral joint. At this point, the rib has a bulge, called the rib's "head". The stellate ganglion, so called because of its star-shaped aspect, is located just above the rib's head. When

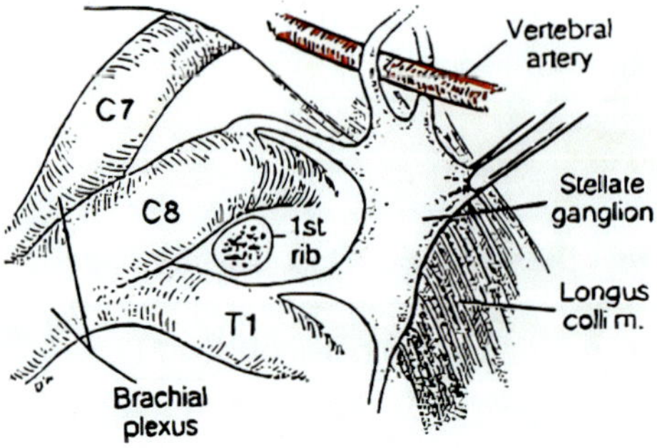


Figure 9.4 Stellate ganglion and brachial plexus.

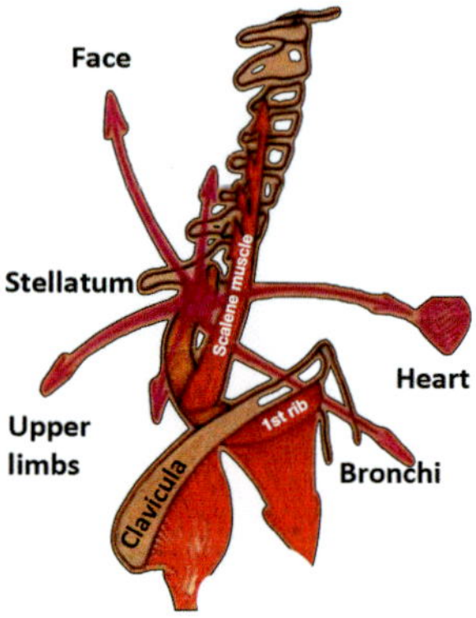


Figure 9.5 Stellate ganglion and first rib.

dissected, the stellate ganglion measures approximately 2.5 cm × 1.0 cm × 0.5 cm. It is present on both the right and left sides but has a right/left asymmetry (**Figures 9.4** and **9.5**).

The stellate ganglion participates in the autonomic innervation of the head, the face, the upper limb, the heart, and the bronchi, but also influences the entire sympathetic latero-vertebral chain.

Sometimes, trauma or a bad position can result in a slight ascension of the first rib, irritating the stellate ganglion. This leads to discharges of Noradrenaline in the innervated territories, creating a complex functional pathology.

### 9.4.2 Symptoms Related to First Rib Syndrome

The onset is always abrupt. The patient will describe several symptoms and specify that they appeared on a precise date. "Since 19 February 2018, I have started to feel unwell". Usually, the patient says that he has consulted many physicians, and that none of the therapies he has tried have improved anything. The symptoms described do not usually fit into a classical nosological framework. They consist of general functional disorders, such as:

- tachycardia
- cardiac erethism
- cardiac rhythm disorders
- chest discomfort
- feeling breathless
- anxiety
- pseudo-asthma
- constipation and sometimes diarrhoea, which can only be explained by a nicotine effect
- instability ataxia
- lipothymia
- trigeminal neuralgia
- fatigue

### 9.4.3 Objective Signs of First Rib Syndrome

A small number of objective signs are necessary to make a diagnosis.

- *Asymmetry of the radial (resting) pulses*: Examination of this condition consists of comparing the intensity of right and left radial pulses at rest (the RAC is not implied here). Although not pathognomonic, this is an essential sign for the diagnosis. The practitioner stands face to face in front of the patient and takes both radial pulses simultaneously (**Figure 9.6**). Both right and left pulses must be taken with identical pressure.
    - Generally, pulses are taken with the thumb positioned at the level of the slope of the radial styloid process (**Figures 4.7–4.9**). Alternatively, pulses can be taken with the index and middle fingers. The idea is to evaluate whether the right and left resting pulses are symmetrical, first when the patient's head is upright, looking straight in front, and then when the head is turned to the right and the left. In the event of irritation of the stellar ganglion due to an ascent of the first rib on one side or the other (colloquially referred to as "blockage of the first rib"), this will lead to an impression of a decrease in the intensity of the pulse on that same side.

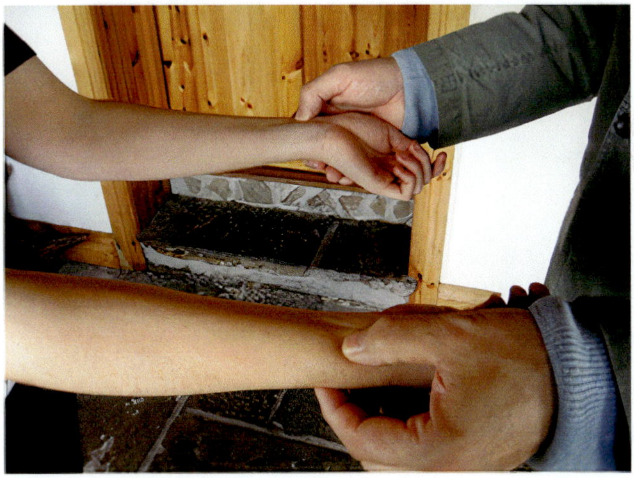

**Figure 9.6** Taking the radial pulse on both sides.

- *Limitation of head rotation on the same side as the first rib blockage.* To objectify this limitation, the practitioner stands behind the patient, places his hands on the patient's shoulders, and asks the patient to turn her or his head to one side and then to the other, asking: "Can you see my hand? My elbow? Or up to my shoulder? To my face?"

- *Pain when pressing on the costo-vertebral joint.* To test this, the patient should be asked to lie on the examination table on the stomach (procubitus), looking down with the chin resting on the table's edge, and the head situated just outside, in front of the table, and both arms hanging on either side. In this position, the first thoracic vertebra is clearly visible and more prominent than the other dorsal vertebrae. The practitioner then applies pressure with his thumb onto both costo-vertebral joints on either side of the first thoracic vertebra. In case of blockage of the first rib, the thumb "sinks in" less deeply and induces pain.
- *Asymmetry of the ascent of the first rib on inspiration* (**Figure 9.7**). To observe this, the practitioner places himself standing up behind the bare-chested patient and asks them to breathe in and out, while at the same time comparing the mobility of the right and left first ribs during inspiration and expiration. In the event of first rib blockage, the mobility of the rib will be reduced on that same side.

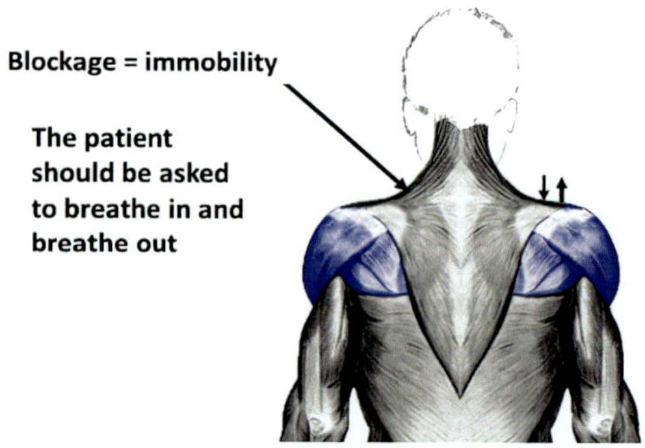


**Figure 9.7** Limitation of ascent of the first rib on inspiration.

### 9.4.4 Diagnosis of First Rib Syndrome

Diagnosis of a first rib syndrome rests entirely on questioning and clinical examination. No additional technical procedure can confirm the diagnosis.

### 9.4.5 Treatments of First Rib Syndrome

Various alternatives can be considered for treating the first rib syndrome.

#### *9.4.5.1 Osteopathic Manipulation*

This technique was taught in Lyon by Dr Edouardo Torti from Argentina in 1997. The patient lies in ventral procubitus on an elevated table and rests the chin on the edge of the table while dropping both arms on either side of the table, as described above. The practitioner stands at the patient's head and pushes on the first rib with the flat of the elbow. To do this, he will bend over, placing one foot forward.

Manipulation of the first rib syndrome on a patient sitting on a chair has been occasionally practiced during the past. However, it is not highly recommended, considering the risk of undesirable consequences, such as vascular problems.

#### 9.4.5.2 Auto-Manipulation

The process consists of the following sequence (**Figure 9.8**). Asked to sit in an armchair, the patient begins by breathing in fully, holds the breath, and pulls the upper part of the body up, with elbows straightened and arms leaning on the arms of the armchair, as shown in the figure. The patient maintains apnoea in this same position for a few seconds and then sits back slowly while breathing out. This exercise should be repeated about ten times a day.

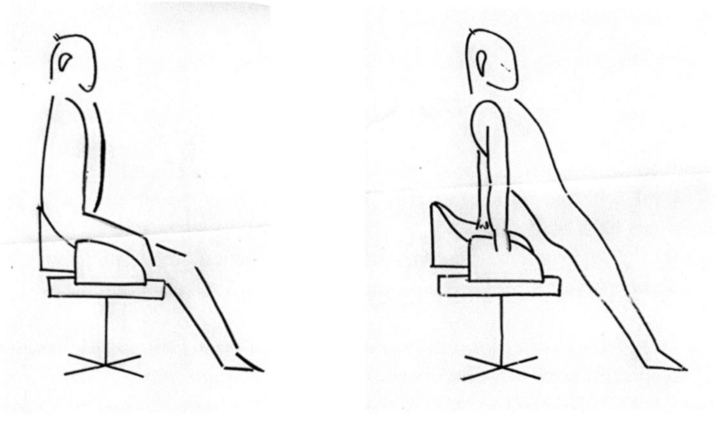

**Figure 9.8** Auto-manipulation of the first rib.

### 9.4.6 Auriculotherapy

Auriculotherapy remains the most effective means of treating a first rib syndrome. On the *mastoid aspect* of the homolateral ear, at the lower part of the *posterior anthelical groove,* level C7/D1, it is possible to find by way of electrical detection a point representing the ***first rib*** (**Figure 9.9**).

On the *external aspect* of the homolateral ear, one can detect a point representing ***the stellate ganglion***, located on the basal part of *the wall* (representing the sympathetic paravertebral ganglionic chain) at level C7/D1. Moreover, the ***first rib*** is represented

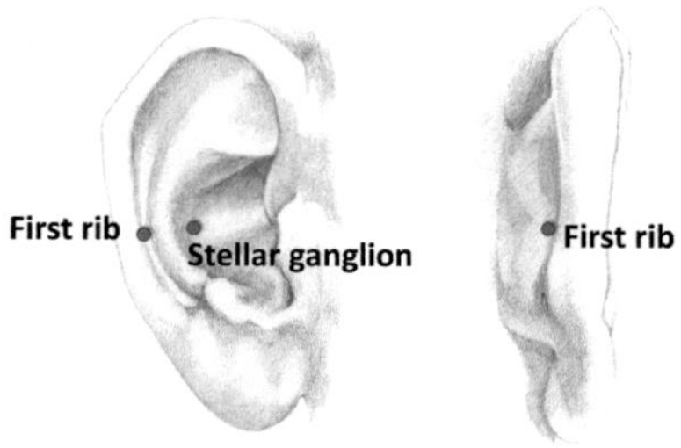


**Figure 9.9** Auricular treatment of first rib syndrome.

not only on the mastoid aspect as just described but also on the *external aspect*, located at the lower part of the *scaphoid fossa*, at the same C7/D1 level (**Figure 9.9**).

All these points can be treated with an SPN (semi-permanent needle). The aim is to relax muscle contractures in the costo-vertebral region and remove compression of the stellate ganglion. Following treatment, one can expect the right and left radial pulses to become symmetrical again.

## BIBLIOGRAPHY

1. Bourdiol René. *Elements of auriculotherapy*. Maisonneuve 1980
2. Nogier Paul, with the collaboration of BOURDIOL René and Bahr Frank. Loci auriculomedicinae 1975
3. Nogier Paul. *The problem of the first rib*. Journal Auriculomedicine n°3. April 1976.
4. Nogier Paul. *First rib. Self-manipulation*. Journal Auriculomedicine n° 29. October 1982
5. Nogier Paul. *From auriculotherapy to auriculomedicine*. Éditions Maisonneuve. 1981
6. Nogier Raphaël. *Health through the ear*. Editions Mango 2018
7. Nogier Raphaël. *How to look for an ear point? The search and treatment of a first rib. The search for and treatment of a disruptive scar*. Xth International Symposium of Auriculotherapy. Lyon, June 4–6, 2021

CHAPTER 10

# The RAC Exhaustion Phenomenon
## *Dental Foci and Pathological Scars*

**Raphaël Nogier**

## 10.1 INTRODUCTION

Although not widely taught, the phenomenon of exhaustion can be seen as one of the key points for understanding the RAC.

Usually, the RAC response following stimulation is inexhaustible in a healthy individual. When a sufficiently powerful flash of light is projected onto an individual's bare chest, a vascular reaction is obtained almost instantaneously. It lasts three pulses, the first more intense and perceptible than the following two. This phenomenon can be repeated ad libitum. After each flash, a RAC appears.

However, the reaction runs out in various pathologies after one, two, three, or ten stimulations. If the light stimulation is suspended for a few moments and then resumed, the RAC will reappear before running out again when stimulations are repeated.

### 10.1.1 What Causes the RAC to Run Out after Repeated Stimulation?

The vascular reaction can be subject to exhaustion after repeated stimuli if there is a permanent irritative element at some part of the sympathetic network, also called a *disruptive focus*. Up against such an obstacle, the sympathetic system is compelled to resist relentlessly and consequently becomes exhausted [6]. Here is a demonstrative example.

A few years ago, a 26-year-old woman, a specialised educator, came to my practice, describing three different symptoms: intense and unexplained fatigue, tachycardia, and a very incapacitating pseudo-vertiginous instability when standing, to the point of being unable to work. The symptoms had begun two years earlier, for no apparent reason, and had led her to consult her GP, an ear-nose-throat specialist, a neurologist, and a cardiologist. After numerous investigations, which all turned out to be normal, she was advised to see a psychiatrist. However, she preferred to consult me.

On questioning this patient, it appeared to me that she did not have a neurotic profile. Her pulse was distinctive and well-perceptible. It was rapid, at approximately 100 beats per minute. I began the examination with a white light test. The flashes did

DOI: 10.1201/9781003753629-10

produce a RAC; however, by repeating them, the reaction became gradually less intense before disappearing altogether.

I asked her if there were any scars on her skin, as this could be a cause of RAC exhaustion. She was visibly pleased with my question, as she indeed had a scar she had not told me about when I initially questioned her. It was a small scar following right inguinal hernia surgery, horizontal, 2 cm long, red-coloured, hot, tense and very painful when touched. The operation had been performed two years earlier, shortly before the onset of the symptoms. Considering the pathologic aspect of the scar, I referred the patient to a dermatologist who merely prescribed a soothing ointment. Three weeks later, finding something was abnormal on her scar, she went to an emergency hospital unit, where a physician proceeded to remove an unabsorbed surgical thread several centimetres long (**Figure 10.1**).

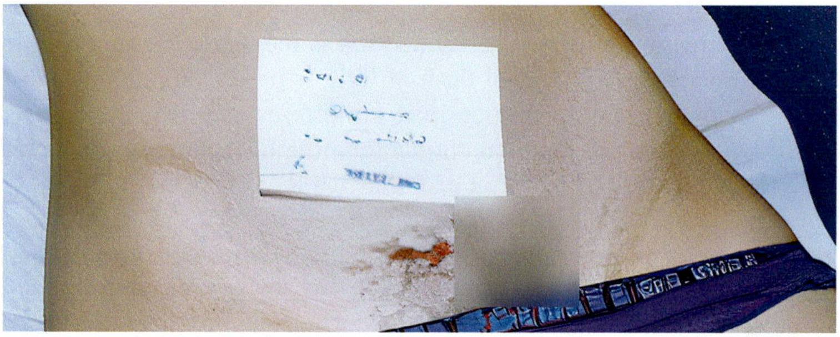

**Figure 10.1** Pathological scar after hernia repair.

### 10.1.2 What Happened Following Removal of the Unresorbed Thread?

As a result, the instability, tachycardia, and fatigue all vanished immediately. Hence, there was an obvious relationship between the unabsorbed thread in the hernia scar and the clinical signs. This case is also interesting because the symptoms for which the patient consulted were so prominent that she forgot to mention the scar despite the pain.

### 10.1.3 What Can the Relationship Be between an Unabsorbed Surgical Thread, and Fatigue, Tachycardia and Instability?

This, of course, is the relevant question, which can be answered by saying that the solution was found thanks to the radial pulse, since after the removal of the thread, the RAC exhaustion phenomenon disappeared, meaning that each flash of light projected onto the skin was again followed by a normal RAC reaction.

Most likely at the root of all this lies the sympathetic system, which innervates the radial artery, produces the vascular response RAC, and innervates the skin.

The sympathetic system partly controls the cardiac frequency and is responsible for the functional regulation of many organs. This can explain the symptoms of instability and fatigue in the case of this young woman. Constant irritation of the skin by the presence of a surgical thread undoubtedly led to permanent overstimulation of the sympathetic system, which was no longer capable of managing its normal functions, thus leading to the tachycardia, instability, and fatigue she was suffering from.

The consequences of RAC exhaustion are multiple, due to impairment of the sympathetic system, the role of which should normally consist in managing the body's reactions when faced with physical effort, stress, or aggression. This reduces the capacity to adapt to any kind of stress: viral, bacterial, thermal, emotional, etc. The sympathetic system can no longer fulfil its regular role because it is constantly up against a permanent source of irritation.

### 10.1.4 What Are the General Symptoms and Signs Related to RAC Exhaustion?

RAC exhaustion can be found in many pathologic conditions, whether functional or organic, without necessarily being able to determine whether it is a cause or a consequence.

In functional conditions, we can find symptoms such as unexplained fatigue, vertigo, tachycardia, as we have just discussed, but also menstrual cycle and fertility problems, transit disorders, migraine, non-migraine headaches, recurrent infections, and chronic urticaria. In the organic field, let us mention recurrent polyps of the bladder.

### 10.1.5 Technique for Diagnosing RAC Exhaustion

RAC exhaustion can be diagnosed using *a modified white light test.* It is a sort of stress test applied to the RAC response. As described in the previous chapter, the patient lies supine on the examination table, bare-chested, eyes indifferently open or closed. The practitioner is placed behind him, taking his left radial pulse. The pressure he exerts with his finger (thumb or index and medius) on the radial artery should be "mid-deep", neither too strong nor too light (see **Figure 13.2**). The practitioner then triggers a flash of white light onto the patient's chest, immediately inducing a RAC response.

Whereas a basic white light test would consist of counting the number of RACs (normally three), in the case of a RAC exhaustion test, one does not wait for all three responses. Instead, *immediately following the first RAC reaction*, one repeats a second flash of white light and then again a third flash immediately after the first RAC response, and so on, up to ten flashes. If the patient has a normal reaction, the same intensity of RAC response will be maintained indefinitely after each flash (**Figure 10.2**).

Flash → **RAC** / Flash → **RAC** / Flash → **RAC** ... -> 10th Flash

**Figure 10.2** Normal RAC response. No exhaustion.

By contrast, in the case of RAC exhaustion, the *intensity of the first RAC responses after each flash will gradually fade out* more or less quickly from the first to the last of the series of ten RACs (**Figure 10.3**).

Flash → **RAC**, Flash → **RAC**, Flash → **RAC**, -> Flash → **RAC**

**Figure 10.3** RAC exhaustion.

## 10.2 CAUSES OF RAC EXHAUSTION: THE NOTION OF DISRUPTIVE FOCUS

Finding a RAC exhaustion then implies looking for a **disruptive focus**, essentially a **dental focus** and/or a **pathological scar**.

## 10.3 THE NOTION OF DENTAL FOCUS

If exhaustion of the RAC occurs rapidly (after two or three flashes), this will often indicate the existence of a dental focus.

### 10.3.1 Definition

A dental focus is a particular type of dental pathology, painful or not, visible or not, implying radiological signs or not, present or past, and which has the property of being linked to a pathology at a distance, seeming a priori to have no connection with the dental focus [8].

The notion of dental focus should not be confused with that of an infectious focus.

The concept of dental focus has existed for a long time and has been mentioned by many authors. We speak of a dental focus only if the following three characteristics are present:

- Generally, the dental pathology is silent.
- Pathological information of dental origin will disturb the sympathetic system, mainly implying one target organ.

- One or several target organs (e.g., shoulder, stomach, Achilles tendon, etc.) can be implied, expressing pathology such as pain. The target organ is an important point. One cannot speak of dental focus without a pathology induced at a distance.

### 10.3.2 In Terms of Pathology, a Dental Focus Can Be

- a wisdom tooth, impacted or not
- a supernumerary tooth
- a cyst or an apical granuloma
- the presence of intraoral galvanism
- maxillary sinusitis
- iatrogenic pathology (poor filling of a canal or the presence of a nerve puller which has been left inside the canal following a fracture of the equipment)
- a gingival scar after dental avulsion

### 10.3.3 Clinical Signs of a Dental Focus

Nothing is more clinically diverse than the general impairments related to a dental focus. Virtually anything can be implied. The symptoms described by the patient are functional and related to the sympathetic system, as mentioned in **Table 10.1**.

**Table 10.1 Clinical Signs of a Dental Focus**

| General signs | Psychiatric signs | Cardiovascular signs | Infectious signs |
|---|---|---|---|
| Severe fatigue<br>Balance disorders<br>Headache | Anxiety depression | Blood pressure disorders<br>Tachycardia | Recurrent infections<br>Sore throat<br>Ear infections<br>Lung infections<br>Urinary tract infections<br>Digestive disorders<br>Emesis |

**Example**

Samantha, a 27-year-old woman, is referred to me by her general practitioner. She suffers from a problem of emesis that has been waking her up at about 2 am every night, ever since she was a teenager. She tells me that she lost her mother when she was 12 years old. She has consulted gastroenterologists, neurologists, internists, and a psychiatrist. None of these specialists has found any definite pathology. When examined with the white light test, the first flash is followed by a normal RAC response, whereas the second flash produces no RAC at all. Such rapid exhaustion of the vascular response is often related to a dental focus. In this case, a focus is detected on tooth number 25, which will be treated by an auricular point on the contralateral ear. As a result, the

RAC immediately becomes stable again, and the exhaustion phenomenon disappears. Clinically, the emesis subsided the night after the session. Five years later, I saw Samantha again. Only once had she vomited in the meantime.

This case is, of course, unusual because dental foci are not always as spectacular. Generally, they are characterized by common everyday conditions that might not particularly attract the physician's attention, such as fatigue, chronic pain, transit disorders, headaches, migraines, etc.

In Samantha's case, there was:

1. A dental pathology, consisting of a devitalised tooth
2. A pathological information on the patient's ear, located on the representation of the trigeminal nerve. This point was treated by auriculotherapy
3. A target organ: the stomach

### 10.3.4 Pathophysiology of Dental Foci

Dental pathophysiology can be explained by a malfunction of the sympathetic system. The trigeminal nerve innervates all the teeth, and it is conceivable that an irritative factor located on the trigeminal nerve could entail general disorders.

### 10.3.5 How Does One Diagnose a Dental Focus?

It is very difficult, if not impossible, to diagnose a dental focus without using the vascular response RAC. A dental focus represents a functional pathology, most of the time undetectable by imagery. Furthermore, it is not necessarily associated with an occlusion disorder, an infection, or dental pain. We are faced with an average patient, the complaints of whom we are used to hearing every day, such as recurrent infection, pain, and fatigue. The patient never complains about their teeth. Only two vague aspects can be considered characteristic: in the first place, no treatment until now has been able to resolve the patient's complaints. Secondly, the condition is chronic and has lasted for several months or years. Both these items of information, when associated, are suggestive.

#### *10.3.5.1 Dental Pressure Test*

The dental pressure test is one of two tests to detect dental focus.

While taking the patient's pulse with the left hand, one searches for a positive RAC while gently applying light pressure with the right index finger across the cheek at the level of each dental root, one after the other. The entire maxillary and mandibular arches must be carefully explored.

Only a focus-bearing tooth causes the pulse to react with a positive RAC when pressure is exerted on its root.

A small focal point will produce, say, 2 RACs, whilst the maximum will not exceed 9 RACs. The number of RACs is essential and must be counted because this is what will allow us to measure the importance of the focus. For example, we will call it a 3-RAC focus, a 5-RAC focus, or a 9-RAC focus. This will be useful because one may come across several teeth that are reactive to touch. In this case, the RAC count for each individual tooth will allow us to compare their importance. The most reactive focal tooth should be treated first.

#### 10.3.5.2 Black-White Rod Test

A disruptive focus, whether on the body or on a tooth, as well as its representation on the ear, can be detected with the black tip of the black and white rod (see **Figure 12.1**).

So, the second method for testing a dental focus implies gradually scanning the black tip across the cheek or lip at a distance of approximately 1–2 cm over the maxillary and mandibular quadrants from one side to the other at the level of the dental roots.

In the event of a dental focus, the examiner will feel a RAC reaction when the extremity of the black rod reaches the area over the root of the tooth which bears the focus.

The technique using the black tip is complementary to the dental pressure technique. We recommend using both, one confirming the other.

### 10.3.6 Reminder on the Identification (Naming) of Each Tooth

Each tooth (**Figure 10.4**) is named by a number containing two digits XY.

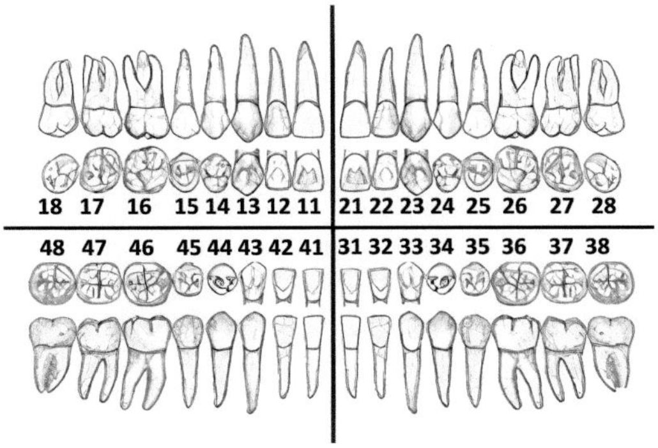


**Figure 10.4** Tooth naming (NB: observe that, as with all anatomical illustrations as viewed from the front aspect, what appears on the *left* side of the *figure* concerns the patient's *right* side, and vice versa for the other side).

The first digit X refers to the quadrant to which the tooth belongs:

1. right maxillary (upper) quadrant
2. left maxillary quadrant
3. left mandibular (lower) quadrant
4. right mandible quadrant

The second digit Y refers to the type and position of the tooth:

1. central incisor
2. lateral incisor
3. canine
4. first premolar
5. second premolar
6. first molar
7. second molar
8. third molar or wisdom tooth

**Example**

Tooth number 37 is the second molar tooth in the left mandibular quadrant.

### 10.3.7 Treating a Dental Focus by Auriculotherapy

Once we have localized a dental focus, auriculotherapy will allow us to neutralize it without difficulty. This consists of removing the pathological information that is emitted by the tooth. The focus must always be treated on the opposite ear, by a point on the representation of the trigeminal nerve, located on the rear border of the contralateral lobule (**Figure 10.5**). A dental focus on the left is treated on the right ear; a dental focus on the right is treated on the left ear.

#### *10.3.7.1 Finding the Auricular Point Corresponding to the Focus*

Technically, locating the auricular point consists of taking the pulse with the left hand while very gently palpating the rear edge of the lobule and the tail of the helix (**Figure 10.5**) between the thumb and index finger of the right hand. Normally, this palpation does not produce a RAC, whereas in the case of a dental focus, RACs occur when the point corresponding to the focus is lightly pressed.

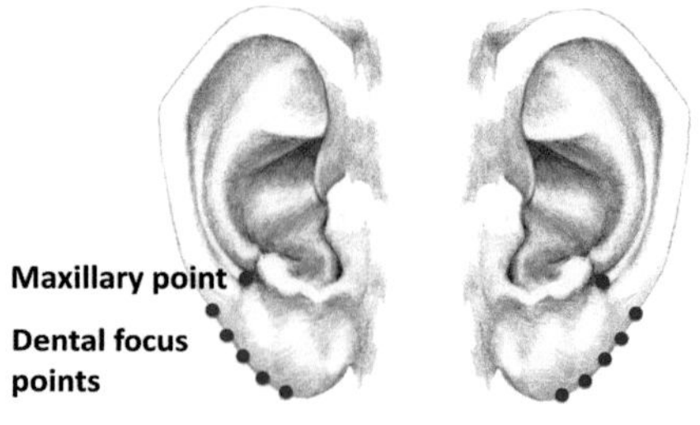


**Figure 10.5** Treating a dental focus, with trigeminal points (second or third branches) on the rear border of the lobule, and a maxillary point at the lower part of the scaphoid fossa.

The number of RACs should be counted. We will find the same number of RACs by palpating the border point and the tooth itself. If, for example, we obtain 5 RACs with pressure on the focal tooth, the same pressure on the corresponding ear point will also react with 5 RACs.

It is possible to confirm these findings with the black tip of the black and white rod. The ear point corresponding to the dental focus will trigger the same number of RACs as the focus itself.

If there are several dental foci, there will be as many points as there are foci. Hence, the need to count the RACs making it possible to identify which ear point corresponds to which focal tooth.

Finally, it is helpful to add the maxillary point, situated at the lower extremity of the scaphoid groove (**Figure 10.5**), to the treatment.

#### *10.3.7.2 Confirming the Point*

Detection of ear points with the pulse reaction remains subjective and, therefore, "examiner dependent". Considering this, after locating a point with the RAC, it is advised to systematically confirm the presence of auricular points by means of an objective technique, such as electrical detection. An auricular point representing a focus is characterized by a lower electrical resistance than the surrounding area. Modern instruments based on differential detection allow reliable and accurate location of ear points.

#### *10.3.7.3 Treatment of the Ear Point*

The points corresponding to a dental focus should be treated with a semi-permanent needle (SPN). For those who do not have this equipment at their disposal, it is possible to use Vaccaria seeds or metal balls, which the patient should stimulate regularly. We recommend not treating these points by projecting light or frequencies. It is preferable to use mechanical stimulation techniques. Auriculotherapy should include the maxillary point, located in the lower part of the scaphoid fossa (**Figure 10.5**).

#### *10.3.7.4 Checking for Absence of RAC Exhaustion*

After the dental focus has been "neutralized", the practitioner will immediately ensure that exhaustion of the RAC has disappeared. A white light test will be repeated to confirm that a stable RAC has been restored.

If, however, it is not the case, there are two possibilities: either the point treated on the ear does not correspond to the focus, or there might exist another dental focus, or maybe a pathologic scar. In both cases, the point(s) should be looked for again by gently palpating the posterior rim of the lobule border between thumb and forefinger, as described earlier.

#### 10.3.7.5 *The Patient Should Be Revisited after Four Weeks*

When the RAC function is restored, the patient often experiences an increase in symptoms during the following 48 hours: exacerbation of fatigue, pain, etc. After that, however, the symptoms will subside and may, at best, be completely resolved within a few days. This improvement may last for a month or more. We advise seeing the patient again within 30 days after the first session to check for a possible relapse of RAC exhaustion, in which case the patient should be treated again and thereafter seen every month until the phenomenon has disappeared. It may take several sessions to treat a dental focus.

### 10.3.8 When Should the Dentist Intervene?

Calling on the dentist will be necessary whenever auriculotherapy is not sufficient to stabilise the RAC reactions. If the exhaustion phenomenon returns systematically despite half a dozen sessions with auriculotherapy, the patient should be referred to a dentist for local treatment. Generally, we tend to send our patients to the dentist only if we are unable to neutralise the dental focus. On the other hand, dental treatment alone may not be sufficient, in which case it is suitable to treat the informational aspect of the dental focus with auriculotherapy. While the dentist will treat a lesion, auriculotherapy will deal with a disturbed function *(functio laesa)*[1] dental focus implies three different levels of intervention

- The **tooth itself**: from an anatomic-pathological point of view, a focus can be due to a granuloma, a cyst, a iatrogenic pathology, an impacted wisdom teeth, a supernumerary teeth, or a maxillary sinusitis. In all these cases, the dentist or the ear-nose-throat (ENT) specialist will be able to intervene. In many situations, however, no visible or radiological pathology is found.
- The **pathological information** linked to the tooth we can treat with auriculotherapy, as mentioned above.
- The **target** may be a joint, e.g. a shoulder, a tendon, maybe Achilles tendon, an organ, e.g. the stomach, or indeed any part of the body. Auriculotherapy will aim to treat the point corresponding to the target.

## 10.4 DISRUPTIVE OR PATHOLOGICAL SCARS

So-called disruptive or pathological scars are the second known cause of RAC exhaustion. In this type of depletion, the RAC usually holds out slightly longer than for a dental focus. Whereas for the latter, the RAC will become exhausted after one, two, or three flashes of light, the RAC tends to continue through five, six, seven flashes or more, before showing exhaustion in the case of a disruptive scar (**Figure 10.6**).

### 10.4.1 Definition

The term *disruptive, or pathological scar,* can refer to any scar located on the skin, but also on an internal organ, that will induce a pathology at a distance,

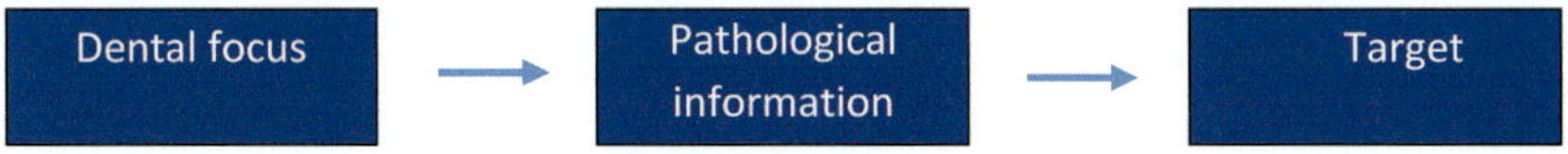


**Figure 10.6** Disruptive or pathological scars.

with no obvious connection to the scar. The reader might well be surprised by the notion of scar in relation to organs. But with auriculotherapy, we know that a damaged organ, such as the liver after hepatitis, the pancreas after pancreatitis, or the prostate after prostatitis, can create disorders comparable to a skin scar. It seems that when an organ has undergone significant tissue reorganisation, with the formation of fibrosis, a genuinely disruptive scarring process may well follow.

Scars liable to cause loco-regional pain have been extensively described by the French surgeon René Leriche, who devoted part of his life to the study of the sympathetic system. In his book *La chirurgie de la douleur (Surgery of Pain)* [2], he reports the fact that infiltration of certain skin scars with procaine has produced remarkable effects on loco-regional pain that appeared following a scarring process. Particularly interesting in René Leriche's presentation is the fact that scar-related disorders can occur months or even years after the trauma that initially caused the wound.

In the same period, the German physician Ferdinand Hunecke noticed that infiltrating procaine on a scar located on the leg resulted in relieving the patient of shoulder pain. As a result of this observation, he became interested in the effects produced by scars and developed *neural therapy*, a method that focuses on treating scars.

Wounds on the skin, and consequently the scars that result from them, modify the behaviour of the sympathetic system. Proof lies in the fact that infiltrations of sympathetic ganglions (the stellar ganglion if the scar is located on the upper limb or the D12-L1 lumbar ganglion if the scar is located on the lower limb) produce the same effects as infiltrations of the scar itself (René Leriche) [2].

Paul Nogier, although he did not himself discover the phenomenon of disruptive scars, nevertheless improved Leriche's and Hunecke's concepts by proposing to treat disruptive scars not locally with procaine infiltrations but by auriculotherapy. Indeed, treating scars using the ear brings real progress in that it seems more effective than local treatment. In addition, it makes it possible to treat scars located on an organ inaccessible to procaine infiltrations.

### 10.4.2 Clinical Signs That May Be Induced by a Disruptive Scar

See **Table 10.2**.

**Table 10.2 Clinical Signs Induced by a Disruptive Scar**

| | |
|---|---|
| General signs | Severe fatigue<br>Balance disorders<br>Headache |
| Neuropsychiatric signs | Pain/anxiety/depression |
| Cardiovascular signs | Blood pressure disorders/tachycardia |
| Infectious signs | *Repeated infections*: sore throats, ear infections, lung infections, urinary tract infections |
| Digestive signs | Vomiting<br>Motion disorder |
| Rheumatological signs | *Joint pain*: shoulder, elbow, knee tendonitis |
| Skin signs | Chronic urticaria |
| Gynaecological signs | Infertility |

### 10.4.3 Pathophysiology of a Disruptive Scar

It is difficult to assert with certainty the physiopathology of disorders related to disruptive scars. It seems that, as with a dental focus, the orthosympathetic system lies at the root of the disorders. Indeed, the entire skin is innervated by the sympathetic system. Understandably, a scar can become an irritating factor towards the sympathetic system, prone to disturb it continuously and creating the phenomena of RAC exhaustion. The same applies to scars on visceral organs, all of which are also innervated by the orthosympathetic system [4].

### 10.4.4 Aspects of a Disruptive Scar

Fortunately, not all scars are disruptive. But in principle, any scar can be or can become disruptive (see **Figures 10.7–10.9**). There is no infallible way of knowing

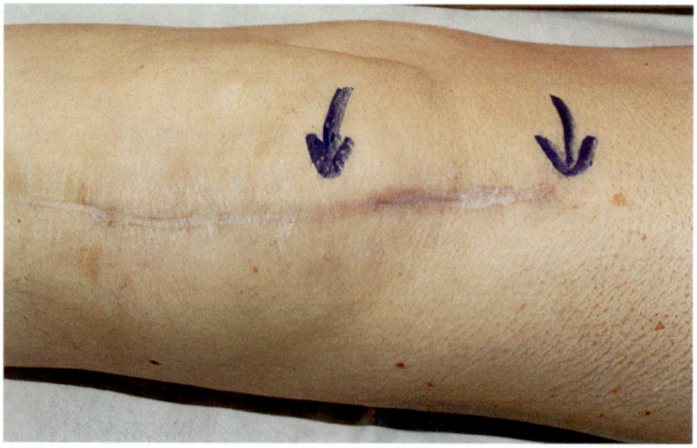

**Figure 10.7** Scar following knee replacement. The portion of the scar between the arrows is pathological.

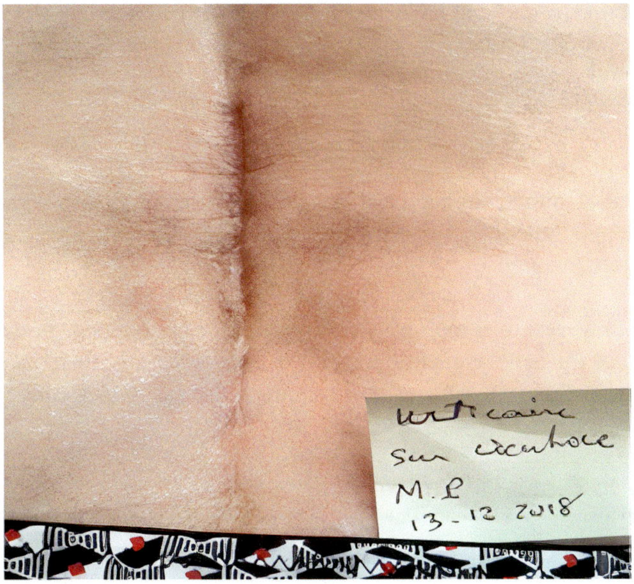

**Figure 10.8** Surgical scar on lower back at level L5-S1, having resulted in chronic urticaria, treated with antihistamines for two years.

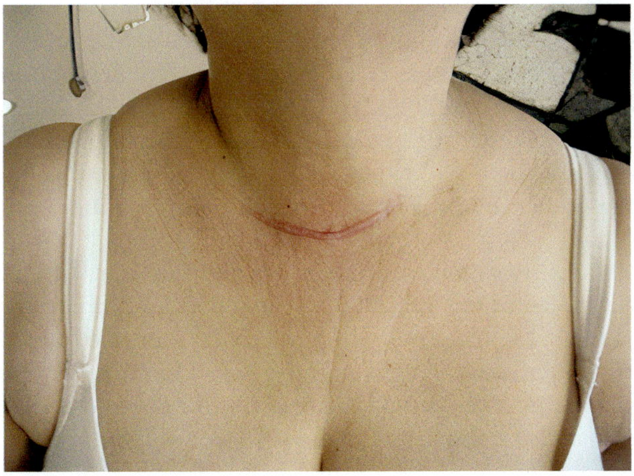

**Figure 10.9** Disruptive scar after thyroidectomy, leading to fatigue and significant weight gain.

whether a scar is a source of problems. Diagnosis requires a clinical approach based on questioning the patient and examining the scar itself, with or without using the pulse reaction.

Locally, a disruptive scar can have any of the following characteristics:

- Horizontal
- Red-coloured
- Hot
- Tense
- Dysesthesia (abnormal decrease or increase of sensitivity)
- Painful (spontaneously or by touch), or possibly insensitive
- Sometimes swollen

Surprisingly, however, in some rare situations, a scar may appear perfectly normal, showing none of the aspects mentioned above, and yet clearly turn out to be disruptive. Detection of this type of scar will require pulse reaction testing, as described below.

### 10.4.5 How to Test a Disruptive Scar

Clinical evaluation of a scar can be done using one of the following three testing methods.

#### *10.4.5.1 Testing the Scar by Lightly Grazing It with Cotton Wool*

Initially, this test does not require taking the pulse. It consists merely in finding out whether the patient feels dysesthesia or pain when the examiner applies light touch with cotton along the whole length of the scar or only on part of it. The patient is asked to compare and say if there is a difference in sensation between touch on a healthy part of the skin and on the scar itself. If the scar is normal, grazing it with cotton will give a sensation no different from that of a healthy portion of skin. If the scar is disruptive, grazing it will either cause an unpleasant and sometimes painful sensation or may, on the contrary, be felt as insensitive.

The second part of this same test (lightly grazing the scar with cotton wool) is carried out with the pulse reaction. If the scar is normal, grazing over it (in addition to not being felt as unpleasant) will produce a response of one or two positive RACs, as on any other healthy portion of the skin. On the other hand, if the scar is pathological, grazing it will produce a *negative* RAC over a variable number of beats, proportional to the degree of pathology (see Chapter 16, pages 194–195).

#### *10.4.5.2 Testing the Scar with the Black Rod or the Black Test Ring*

This test also requires the use of a pulse reaction. It is the most reliable method for detecting a pathological scar. Having over 40 years of experience, it is of daily use. While taking the pulse with his left hand, the examiner, with his right hand, slowly "scans" the end of the black rod or the black test ring (see **Figures 12.1** and **12.8**) over the scar at a distance of approximately one centimetre (see **Figure 12.14**). In the case of a disruptive scar, a *positive* RAC will be observed. It is necessary to count the number of RACs to obtain an indication of how pathological the scar is. It should be noted that most often, only part of the scar produces RACs. A scar is rarely pathological on its entire length. We have often noticed that in the case of a sutured wound, the resulting scar is reactive on the portions that have been sutured.

In short, grazing a pathological scar with cotton will produce a **negative RAC**, whereas testing the same pathological scar scanning with the black rod or test ring over the scar will result in a **positive RAC**. Generally speaking, the diagnosis of a disruptive scar may be summed up according to **Table 10.3**.

**Table 10.3 Characteristics of Scars, Normal and Pathological**

| Type of scar | Aspect | Light touch | Black rod/test ring over the scar |
|---|---|---|---|
| Normal | **Normal** | **Positive RAC** | **No RAC** |
| Pathological | **Red, swollen possibly normal** | **Dysesthesia/Painful negative RAC** | **Positive RAC** |

## 10.4.6 How Does One Treat a Disruptive Scar?

### *10.4.6.1 Testing the Ear with the Black Rod*

In my opinion, the best way to treat disruptive scars is auriculotherapy. Many authors have described the effectiveness of local infiltrations with procaine. Having experienced them, it appears to me that treatment by means of the ear is more rapidly effective and, above all, the effects last longer. Additionally, auriculotherapy has the possibility of treating organ scars, which is not the case with local infiltrations. Two ear points should be detected and treated:

1. The border point corresponds to the scar itself,
2. A point on the base of the wall, located on the radius of the scar, corresponding to the sympathetic ganglion innervating the dermatome in which the scar is located.

*Skin scars*, in general, are represented on the summit of the border of the helix (**Figure 10.10**). First, it is necessary to define in which somatic dermatome the scar is located. One can then localize the level of the scar's representation on the border of the helix by drawing a straight line starting from the zero point and extending towards the border, passing through the auricular representation of the vertebra corresponding to the affected dermatome, finally ending up on the correct level of the

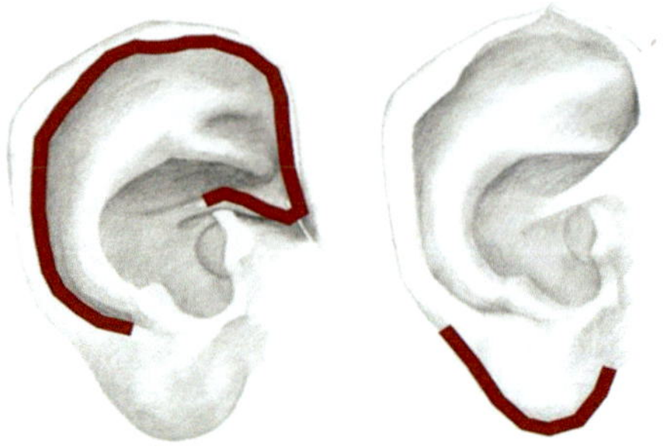

Figure 10.10 Schematic representation of scar locations on the ear.

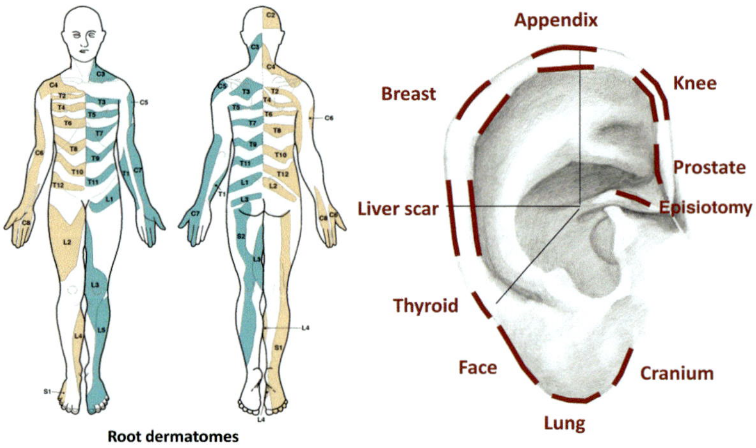


Figure 10.11 Auricular representation of scars according to dermatomes.

border of the ear (**Figure 10.11**). This region of the border is then explored with the black rod to detect (by a positive RAC) the exact point (or line) corresponding to the scar. Normally, this exploration should not trigger a RAC. If there is a disruptive scar, a positive RAC reaction will be obtained and should be counted.

*Organ scars* are also represented on the border, on the extension of the auricular radius that passes through the organ. *The navel* is also a scar and, indeed, fairly often turns out to be disruptive. It can be readily treated by three points situated on a straight line: (1) the border, (2) the base of the wall (sympathetic ganglion), and (3) the zero point.

All scar and sympathetic ganglion points should be confirmed using an electrical detector (see exceptions below) and treated with an SPN (semi-permanent needle).

*N.B.: In the region of the ascending branch of the helix, where the anal, vaginal, and lower abdominal scars are to be found, it is technically impossible to locate the points with an electrical detector. The edge of the ascending branch is rather sharp, making it impossible to apply the detector correctly. Consequently, an exception is made to the rule of always confirming by electrical detection, points found with the RAC.*

### 10.4.7 Miscellaneous Representations of Scars on the Ear

#### *10.4.7.1 Facial Scars*

Scars on the forehead, the cheek, and the chin are treated on the rear border of the lobule. This representation corresponds to the three branches of the trigeminal nerve. Incidentally, the second and third branches of the trigeminal nerve also bear the representations of dental foci. There again, the treatment must be contralateral.

#### *10.4.7.2 Thyroidectomy Scar*

It is located on the C2 dermatome on the front wall of the neck (**Figure 10.9**). It is a scar more frequently found in women, as indeed it is essentially women who suffer from thyroid disorders. General disturbances such as fatigue, weight gain, or depression are often associated with this type of scar. Patients, as well as their physicians, will frequently tend to attribute the cause of these symptoms to incorrect dosage of the replacement therapy. However, in this type of situation, exhaustion of the RAC makes it possible to evaluate the impact of the pathological scar, and the black rod test will allow us to locate which part of the scar is reactive. If only one side reacts, the border at the level of C2 will be treated on the contralateral ear, whereas both ears are to be treated if both sides of the scar are reactive. As a rule, contralateral treatment is performed whenever the impairment is located above C3.

#### *10.4.7.3 Liver Scar*

The representation of this scar can be found on the helix of the right ear between levels C6 and T2. This is an important localisation that we treat for many liver impairments capable of causing RAC exhaustion, such as [1]:

- **Viral hepatitis**, **A**, **B**, **C**, and **toxic hepatitis**: At their onset, the different varieties of hepatitis are all accompanied by a depletion of the RAC, which can last for weeks or even years. Usually, the scar point(s) can be found very easily, and treatment with an SPN will dramatically improve the fatigue.

- **Infectious mononucleosis**: Whether in the acute or chronic phase, treatment of the liver scar by auriculotherapy is the treatment of choice for IMN. Fatigue, which can last for a very long time after a viral sore throat, is rapidly diminished after treatment of the liver scar.
- **Chemotherapy treatments**: Cancer is, unfortunately, a frequent reason for consultation in auriculotherapy. Although it does not affect the development of cancer, it nevertheless does have a beneficial effect on tolerance to chemotherapy. It reduces the digestive signs and the fatigue caused by chemotherapy treatments, which are systematically accompanied by a RAC exhaustion. In contrast, the RAC is not affected by the majority of cancers. In practical terms, it is important to see the patient as soon as possible after the first treatment and before each subsequent treatment in order to check the liver scar.
- **Certain radiotherapy treatments**: In some radiotherapy treatments, RAC exhaustion occurs after several sessions. This exhaustion generally occurs simultaneously with the onset of fatigue. Also, in this case, can the hepatic scar point be found, as can points corresponding to the organ, such as prostate or breast.
- **Breast scars**: They are located on the border between the T4 and T7 levels. RAC exhaustion due to scars is more often linked to cosmetic surgery than to cancer surgery scars. In these cases, it is important to examine the scar(s) involved with the black rod. Very often, it is found that several fragments of the scar react to the black rod and must, therefore, be treated on the homolateral ear.
- **Hysterectomy, caesarean section, episiotomy, and prostatitis scars**: These scars are to be found along the rim of the ascending branch of the helix (**Figure 10.11**). Technically, considering that it is difficult or impossible to apply an electrical detector to this part of the ear, these points must be located using only the black rod with the pulse reaction. One can then treat by inserting an acupuncture needle 20 mm long, not vertically but parallel to the rim of the ascending branch. The needle should remain for about thirty minutes before removal. This location can also be used for post-natal care in the event of post-partum depression in which RAC exhaustion can be observed. With men, scars due to prostatitis can also be found in this area, leading to significant fatigue not only in the acute phase but also in the chronic phase, with exhaustion of the RAC. In all these situations, the ascending branch of the helix should be examined with the pulse and the black rod in search of a scar point.

## 10.5 OTHER DISRUPTIVE FOCI

In 95% of cases, RAC exhaustion can be treated with border points. However, it may sometimes occur that no border points can succeed in restoring a normal

RAC. In such cases, it is necessary to search for other points on the ear with the pulse and the black rod [5], starting from the periphery of the ear and following a spiral course towards the centre. In a very small number of cases, points are found on the anthelix or inside the concha. Could they possibly correspond to disruptive lymph nodes?

## 10.6 CONCLUSION

The search for RAC exhaustion is, without doubt, essential for reliable testing using the pulse. This process implies referring to a precise protocol. It is important to remember that to ensure a valid RAC examination, one must first check its reliability.

## NOTE

1. A concept important for us, described by Cornelius Celsus, a physician as far back as the 1st century (AD), according to Dr Marc Vandebrecht.

## BIBLIOGRAPHY

1. Bourdiol René. *Elements of auriculotherapy*. Maisonneuve 1980
2. Leriche René. *La chirurgie de la douleur*, 2nd edition. Masson & Cie 1939 (pages 399–418)
3. Nogier Paul. *Le traité d'auriculothérapie*. Éditions Maisonneuve. 1969.
4. Nogier Paul in collaboration with Raphaël Nogier. *The man in the ear*. Éditions Maisonneuve. 1979
5. Nogier Raphaël. *La photoperception cutanée*. Éditions Haug 1994
6. Nogier Raphaël. *The exhaustion phenomenon of the VAS*. IVe Symposium of Auriculotherapy Puerto Rico 2002. Annales du Glem 2002. Pages 73–76
7. Rouxeville Yves. *Panorama of auriculotherapy and auriculomedicine*. Springer 2000
8. Vulliez Chantal. *Auriculotherapy and oral pathology*. Sauramps Médical 2020

# CHAPTER 11

# Introduction

**Anthony de Sousa**

## 11.1 FOREWORD

In the preceding chapters, we have attempted to review different aspects of the vascular response, a clinical phenomenon unheard of until a few decades ago. After recounting how it was discovered, discussing the physiological and experimental aspects, and describing how it can be perceived merely by touch, we have endeavoured to understand its significance, showing how this reflex is fundamentally an expression of the sympathetic system.

We are now in a position to present the techniques and applications that depend on pulse assistance. Whether in the specific field of auriculotherapy or general clinical practice, these applications have in common to be designated by the term ***signal medicine***.

This fourth part will be devoted to the classical techniques discovered by Paul Nogier, whereas in the fifth part, Raphaël Nogier will present the techniques and reflections that he himself has developed over the last few years. In the sixth part, Chantal Vulliez will discuss how the vascular signal can be applied to the field of dental medicine.

To feel at ease with the following chapters, the reader should be familiar with the fundamental principles of *auricular mapping* and *general auriculotherapy* (auriculotherapy *without* pulse assistance). Various reference books are mentioned at the end of this chapter. Theoretical and practical training is also offered by various medical associations and universities in many countries.

## 11.2 A WORD ON TERMINOLOGY

Out of respect for the opinion expressed in the past by Paul Nogier, we now consider the term "Auriculomedicine" to be unsuitable and prefer to replace it with the expression **signal medicine**, which he himself had imagined, and also by the more recent designation: **pulse-assisted auriculotherapy**.

## 11.3 THE CHOICE OF TECHNIQUES

During the 45 years of his activities as a researcher, Paul Nogier produced an impressive number of observations and discoveries, driven by an irresistible passion for


DOI: 10.1201/9781003753629-11

research and an unrelenting work power. Indeed, at times, he would facetiously describe himself as a "research bulldozer".

Amidst the vast corpus of knowledge inherited from Paul Nogier's written and oral works, we have been compelled to make choices regarding the techniques presented in this book. In view of the complexity and difficulty of some of these notions and also considering certain contradictions that have appeared over time, we have selected the techniques that seemed to us representative of the spirit of the method and which, in the light of experience, have proved most appropriate from the point of view of diagnosis, treatment, and efficiency. We have occasionally taken the liberty of simplifying the description of certain techniques, depending on the practical aspects of their application. Our aim was not so much to be exhaustive, but rather to clarify. And above all, we have endeavoured to provide support that would prove accessible to practitioners wishing to learn these techniques. Finally, our choices have undoubtedly been influenced by several years of teaching, in which the ever-rewarding contact with students has given us the opportunity to learn a great deal from their enthusiasm as well as from their difficulties.

## 11.4 GENERAL REMARKS ON PULSE-ASSISTED MEASUREMENT AND DIAGNOSIS

The purpose of an examination in the context of signal medicine and pulse-assisted auriculotherapy is to perform a clinical *screening*, in other words, a set of *diagnostic measurements* usually leading to a therapeutic choice, whether it be auriculotherapy, general medicine, or possibly other techniques. A few comments may help to understand the specificities of the process:

- From a methodological point of view, it should be noted that the development of diagnostic techniques related to signal medicine did not arise in connection with individual pathologies or nosological entities, as is more often the case with medical research. Pulse-assisted techniques stemmed from a much wider research process, both fundamental and applied, entirely based on the discovery of the vascular response. The RAC is the common denominator of all the techniques involved, each one eventually leading to various clinical applications.
- It may be interesting to note that the semiological parameters that can be measured by the pulse are of two kinds. On the one hand, they may concern clinical notions and symptoms well known in classical medicine, such as digestive or locomotor disorders, sleep problems, or neuromodulators. But in addition, the method has enabled us to discover a number of original parameters which, at present, *can only be explored by way of the pulse reaction,* for example, those resulting from application of specific pressures to the skin or exposing the skin to light, or yet other techniques which will be discussed later.

- The order of presentation of the techniques has been designed with the intention of integrating them into clinical practice in a progressive and didactic manner. Several examination protocols are included at the end of various chapters to guide the examiner with the sequences to follow according to the clinical situation.
- Finally, some techniques can be applied to virtually every patient, whereas others may be selected because of the specifics of the situation. While the complexity of an examination may vary considerably, experience shows that a simple and coherent approach can be as effective as an exhaustive investigation.

## BIBLIOGRAPHY


### Article on Pulse-Assisted Auriculotherapy

1. Rouxeville Yves. We prefer "Pulse-assisted Auriculotherapy" to "Auriculomedicine", Annales du Glem 2020–2021

### Reference Books on General Auriculotherapy, without Pulse Assistance

2. Nogier Paul. *Introduction pratique à l'Auriculothérapie* (Maisonneuve) 1980
3. Nogier Raphaël. *A Guide to Auriculotherapy* (Mango) 2018
4. Nogier Paul and Raphaël. *The Man in the Ear* Part One (Maisonneuve) 1979
5. Rouxeville Yves. *Auriculotherapie, Clinique et Pratique* (SATAS) 2016

CHAPTER 12

# Instruments Used for Measurements with the Pulse Response

**Anthony de Sousa**

## 12.1 INTRODUCTION

Following the discovery of the vascular response and the development of associated signal medicine techniques, a range of original instruments has gradually emerged, capable of triggering a RAC under a variety of conditions. This chapter will review some of the main instruments currently in use today before describing the techniques themselves in later chapters.

These instruments are nearly always used in conjunction with the pulse reaction (with one exception, when *imposing* a test ring [TR], as described below).

They can be grossly divided into three categories:

- Instruments used for detecting or analysing an ear point. These include ear point detectors, spot lamps (white and colour), and frequency generators.
- Instruments designed to measure the organism's reaction to specific information or parameter. This is done by approaching or bringing into contact with the ear or other parts of the skin, instruments such as TRs, colour filters, or white or colour broad-beam lamps while measuring the pulse reaction with the other hand.
- Instruments known as pressure rods consist of a spring-loaded metal rod. They act by direct contact applied onto the skin of the ear to exert a specific pressure and measure the resulting pulse reaction.

## 12.2 EAR POINT DETECTORS

In addition to the detection of ear points through pain induced by local pressure or by measurement of electrical impedance, ear points can also be detected by way of the RAC. The simplest detectors used for this purpose are elongated instruments, usually bearing two opposed pointed cones at one end (**Figures 12.1** and **12.2**). The idea is to scan the tip of the cone perpendicular across the ear's surface at a variable distance, between a few millimetres and two centimetres. When the cone tip is over a pathological point, it triggers an RAC. The scanning gesture may concern the whole ear surface or a limited part, depending on what one is searching for (Chapter 14).

DOI: 10.1201/9781003753629-12

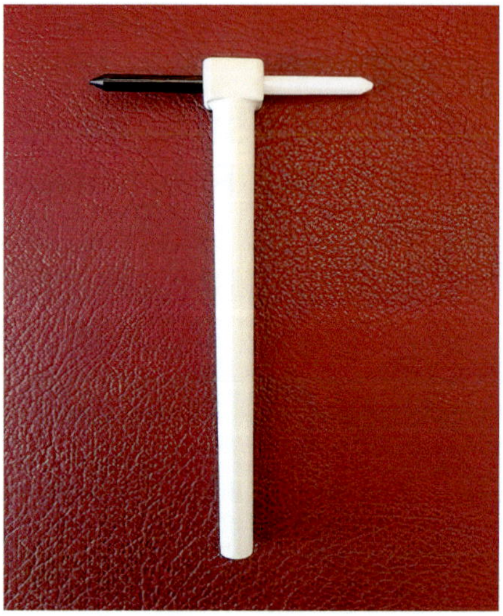

**Figure 12.1** The white-black detector, also called the black and white rod (Sedatelec).

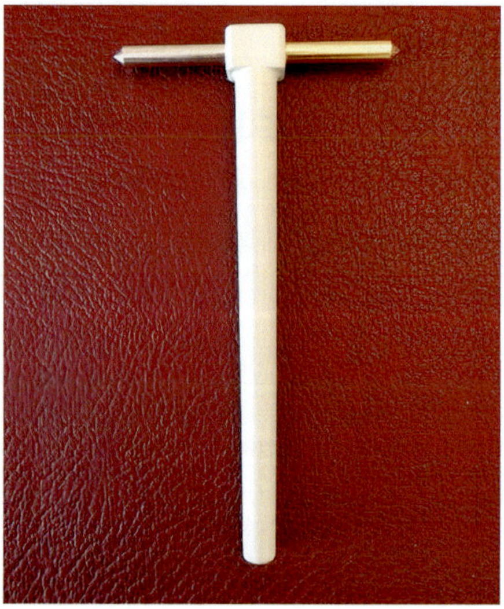

**Figure 12.2** The gold-silver detector (Sedatelec).

The mechanism involved is not yet fully understood. By analogy with the variation in electric resistivity of an ear point in comparison to its surroundings, it can be assumed that the electromagnetic field, normally generated on the skin surface, may, in the same way, be modified locally due to the presence of a pathological point. So, when the tip of a cone appears in such a modified field, along with a reflection phenomenon implying photoemission and/or photoreception (Chapter 8), one can imagine that the whole process induces a micro-stress capable of triggering an RAC.

The two main detectors based on this principle are the white-black detector and gold-silver detector:

- The **white-black detector** (Sedatelec), also referred to as the **black-and-white rod**, is shown in **Figure 12.1**. This detector is a basic instrument for detecting pathological ear points and fine-tuning their location [1]. Both white and black sides have a pointed cone at the tip.
- The **white rod** is required for the detection of most ear points. White colour is emissive and causes most pathological ear points to react through photoreception. Incidentally, the white rod can also be used for scanning an area of the body, e.g. the abdominal wall, in search of a RAC over an impaired organ.
- The **black rod** is used more specifically to detect reactive foci (mostly dental foci and pathological scars). As the black colour is absorbent, the black

rod will "respond" to photoemission over a focus located on the soma and its expression on the ear. Furthermore, the black rod responds to points located on lines called ear boundaries (Chapter 17).

The **gold-silver detector** (Sedatelec), similarly designed for detecting ear points, comprises a gold rod on one side and a silver rod on the other (**Figure 12.2**), both ending as a pointed cone. Despite its effectiveness, this type of detector is seldom used nowadays. Historically, it goes back to a time when, still under the influence of Chinese acupuncture, Paul Nogier was working with the paradigm of determining whether ear points were to be tonified or dispersed according to their reaction to the gold or silver rod. Consequently, the points were then treated with gold or silver needles.

**Example**

Applying this type of analysis to the case of sciatic neuralgia, one would be likely to detect, first, a vertebral point located on the anthelix at the level of representation of L5-S1, reacting to the *gold rod*. Secondly, one would probably find a point on the border of the helix, located at the level of representation of the sensory and/or motor nervous roots of the same L5 or S1 segment and responding to the *silver rod*. Accordingly, these two points will be treated either by tonification or by dispersion, with extemporaneous gold or silver needles designed for repeated use. However, for obvious reasons of sterility and cost, this type of needle has been virtually abandoned today in favour of single-use or semi-permanent steel needles.

## 12.3 WHITE LAMPS

A **source of white light**, such as an ordinary pocket lamp, or a wide-angled white light, can elicit a RAC when briefly projecting light on the skin, e.g. on the arm, chest, or forehead, for approximately one second. As such, it can be used to calibrate the RAC (see Chapter 13).

The **variable light lamp**, or **Heine's lamp** (Sedatelec), offers the possibility of progressively increasing or decreasing the intensity of light [1] and has two main uses. First (**Figure 12.3**), using wide-angle light (without cap) over any skin area of the body, when increasing the light intensity, a moderately intense RAC is observed when the intensity reaches maximum. After decreasing the intensity until total extinction, a characteristic, single, and strong RAC will follow, called a *rebound*. This so-called "rebound at extinction" can also be used to calibrate the RAC.

A different use of Heine's lamp (**Figure 12.4**) does not involve variation of lighting. With intensity set at maximum, a small cap with a narrow hole is placed on its end. The resulting spot-type illumination can be used similarly to the white rod for detecting ear points.

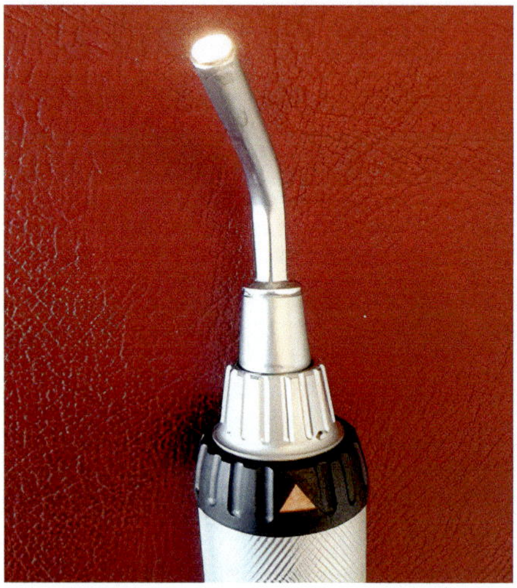

**Figure 12.3** Heine's lamp, without cap, used for variation of light intensity (Sedatelec).

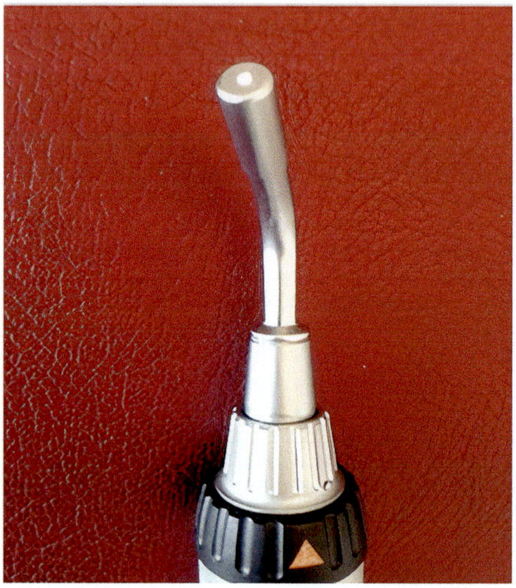

**Figure 12.4** Heine's lamp mounted with a cap for ear point detection (Sedatelec).

## 12.4 THE BLACK PRESSURE ROD

As opposed to instruments such as the black and white rod, which function by interacting with the electromagnetic field over the skin surface, causing the pulse to react when applied at a distance from the skin (a few millimetres), the black pressure rod (**Figure 12.5**) is designed to produce a RAC by exerting direct pressure in contact with the skin, thus bringing into play various skin mechanoreceptors. Similar in appearance to the blue pressure rod used for point detection by inducing local pain (and which delivers 250 grams/mm$^2$), the black pressure rod consists of a metal rod mounted on a spring inside a metal tube) and produces a pressure of 140 grams/mm$^2$ when fully compressed and approximately 70 grams/mm$^2$ when compressed halfway.

This instrument is not designed for ear point detection. It is used to exert a specific pressure on the skin surface of the ear, capable of eliciting a rhythmic reaction of the RAC (Chapter 16).

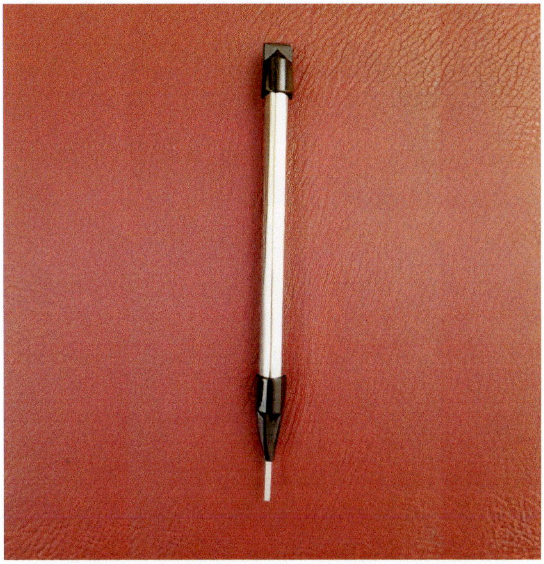

**Figure 12.5** The black pressure rod (Sedatelec).

## 12.5 TEST RINGS (TRs) AND COLOUR FILTERS

These are instruments widely used for the measurement of a great number of parameters. They are designed to embody or express an element or information to which the organism's reaction (RAC) can be measured [1]. Basically, a TR is a container. It can be described as a small, flat, round rubber ring capable of holding the content that is to be tested in between two polycarbonate transparent discs (**Figure 12.6**). The ring is connected to a tab, which allows the TR to be handled and identified by a label. The content is usually in the form of a tablet, powder, liquid (absorbed within a small blotter), or a particular colour. An empty TR must be perfectly neutral, that is, not causing itself any RAC reaction, so that the pulse will only react to the contents of the TR.

Initially, Paul Nogier began his experiments by placing the content to be tested between the slide and the lamella of a microscope. However, since both are made of glass, and glass is not neutral towards the organism, this created an artefact interfering with the pulse reaction. It finally took a long period of research before the neutral device we use today was found.

### 12.5.1 Main Categories of Test Ring Contents

Two examples of TRs commonly used today include:

- The **white/black TR** has two sides, one white and one black, analogous to the white-black rod.

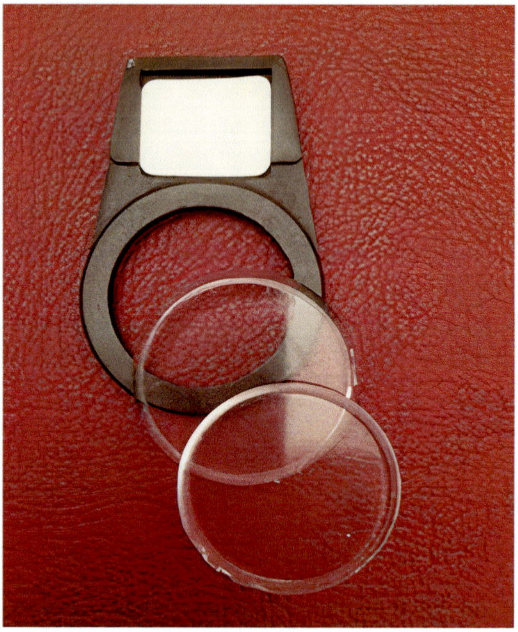

**Figure 12.6** The "empty" TR (Sedatelec).

- The **white side** (**Figure 12.7**) is used primarily to measure the distance (from the ear) at which the TR induces a RAC, a distance called *the reactive level* (**Figure 13.3**).
- The **black side** (**Figure 12.8**) causes the pulse to react when placed over a reactive focus on the body, e.g. a pathological scar or a dental focus (Chapter 10).

- **Colour filters**, often referred to merely as filters (**Figure 12.9**), form a wide variety of TRs called filters because in between the two polycarbonate discs lies a layer of coloured gelatine (Wratten Kodak or Lee), which is translucid [4]. A filter can sometimes contain several coloured gelatines. Due to their diversity, colour filters are widely used in pulse-assisted auriculotherapy techniques [5] (Chapter 18).

At the end of the 1960s, it was Paul Nogier's mastery of the pulse reaction that enabled him to discover that electromagnetic radiation of light could be empirically found to express a resonance with a specific biological function, system, or organ when filtered through a coloured gelatine, according to the responses obtained on the pulse. The gelatine filter colour corresponding to a specific resonance would be physically characterized by its absorption spectrum. These resonance properties eventually opened the way to medical applications, with the possibility of assessing

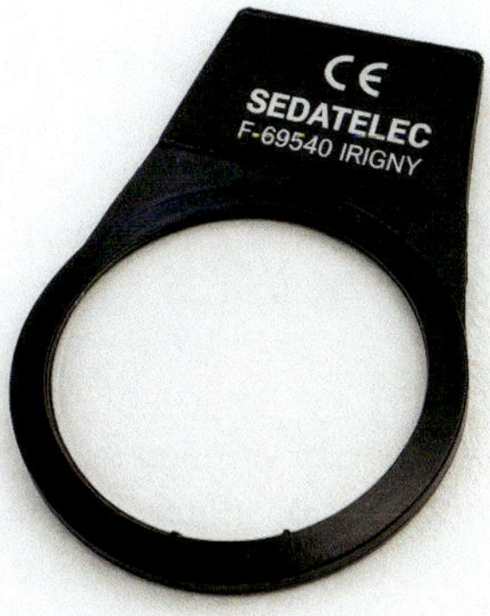


**Figure 12.7** The white side of the black and white TR (Sedatelec).

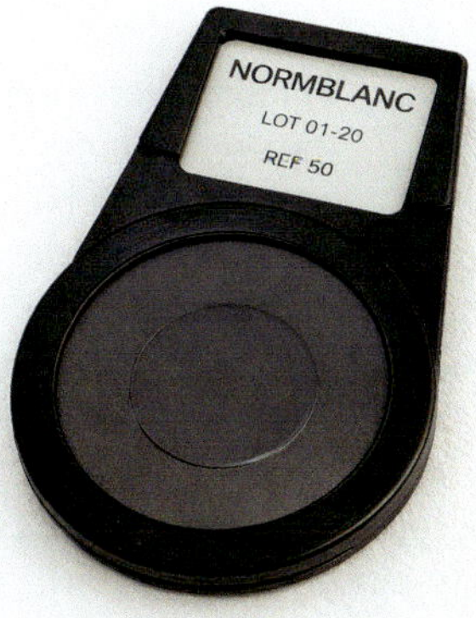


**Figure 12.8** The black side of the black and white TR (Sedatelec).

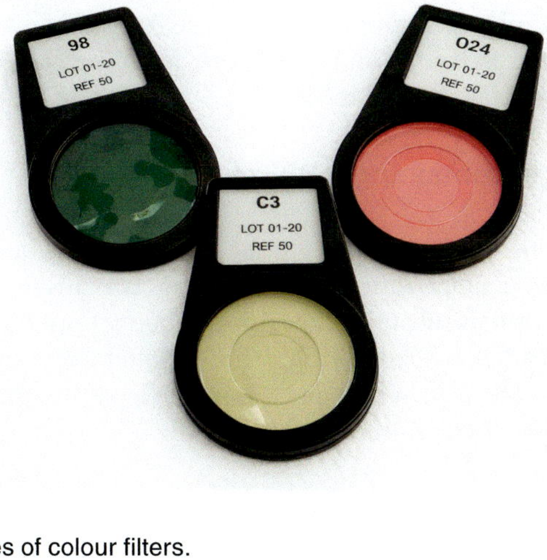


**Figure 12.9** Examples of colour filters.

whether the state of the function or organ concerned was normal or pathological, depending on how the pulse reacted to the filter.

For example, Wratten Kodak Red 25 gelatine provides information on the endodermal, digestive, and respiratory systems.

Perhaps surprisingly, coloured gelatines were originally produced industrially for photography and theatre stage lighting purposes, quite far from the medical applications to which Paul Nogier was led empirically. However, this was the start of several years of intense research.

***Nota Bene*:** Colour filters were first manufactured by **Wratten Kodak** (WK) Company, for the use of photography and theatre lighting. A completely different use arose by chance, when Paul Nogier discovered that, analysed with RAC techniques, many of these colour filters unexpectedly demonstrated resonating properties with biological functions or parameters. For example, filter WK Red 25 has resonating properties with endodermic organs and tissues.

Unfortunately, Wratten Kokak has drastically slowed down or stopped its production of colour filters, because of lack of demand for its initial applications. The Sedatelec company in Lyon, France, still provides colour filters, but they are obliged to find them with a different manufacturer, called **Lee**.

**Lee** uses another nomenclature (e.g. Lee 204) and the filters are not produced with the same exact spectrum but for all filters mentioned in the book there are corresponding Lee filters. Since the original research was made using the WK filters, we use WK filter numbers in the book.

Information can be obtained from Sedatelec, as to the latest updated correspondences between Wratten Kodak and Lee filters, from the point of view of their significances when using the arterial reflex.

### 12.5.2 Test Rings Containing a Substance

As with colour filters, a TR containing a substance (solid, liquid, or powder), when placed close to or in contact with the skin, will induce a RAC reaction, depending on the significance of that substance towards the body. Liquid substances are sometimes, but not always, absorbed within a little blotter paper inserted between the two polycarbonate tablets. As a rule, practitioners can easily manufacture most TRs containing a substance by themselves.

The most used contents of these TRs include:

- A **biological substance**: Such as a neurotransmitter, e.g. noradrenaline or acetylcholine (**Figure 12.10**).
- **Nutrients**: These TRs are used for screening food hypersensitivity (Chapter 27).
- **Medication**: The RAC can provide a general idea of the importance of positive reactions, potential side effects, and toxicity of any medication, thus providing an aid for personalised prescription (Chapter 23).
- **Tobacco, alcohol, and other drugs (Figure 12.11)**, making it possible to assess the degree of dependence of a subject undergoing withdrawal and to monitor the evolution of the dependence factor (Chapter 24).

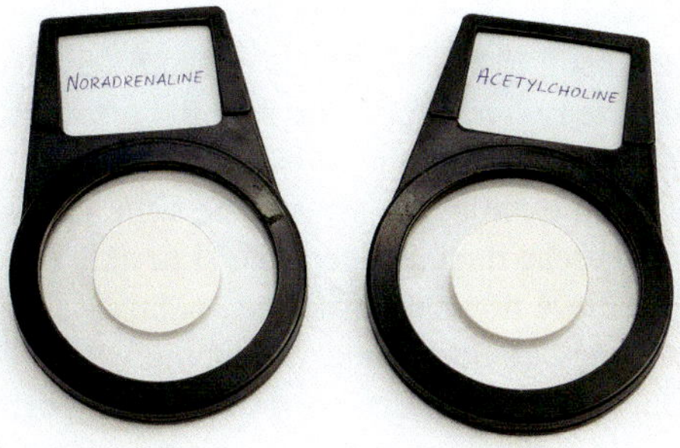


**Figure 12.10** TRs containing noradrenaline and acetylcholine on a small round blotter.

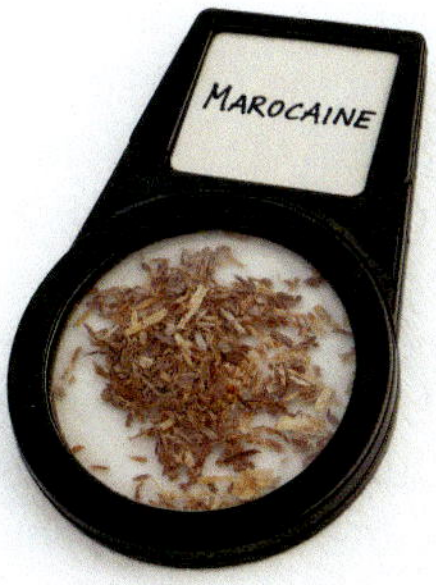


**Figure 12.11** TR containing tobacco.

The **polaroid**, **or reticulate filter**, is an optical system consisting of a polarised network [1] formed by a transparent nitrocellulose film with microscopic crystals of elongated shape. The crystals are all aligned along a specific axis, resulting in polarisation. Only light with a polarisation vector aligned with this axis will pass through the filter. It follows that a double polaroid, where the axes are perpendicular to each other, causes total extinction to the passage of light (**Figure 12.12**).

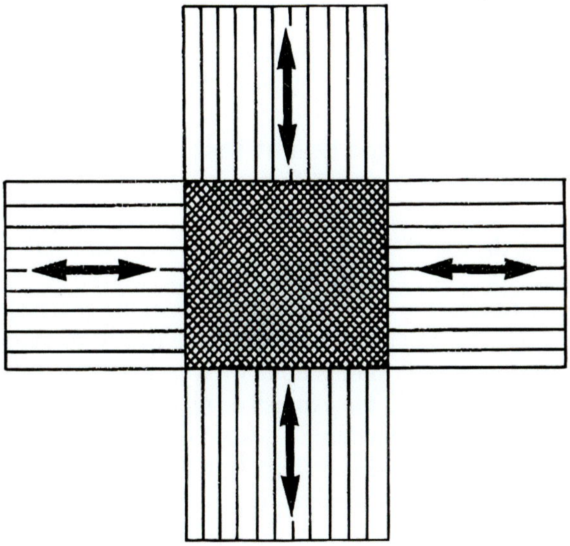

**Figure 12.12** Crossing two polaroid filters with their axes at 90° produces light extinction at their intersection (central part).

Using the pulse reaction, Paul Nogier noticed that the skin itself naturally contains polarised networks. This can be observed by placing a simple polaroid filter on the skin of the forearm. It will produce a strong RAC if the axis of the filter is parallel to that of the network within the skin. The two networks are said to "resonate". This simple technique enabled Nogier to point out that the axis of the network within the skin can vary physiologically. When the patient is awake, the skin axis appears longitudinal, parallel to the forearm, whereas during sleep, the skin axis rotates by 90°, becoming transversal. Apart from these normal variations, polarised networks within the skin may also undergo pathological alterations, producing various odd or chaotic aspects. Techniques based on polarised filters are primarily experimental and are not currently applied to clinical situations, with the following exception:

- A **double polaroid filter at extinction**, placed on the skin, and whatever its orientation, will inter-react with the networks inside the skin, thus creating a minor but very definite stress, causing a strong RAC. Many practitioners use this property to calibrate the pulse at the beginning of an examination. The technique simply consists of placing the filter in the middle of the thorax (sternum), thus triggering a well-individualised pulse reaction, usually over two or three cycles (Chapter 13).

### 12.5.3 Terminology Regarding Test Rings

In the jargon commonly used by practitioners using signal medicine techniques, a convenience of language tends to favour an improper use of the term "filter" when referring to TRs in general. This habit may be considered acceptable in practice. However, a preferable and more rigorous terminology would be if the term "filter" were reserved for colour filters and polaroid filters, so called precisely because they are transparent, which is not the case for many other types of TRs. Language habits are often difficult to change!

### 12.5.4 Basic Principles on the Use of Test Rings (TRs) and Colour Filters

Generally speaking, the use of TRs involves one of two main applications:

- **Assessing** or **testing** the organism's reactions to the contents of a test ring using the RAC. This can be carried out on the **ear** or the **soma**.
- **Imposing** the TR on the skin is done *without using the RAC*. The object is to bring out, on the ear, the expression (also referred to as selection) of test ring-dependent information that would not have appeared spontaneously without imposing the test ring [3]. It consists of merely placing the TR on the arm or chest (at inspiration).

### 12.5.5 Assessing a TR on the Ear: Three Basic Techniques

These techniques all require using the pulse reaction (RAC).

- **Approach the TR** in line with the ear (**Figure 12.13**) gently and at moderate speed to determine whether this movement induces a pulse reaction and, more precisely, at what distance from the ear. The movement starts from a distance of 60–40 cm or less, depending on what is being tested.

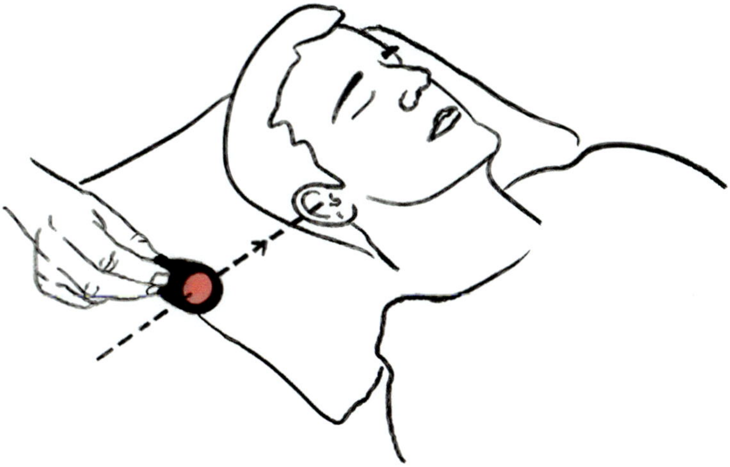

**Figure 12.13** Approaching a TR or filter in line with the ear.

- **Direct contact of the TR** against the ear. An initial contact is known as "**the first contact**", followed by a repetitive contact (two or three repeated contacts within about half a second), known as "the second contact". The TR is then held in contact with the ear for a few seconds while the number of RACs is counted. The determining factor will be the difference between the number of RACs triggered after the first and second contacts:
  - A positive difference (more RACs at second contact) expresses hyperreactivity or allergy, depending on what is tested, e.g. hypersensitivity to a substance or side effects of a drug within an individual patient.
  - A negative difference (fewer RACs at second contact) expresses hyporeactivity or insufficient action, e.g. of a drug.
  - The same number of RACs at first and second contacts expresses indifference.
- **Rapid pull out** from the ear. Starting from the ear, the gesture consists of abruptly removing the TR in line with the ear ("as if the organism were suddenly deprived of a substance that would have had a positive effect"). The pulse may respond with a strong RAC. If so, the number of RACs will be proportional to the importance of the supposedly beneficial effect, e.g. the positive effect of a drug on an individual patient.

### 12.5.6 Assessing a TR on the Body (Soma)

This can be carried out by **direct contact**, for example, on the arm, the chest, or the head, to assess the organism's reaction to the contents of the TR (e.g. a neurotransmitter). Or it can be carried out by **scanning** the TR at a distance of one to two cm from the skin, for instance, over the chest or abdomen (**Figures 12.14** and **4.4**), to locate any kind of functional or organic pathology, for example, a stomach problem, the location of an osteopathic blockage on the spine (**Figure 4.5**), a dental focus or a pathological scar (Chapter 10). A positive RAC occurs when the TR reaches the pathological region.

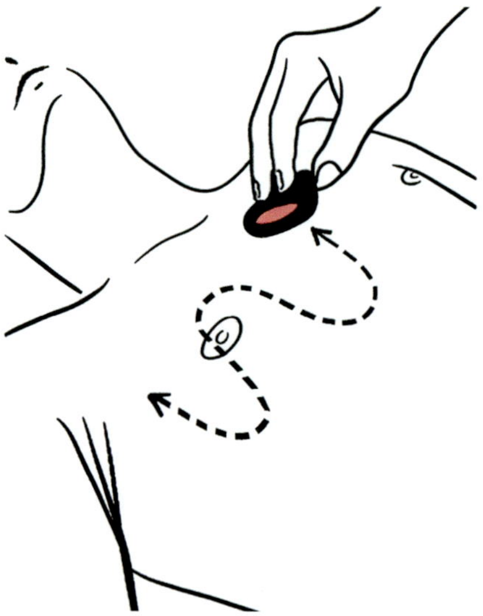

**Figure 12.14** Scanning a TR over the chest.

### 12.5.7 Imposing a Test Ring

This technique is the only one not require taking the pulse. It consists merely of placing the TR on the body to select or bring out specific information on the ear that would not otherwise be expressed.

The TR is placed at inspiration, usually on the arm or **chest**. Placing it on the arm will *enhance* the expression of the selected information, whereas putting it on the chest will *inhibit or reduce* its expression (Chapter 13).

## 12.6 COLOUR LAMPS

Whereas colour filters induce a RAC through photoemission when placed on a wide territory on the ear or the body, by contrast, colour lamps (**Figure 12.15**) also contain

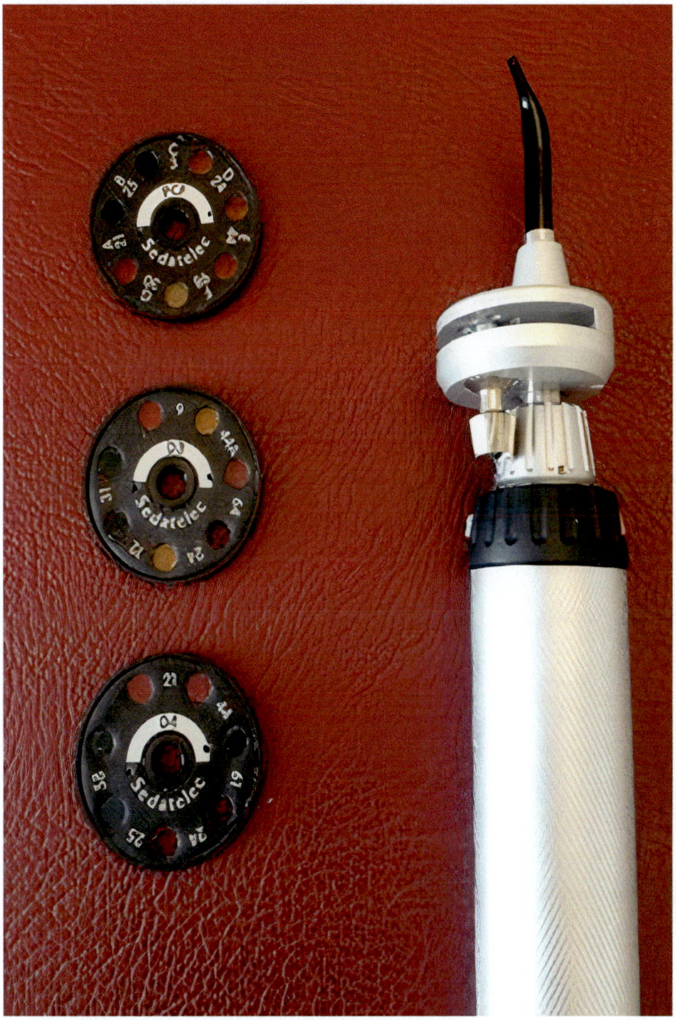


**Figure 12.15** Lamp with discs containing various colour gelatines.

colour gelatines but are designed to act as spotlights and project more precisely onto ear points [1]. In this case, a RAC will be triggered by photoreception (Chapter 8).

A recent version of the colour lamp (**Figure 12.15**) is built on the same principle as Heine's lamp (**Figure 12.3**). The colour gelatines are smaller than those in a colour filter and arranged in a circle within a small disc. The disc is inserted into a slot in front of the light bulb, and by simple rotation of the disc, it is possible to choose the specific colour with which one expects to detect a point.

## 12.7 FREQUENCY GENERATORS

Frequential stimuli are widely used in pulse-assisted techniques. Two main frequency systems have been extensively explored: first, during the seventies, the ***fundamental frequencies***, discussed in Chapters 8, 20, and 21, and later, during the eighties, ***beat frequencies*** described in Chapter 26.

Over the years, several types of generators have been used to explore fundamental frequencies. Today, we primarily use generators in which both frequency systems are incorporated, for example, the GL+ (Micropad), shown in **Figure 12.16**.

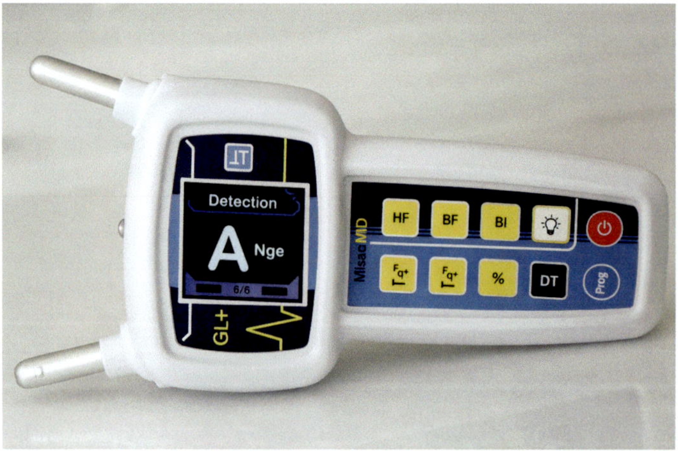


**Figure 12.16** The GL+ (Micropad).

Finally, the **Premio 40** (Sedatelec) (**Figure 12.17**) and the **Microlight** (Micropad) (**Figure 12.18**) can deliver both colour (spot or broad) and frequency stimulations (fundamental and beat frequencies).

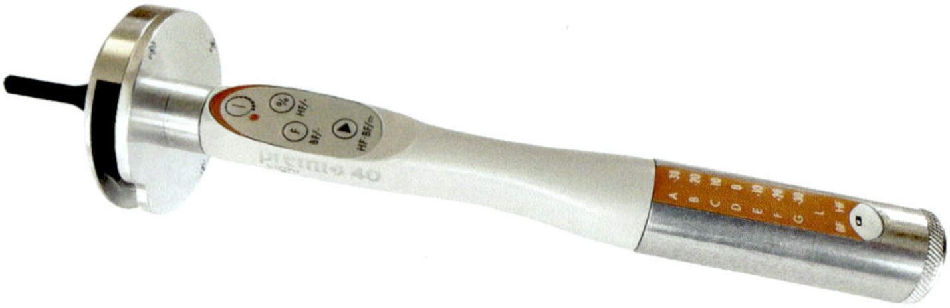

**Figure 12.17** The Premio 40 (Sedatelec).

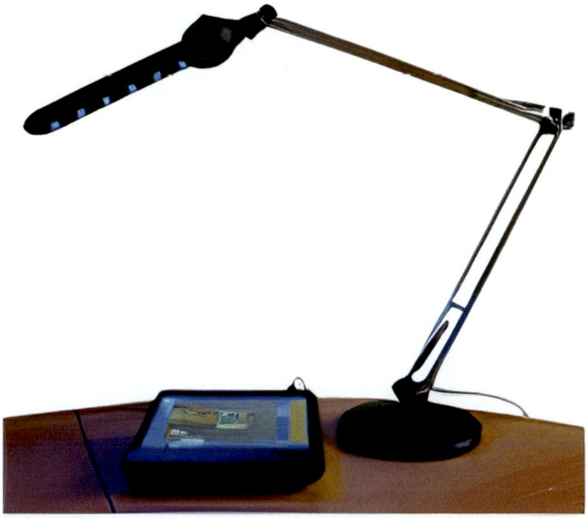

**Figure 12.18** The Microlight (Micropad).

## 12.8 CONCLUSION

This introduction to the main categories of instruments used in pulse-assisted techniques is, of course, not exhaustive. During the following chapters, we occasionally mention other types of instruments.

## BIBLIOGRAPHY


1. Nogier PauL. *From Auriculotherapy to Auriculomedicine* (Maisonneuve) 1981: 47, 81, 85, 133, 140
2. Nogier Paul. *Advanced course in Auriculomedicine*, Lyon 1981–1994
3. Nogier Paul. *The mechanism of action of a filter placed on the skin.* Revue Auriculomédecine 1977, 8.13
4. Nogier Paul. *Les filtres.* Revue Auriculomédecine 1981, 23.35 and 24.27
5. Rouxeville Yves. *Auricular Acupuncture* (Sauramps médical) 2000, 111–118

CHAPTER 13

# Initial Stages of Examination in Pulse-Assisted Auriculotherapy

**Anthony de Sousa**

Considering the subtlety of the vascular response (VR), it is worth initiating a pulse-assisted examination in a precise and structured manner. The following initial stages should be undertaken systematically, especially when examining a patient for the first time.

## 13.1 PRELIMINARIES

- **Clinical examination**: pulse-assisted techniques and auriculotherapy form a medical specialty with the same requirements as any other. In principle, all examinations and treatments in this field should begin with appropriate history-taking, clinical examination, and adequate consideration of the medical diagnosis.
- **Positioning**: various positions for patient and practitioner during examination are illustrated in Chapter 4. They depend, of course, on the type of problem to be treated. Careful positioning will help ensure good pulse perception quality and make the patient and examiner comfortable and relaxed. As the examination progresses, the patient may unconsciously become a little tense after a few minutes, thus making the pulse less perceptible. So, they should be reminded to relax as often as necessary.
- **Evaluation of the resting pulse**: the resting pulse (steady state pulse, with no skin stimulation) can be considered as the "carrier wave" of the RAC, and as such, deserves to be briefly assessed at the onset of examination, before coming to the stage of perceiving the RAC itself. Is the rhythm regular? If not, as in the case of fibrillation, it does not necessarily suppress the RAC but can make it more difficult to perceive. Bradycardia will have the minor drawback of slowing down the sequence of VRs. A soft pulse may suggest a drop in vitality or may result from a pathological condition, whereas a sharp pulse suggests a state of nervous hyperreactivity or allergy. By and large, taking the pulse to work with the RAC may occasionally offer an unexpected opportunity to come across a cardiovascular situation of which the patient may be unaware and should possibly be referred to a specialist. A frequent example is that of atrial fibrillation.


DOI: 10.1201/9781003753629-13

- **It is also interesting to compare left and right radial pulses** (**Figure 9.6**). *Asymmetry* of the radial pulse may be due to an *anatomical* condition, or may be of *functional* origin, often due to an osteopathic blockage of the *first rib* on the side on which the pulse is less ample (**Figures 9.4–9.6**). Furthermore, the amplitude of the resting pulse will usually be found to decrease even more when the head is turned to the same side. If the pulse is weaker on the side where one would expect to take it, one may consider working with the corresponding pulse on the opposite side. In this case, the patient's forearm has to be crossed over the anterior wall of the chest (**Figure 4.2**), a less convenient but possible position.

## 13.2 PERCEPTION OF THE RAC

Following these preliminaries, the examiner is now ready to elicit an arterial reflex triggered by way of one or the other of the following techniques, according to personal preferences:

- Light touch on any part of the skin,
- Exposing the skin to a white lamp preferably wide-angled over the chest and/or abdomen,
- Placing a double polaroid filter at extinction onto the chest,
- Approaching a white test ring in line with the ear.

To describe as clearly as possible the subjective sensation resulting from a VR, in other words, "what it feels like", perception of the RAC is a mental act of **discrimination**, or **comparison**, between two tactile sensations of **different intensities** (**Figure 13.1**), between the "hardness" of the pulse at rest (*steady state,* blue

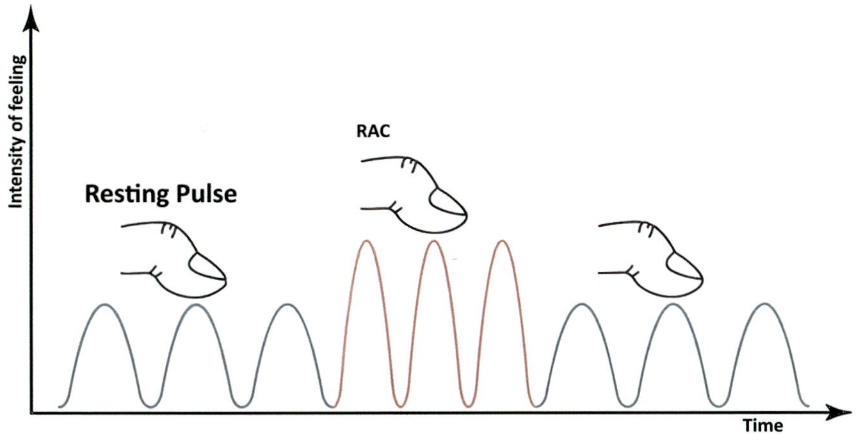


**Figure 13.1** Schematic representation of what a RAC "feels like". Blue curves: intensity of the pulse at rest (steady state). Red curves: intensity increased by a positive RAC.

curves on the figure), and the hardness of the pulse when increased, under the effect of a positive RAC (red curves). A frequent analogy can be imagined with the sensations of hardness obtained by pressing one's finger on a bicycle tyre, first when the pressure is low and then when the pressure has been increased by pumping air into the tyre.

Naturally, the RAC can also be *negative*, in which case the amplitude of the red curves would be *decreased*. For simplification, this is not represented in **Figure 13.1**.

This mental comparison implies that the brain has consciously "**learned**" the intensity of the resting pulse over approximately three to four cycles to be able to identify the occurrence of an "anomaly" compared to what it has learned. The anomaly consists of a series of beats of different intensity, either stronger (positive RAC) or weaker (negative RAC), due to the skin stimulation. Incidentally, it may be interesting to note that we have already encountered a similar "learning" process in Chapter 6 concerning experimental aspects (**Figures 6.11** and **6.12**) applied to recording techniques using artificial neural networks.

## 13.3 CALIBRATION OF THE RAC

Calibration can be considered as the "fine-tuning" of the examiner's perception of the RAC. A "trial and error" technique consists of finding *at what depth* the finger pressing on the artery feels the *amplest perception of the vascular reflex*. In practice, the examiner stimulates the skin several times while *varying the depth of pressure* of the finger at each trial (**Figure 13.2**). Usually, the optimal depth is about halfway between maximum pressure (obliteration of the artery against the bone) and minimum pressure (the pulse is no longer felt). The finger pressure should be kept constant once the optimal depth has been found.

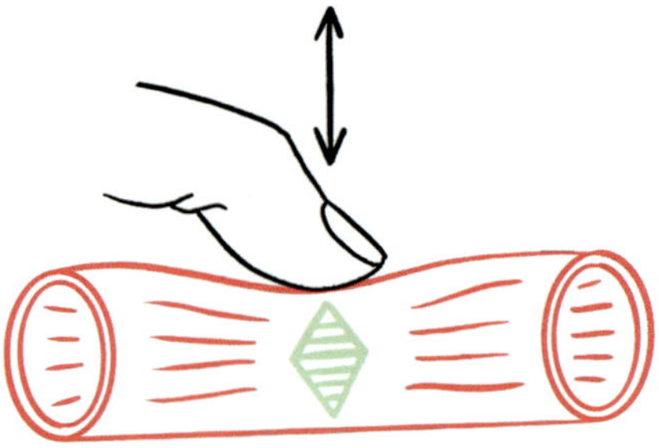

**Figure 13.2** Calibration: finding the optimal depth of pressure for the amplest perception of the RAC.

Despite good stability, the examiner may frequently have to *repeat* calibration over the course of examination and treatment. This is particularly the case when the examiner has to leave the pulse to handle instruments. In addition, a subjective sensation of progressive numbness of the finger in contact with the artery may occur during the examination, leading to decreased perception of the RAC. In addition, the quality of the signal itself may change as a result of treatment. A tense and sharp pulse at the beginning of the examination may become soft and rounded after therapeutic action. Conversely, a rather "soft" pulse at the beginning of the examination is likely to evolve towards a more "tonic" response. All of these situations may require recalibration. With practice, this is easy and almost instantaneous.

Calibration of the RAC also allows:

- Assessing the quality of the VR: Is the RAC response tenuous, soft, difficult to perceive, or, on the contrary, ample, sharp, and easy to feel?
- Deciding whether one feels more at ease taking the pulse with the thumb (**Figure 4.11**) or with two fingers (**Figure 4.13**) after comparing the two.

## 13.4 CHECKING FOR RAC EXHAUSTION

This important step has already been described in detail in Chapter 10. We have seen that the RAC is normally inexhaustible when the same stimulation is repeated indefinitely. In certain pathological conditions, however, the RAC is found to be depleted more or less rapidly because the sympathetic system has become abnormally tired from having to constantly struggle against an irritative factor, typically a dental focus or a toxic scar. Thus, after calibrating the RAC, it is important to check for exhaustion, as described in Chapter 10 (**Figures 10.2** and **10.3**).

## 13.5 MEASURING THE REACTIVE DISTANCE AT THE EAR OSCILLATIONS

The next step in examining a patient involves measuring *the distance at which a test ring causes a RAC, when approached in line with the ear.* It is called the *reactive distance* or *reactive level.* This rests on the assumption that the skin emits an *electromagnetic field* by photoemission. Apparently too weak to be measured instrumentally, this field can readily be felt by way of the pulse reaction [3]. It can be assumed that when the test ring encounters the emitted field, there will be some kind of reflection phenomenon, the emission then turning back towards the skin and producing photoreception. The micro-stress caused by this "mirroring" process will then trigger a RAC. Such a mechanism is presumably similar to what happens when a point detector is scanned over a pathological ear point (see Chapter 10 on Ear point detectors).

The **technique** consists of measuring *the distance* from the ear at which the gesture of approaching a white test ring in line with the ear produces a RAC (**Figure 13.3**). The manoeuvre can be started from a distance of about 25–30 cm from the ear, using a subtle gesture, neither too fast nor too slow, to avoid missing the distance at which the VR appears. On the one hand, the measurement can be repeated not only to ensure its accuracy but also to observe whether the reactive distance is subject to *pathological oscillations*, as described below.

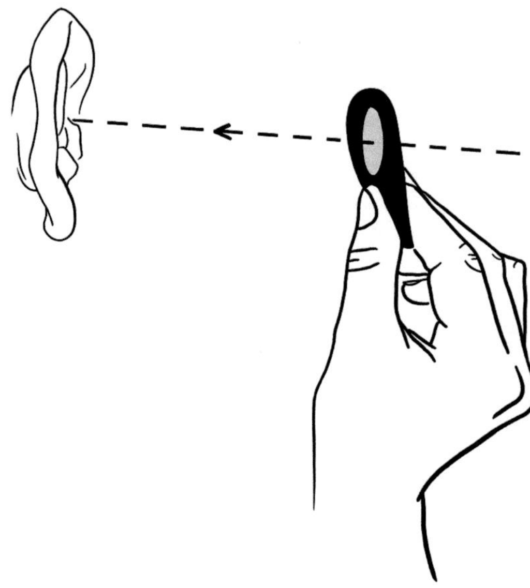

**Figure 13.3** Approaching a white test ring in the axis of the ear.

Paul Nogier considered this electromagnetic field as a kind of physiological radar, comparing it to the *potential energy* of a hydraulic dam. To measure the reactive distance, he began by using a filter with three colours (a Wratten 25-58-44 filter) [4], and later a filter containing seven colours, called the *star* filter, or *colour* programme *filter* (illustrated on the central part of **Figure 18.1**). However, he ended up preferring the *white test ring*, rightly believing that if any of the colours were to be the site of a pathological reaction, this might interfere with the measurement of the reactive distance.

Ultimately, measurement of the *reactive distance* is considered useful at the beginning of the examination, as it is simple to perform and can provide four additional types of information:

- It can be used as one of the techniques for **calibrating the RAC**, as described above.

- It can provide an initial assessment of the **general vitality of the organism**: a RAC obtained between **6** and **10** cm is considered within normal limits. A distance greater than 10 cm is to be interpreted as *hyperreactivity*, whereas a distance of less than 6 cm reflects *hyporeactivity*, fatigue, or exhaustion. Both situations can be observed in functional states as well as in organic diseases.
- It can measure the body's **ability to resist a stress overload**: the technique consists of imposing a colour programme filter (filter containing the seven colours of the "colour programme") on the chest, which induces stress on the organism. The reactive distance is measured before and after imposing the colour programme filter.
    - If the distance remains the same in both conditions, this indicates a good ability to compensate for the overload. If the distance *decreases* after stressing the organism, this suggests a low resistance to overload, a state of fatigue. There may otherwise be an *increase in* the reactive distance, which indicates an underlying hyperreactivity, possibly within an allergic context.
- It allows detection of possible **pathological oscillations**: in this case, repeated measurements of the reactive level show a different distance each time [2], alternating between decrease and increase. The presence of pathological oscillations can compromise the reliability of the remaining part of the examination; it is, therefore, preferable to eliminate them.
    - This can usually be done by treating the *zero point* or *solar plexus point*, located in the middle of the concha on the ascending branch of the helix (**Figure 13.4**). An extemporaneous needle is placed on this point on both sides for one or two minutes, before checking that the oscillations have indeed disappeared. Treatment of the zero point is

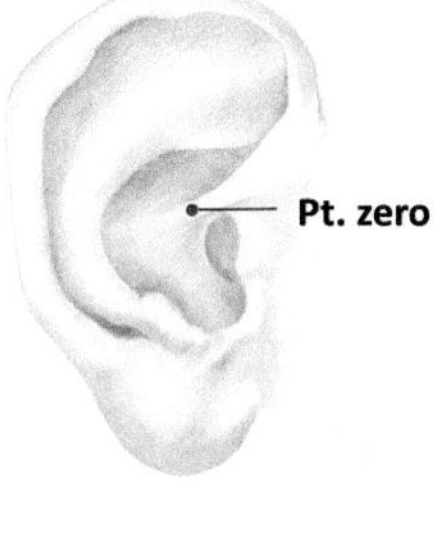


**Figure 13.4** The zero point treating, e.g. oscillations and neurovegetative inversion.

primarily intended to stabilize the conditions of the following part of the examination. Still, it may also produce an immediate therapeutic effect, such as the patient feeling more relaxed (the zero point stimulates the parasympathetic system).

## 13.6 THE TWO TERRITORIES FOR IMPOSITION OF TEST RINGS: THE NEUROVEGETATIVE FORMULA

**Imposition of a test ring** on the skin has been described in Chapter 12. It consists of a particular type of programming that basically gives the possibility of expressing an ear point, a set of points, or any information that may not have been spontaneously accessible without this induction. The imposition of a test ring can be carried out either with the intention of *selecting* or *amplifying* the information it contains or, on the contrary, for the purpose of *dampening or inhibiting* this information.

A typical example of *selection* or *amplification* would be in the case of digestive problems, imposing a colour filter (e.g., Wratten Kodak Red 25) having a *resonance effect* with the digestive field. This would induce the expression of ear points related to the digestive problem, which might not have appeared spontaneously when examining the ear without this imposition.

As for the *dampening* effect, it is less frequently applied, mainly in the case of test rings containing a substance. After *amplifying* the information related to a drug to evaluate its effects on an individual organism, one may then wish to dampen the information to assess the possible consequences of *deprivation* of the drug.

**Two territories**: **periphery and centre**—the possibility of selecting one or the other of these two modalities, *selecting* or *dampening,* is based on having **two separate skin territories** characterised by different neurovegetative tones (**Figure 13.5**):

- The **territory** used for ***selecting*** or ***amplifying*** information contained in a test ring has a sympathetic, adrenergic tone, recognisable by a positive RAC when a noradrenaline test ring (or its analogue Lee 148 colour filter) is placed in contact with this territory. This territory normally occupies the so-called ***periphery***, namely *the four limbs,* **the back, and the sub-umbilical part of the abdomen** (**red in Figure 13.5**).
- **The territory** used for ***inhibiting*** or ***dampening*** the information contained in the test ring, has a parasympathetic, cholinergic tone, responding with a positive RAC when an **acetylcholine** test ring (or its analogue **Lee 328**) is

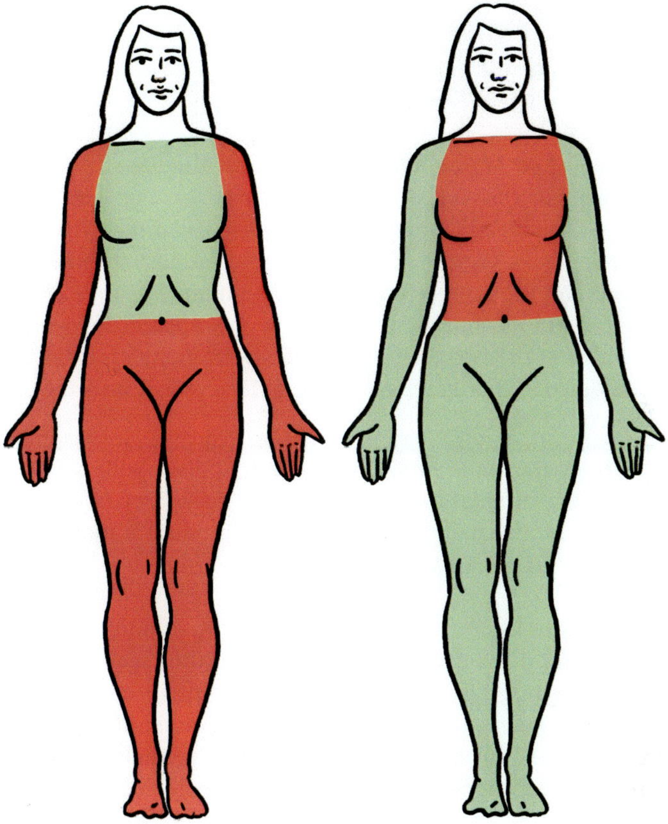

**Figure 13.5** Neurovegetative formula: normal on the left and inversed on the right. In red: territories reacting to *noradrenaline.* In green: territories reacting to *acetylcholine.*

placed on it. This territory is normally located on the *anterior aspect of the chest*, between the clavicles and a horizontal line at the level of the navel. It is called the ***centre*** (**green on the left part of Figure 13.5**).

The location of these two territories corresponds to what is known as a **normal neurovegetative formula** (shown on the left in **Figure 13.5**).

However, many functional or organic disorders result in an *inversion* of these two territories, causing what is called an **inversion of the neurovegetative formula** or **neurovegetative inversion INV** (shown on the right in **Figure 13.5**). In this situation, the noradrenaline (Lee 148) test ring reacts in the ***centre*** and the acetylcholine (Lee 328) test ring reacts on the ***periphery***, that is, on the territories opposite to where they should normally react.

The **technique for determining the neurovegetative formula** is simple. Using the RAC, it takes barely a few seconds:

- **First stage**: a ***Lee 148 colour filter*** (noradrenaline analogue) is placed in brief contact successively with the chest *(centre)*, and then with the arm *(periphery)*. The idea is to compare *the intensity of the RAC* produced by these two contacts. Usually, the filter should produce a more ample RAC when placed on the arm. Note that this technique is *qualitative*; one does not have to count the number of RACs but only appreciate, over one or two RACS, which of the two territories reacts with greater intensity. Note that this technique does not have to be done at inspiration, as is the case for the imposition of a test ring.
- **Second stage**: the same procedure is then applied with a ***Lee 328 filter*** (acetylcholine analogue) successively on the *periphery* (arm), and then on the *centre* (chest). Usually, the filter should produce a more intense RAC when placed on the chest.

If the reaction for both filters is opposite to the norm, it indicates ***inversion of the NV formula INV***. As is the case for *oscillations* of the reactive level (see above), *inversion of the neurovegetative formula* must be diagnosed and corrected at the onset of examination to ensure the reliability of the remaining part of the examination. Both territories must be located according to their normal distribution. Otherwise, the result of imposing test rings will be distorted without the examiner knowing it.

### Treatment of Neurovegetative Inversion

There are two different types of treatment:

- The simplest is the same as for *oscillations* and consists of treating the *zero point* (**Figure 13.4**) with an extemporaneous needle for one or two minutes bilaterally.
- A more analytical approach will help to discover if, apart from the zero point, there could be another cause for the inversion. To do this, the two filters, Lee 148 and Lee 328, are simultaneously imposed (in this case, during inspiration) onto the territories opposite to the one where they should normally react; in other words, imposing Lee 148 (noradrenaline) on the chest and Lee 328 (acetylcholine) on the arm. This double imposition, called "at the opposite", will tend to enhance the neurovegetative inversion and facilitate the expression of a specific causal point

at the ear. This point will be detectable with the white rod and treated with an extemporaneous needle. In both cases, after correction, the test can be repeated to make sure the neurovegetative formula is the right way round, meaning that:

- The territory for ***selecting*** *or* ***amplifying*** the information contained in a test ring is at the **periphery (on the arm)**, as shown in **Figure 13.6**.
- The territory for ***dampening*** *or* ***inhibiting*** the information contained in a test ring is at the centre (on the chest), as shown in **Figure 13.7**.

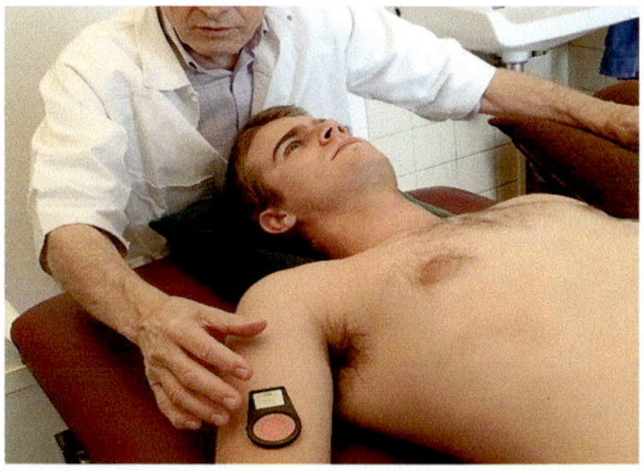

**Figure 13.6** Periphery (arm): *enhancing* information.

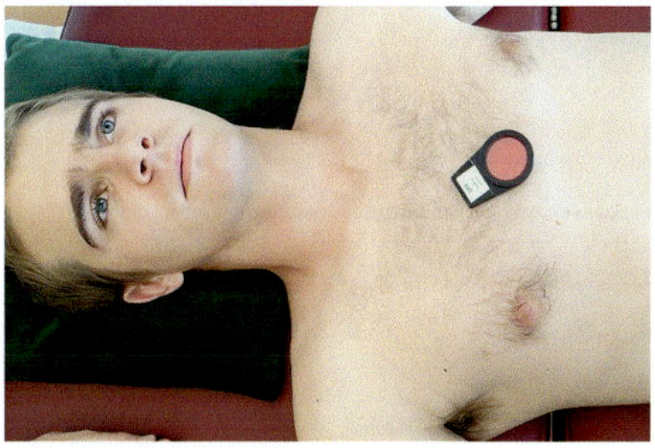

**Figure 13.7** Centre (chest): *inhibiting* information.

### 13.6.1 Comments

- An easier technique for *selection (amplification)* of the information contained in a test ring, when one is unsure of the neurovegetative formula, is to simplify the choice of the territory of imposition of the test ring by making a brief contact of the test ring, first on the arm and then on the chest, to compare the *qualitative* intensity of the RAC on each of the two territories. The site of imposition will simply be the one producing the stronger response.
- The effects of imposing information with a test ring last for approximately one minute, because the body tends to adapt. Beyond this time interval, it is necessary to re-impose the test ring.
- Different responses between the *periphery* and *centre* result from observations with the RAC. However, there is some uncertainty as to the significance of these findings. According to neuroanatomical data, the skin as a whole contains only sympathetic fibres. Therefore, it is unclear why the anterior part of the chest can react preferentially to a cholinergic test ring. For the time being, the contradiction remains unexplained.

## BIBLIOGRAPHY

1. Marignan Michel. *The VAS, or Nogier pulse – Physical, physiological and vascular biomechanical bases* Published in: NOGIER Raphaël: Introduction pratique à l'Auriculomédecine (Haug) 1993
2. Nogier Paul. *Les oscillations*, Revue Auriculomédecine No 10 (1978); 5–6
3. Nogier Paul. *From Auriculotherapy to Auriculomedicine* (Maisonneuve) 1981: 150
4. Nogier Paul. *La perception du signal du pouls*, Revue Auriculomédecine No 28 (1982); 23

CHAPTER 14

# Detection of Ear Points with the RAC

**Anthony de Sousa**

## 14.1 INTRODUCTION

Within the field of general auriculotherapy, that is, *without* using the RAC, the reader will remember that we have at our disposal three classical methods for detecting a pathological ear point:

- *Observation* of an unusual aspect, colour, or morphology of the skin on the outskirts of the point.
- Applying *elective pressure* on the ear with a blue pressure rod (delivering 250 grams/cm$^2$), searching for a hypersensitive region reacting to this pressure by *nociceptive pain*, by contrast with painless surrounding skin, and typically accompanied by a so-called *"grimace sign"*.
- *Instrumental measuring of a variation in the electrical resistance* of the point in relation to its immediate environment, often referred to as the *electrodermal potential*. The variation can be positive or negative.

To avoid a long and tedious examination of the entire ear, the last two methods involve prior selection of a *probability area* based on the examiner's knowledge of the mapping system of the ear and the clinical situation. For example, for a hip problem, the *probability area* would be the summit of the triangular fossa of the anthelix.

## 14.2 PULSE-ASSISTED DETECTION (PAD)

Developed by Paul Nogier in 1966, following his discovery of the RAC, this additional method of detecting ear points is considerably different. By contrast with the above-mentioned comment, the pulse reaction makes it possible to "scan" over the entire surface of the ear (or part of it) with Heine's lamp (**Figure 12.4**) or a white rod (**Figure 12.1**), in a matter of seconds, regardless of prior knowledge of the clinical data or of a probability area. Returning to the previous example, scanning over the ear would make it possible to detect a hip point, even if the patient had not mentioned this symptom.

The **detection technique** can be described as follows. While taking the subject's radial pulse with his left hand, the examiner ***scans*** over the ear with his right hand (**Figure 14.1**) at a distance of about 1 to 2 centimetres, with *a white rod*

DOI: 10.1201/9781003753629-14

(**Figure 12.1**) or with *Heine's lamp* bearing a cap and set to maximum lighting (**Figure 12.4**). The scanning gesture must be applied at moderate speed in order to have time to perceive the RAC, but not too slowly, to avoid artefacts.

This can be done along two perpendicular axes. First, *horizontally* from the upper to the lower part of the ear (**Figure 14.1**), or the other way round, searching for a horizontal *axis* on which a RAC is triggered (**Figure 14.2**, red axis).

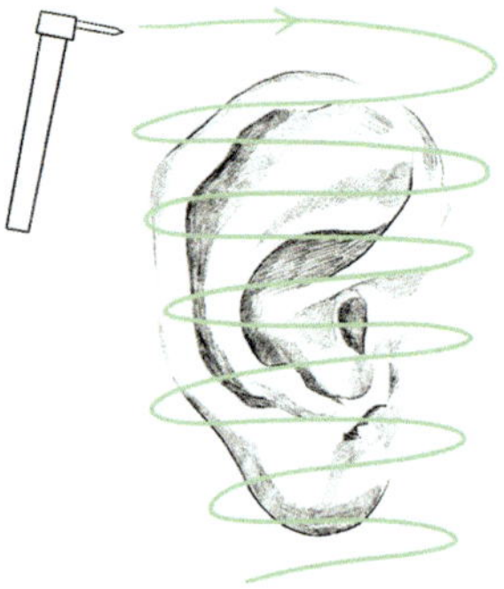

**Figure 14.1** Gesture of scanning over the ear, here with a white rod.

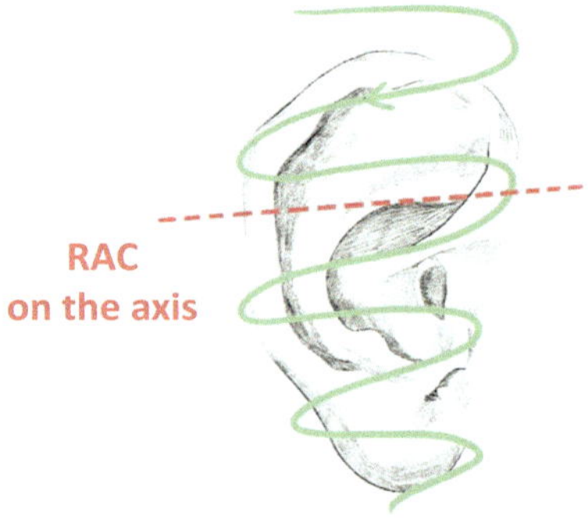


**Figure 14.2** Location of a reactive horizontal axis.

After defining a reactive axis, one will explore it by scanning *vertically*, only along the axis, searching for the point responsible for triggering the RAC (**Figure 14.3**).

By and large, how the scanning gesture is carried out may vary according to personal habits. Many practitioners prefer scanning with a *spiral* gesture (**Figure 14.4**).

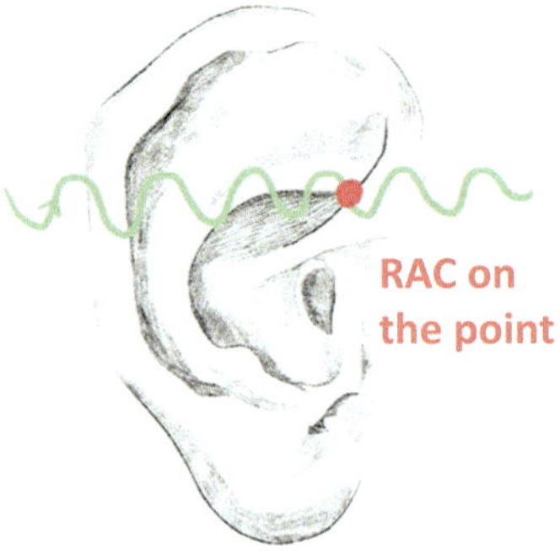


**Figure 14.3** Vertical scanning along the axis to locate the reactive point.

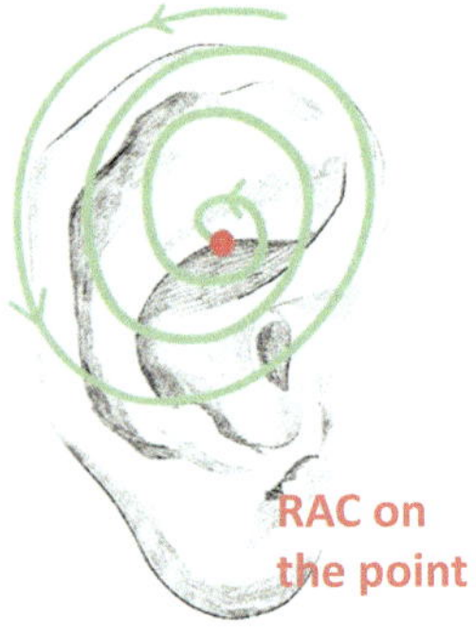


**Figure 14.4** Spiral scanning.

Scanning over the ear can, of course, lead to the detection of *several* axes and points. Remember, only points eliciting a strong RAC should be considered, leaving aside less reactive points. The importance of a point can be assessed qualitatively *by the intensity* of the RAC and quantitatively *by the number* of RACs. So, if several points are detected, their importance can be compared on these two levels.

The **mechanism** by which the tip of a detector located over a pathological point produces a RAC has already been discussed in Chapter 12. The reaction probably also depends on a localised change in the electromagnetic field emitted by the skin in connection with the variation in electrical impedance between an ear point and its surroundings, as mentioned above.

## 14.3 COMMENTS

- **Type of detector used**: In addition to the white rod or Heine's lamp, pulse detection of an ear point can be carried out with any detector adapted to the context, whether it be *a colour lamp, a frequency generator, a black rod*, etc.
- The **area** on which the scanning process is focused may concern:
  - The *external* or the *mastoid (internal)* aspects as a whole, or both
  - Part of the ear, such as a *probability area* (see above), or *a territory* responding to a specific *frequency* (Chapters 20 and 21), or *colour*
  - A specific *ear point,* supposed to exist due to the clinical data
- **Scanning** over the ear may be carried out either:
  - *Without imposition ("on an empty ear")*
  - *With imposition* of a test ring or colour filter *("scanning under imposition of some specific information").* See Chapter 12.
- The **drawback** of pulse-assisted detection is that it is *subjective* and requires experience. Despite its speed and elegance, it may lack precision and reliability. Thus, all four methods mentioned at the onset of this chapter should be practised in close cooperation [3].

## 14.4 HOW DOES ONE PROCEED AFTER DETECTING AN EAR POINT?

Following detection of an ear point, there are basically two options, the choice depending on the clinical problem and the time available.

Having considered the importance of the point in relation to the clinical problem, the first and simplest possibility, in theory, is to **treat it directly**, just as one would do when practicing general auriculotherapy without pulse assistance. Nevertheless, if possible, it will be preferable to use the pulse to determine to what extent the point should or should not be treated directly. The next chapter will describe the technique used to decide whether to treat a point or not.

The second alternative is more typically part of pulse-assisted techniques. It consists of not treating the point directly but integrating it into a diagnostic process using the RAC in the application of the various techniques described in the following chapters, particularly in view of determining factors of *causality.*

From the point of view of the *examination protocol*, it may be interesting to start by scanning the whole ear, regardless of the clinical data, simply noting down the "superficial" points appearing on an empty ear, with the idea of eventually *comparing* these points with those, "deeper down", due to appear later on with various pulse-assisted techniques and programming.

## BIBLIOGRAPHY

1. Nogier Paul. The detection of a pathological point, *Revue Auriculomédecine* 1977, 8–4
2. Nogier Paul. *From Auriculotherapy to Auriculomedicine* (Maisonneuve) 1981: 25, 81, 85
3. Rouxeville Yves. *Livre blanc de l'auriculothérapie*, page 138 (Sauramps Médical) 2020

CHAPTER 15

# Analysis of the Reactive Quality of a Point

**Anthony de Sousa**

## 15.1 INTRODUCTION

Finding a point on the ear does not necessarily imply having to treat it directly. The vascular reflex enables the practitioner to *analyse the reactive quality* of a point and thereby anticipate whether it should be treated or not.

## 15.2 PRINCIPLES FOR TESTING AN EAR POINT

Basically, an ear point can be analysed on a combination of four different concepts:

1. ***Two neurovegetative aspects***: an ear point has the property of bearing two neurovegetative aspects. When Paul Nogier first elaborated this technique, he defined two reactive states, naming them *active energ*y and *reserve energy* [2]. As these notions are somewhat unclear from a physiological point of view, today we are more inclined to refer to the autonomic notions of ***sympathetic*** *and* ***parasympathetic*** aspects of an ear point.
2. ***Two respiration modes***: each of the sympathetic and parasympathetic aspects of a point can be selected explicitly ***according*** to the mode of respiration. During **automatic respiration**, i.e. normal breathing, the organism spontaneously functions under the influence of the ***sympathetic*** *system,* and the ear point expresses a *sympathetic aspect.* However, during voluntary **inspiratory apnoea**, the organism functions under a predominately ***parasympathetic influence,*** and the ear point expresses a *parasympathetic mode.* Consequently, it is possible to *select* the autonomic expression of an ear point by choosing between the two modes of breathing: *automatic respiration* or *inspiratory apnoea.*
3. ***Reactive quality***: when an ear point is treated, it may potentially react, either with a **positive**, so-called "**biotic**" (***therapeutic***) effect or by a **negative**, so-called "**toxic**" effect. This reactive quality of a point can be measured *in both autonomic aspects of the point, i.e. in both respiratory modes.*

   **Technically**, this requires a colour lamp (**Figure 15.1**) on which one can insert a disc containing, amongst others, two punctual colours: **Kodak Wratten**, **blue 44** and **orange 21** colour filters [2], and project them one after the other onto the ear point. One then compares to which colour the

DOI: 10.1201/9781003753629-15 

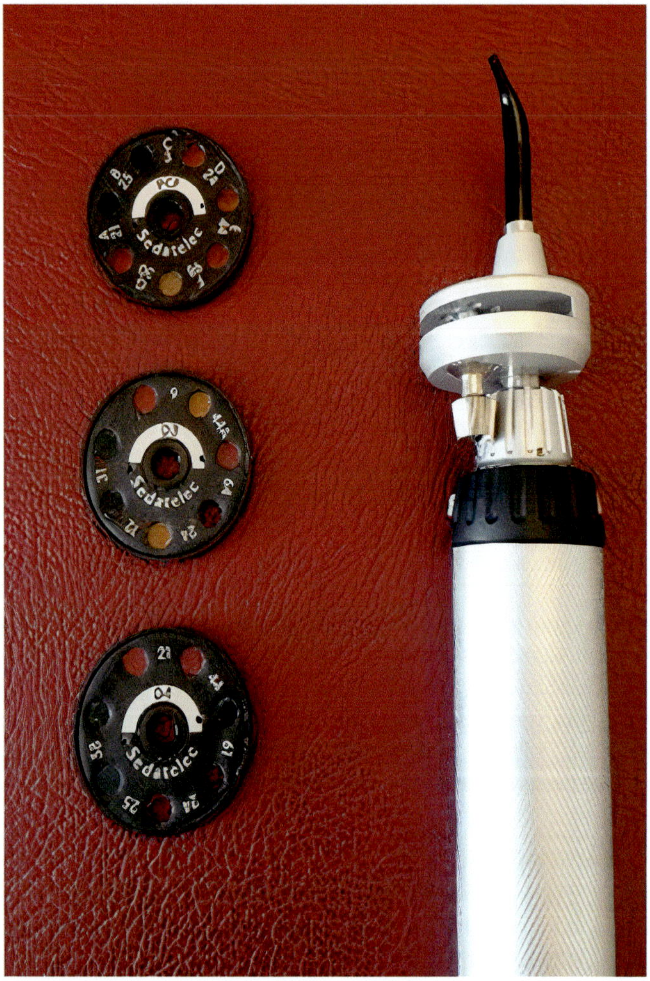

**Figure 15.1** Colour lamp with disks. Each disk contains seven punctual colour filters, totalising 21 colours. One of the discs is inserted into the slot, between the upper part of the lamp and the end cap.

point reacts with the most intense RAC (only qualitatively: so, it is unnecessary to count the RACs). This testing is performed first during automatic respiration (sympathetic aspect) and then during inspiratory apnoea (parasympathetic aspect).

Thus, by examining a point successively in both respiration modes, the following properties apply:

- On its ***sympathetic*** aspect (during **automatic respiration**): if the point reacts to **blue 44**, it expresses a ***biotic,*** *or* ***positive*** character. If, on the contrary, it reacts to **orange 21**, it expresses a ***toxic or negative*** character.

- On its ***parasympathetic*** aspect (during **inspiratory apnoea**): *the two colours take on an opposite value*: if the point reacts to **orange 21**, it is considered ***biotic*** or ***positive***. Whereas if it reacts to blue 44, it indicates a ***toxic***, ***negative*** reactivity.

4. ***Mobile or fixed character of a point***: from the above, it follows that when one passes from one respiration mode to the other, the point should "change colour", switching its reaction from blue to ***orange*** or vice versa. If this is indeed the case, the point is said to be **mobile**. If the reaction to the colour does not reverse, the point is said to be **fixed**. Mobility of a point is normal, whereas fixity is pathological [2].

## 15.3 RECAPITULATION

Combining the four concepts described above, the idea is to compare the intensity of the RAC resulting from projecting **blue 44** and **orange 21** onto the ear point, in turn, first during ***automatic respiration*** (on the ***sympathetic*** aspect), then again during **inspiratory apnoea** (on the ***parasympathetic*** aspect).

**Four situations** are possible. They are listed below in decreasing order from the point of view of treating the point or not. Depending on its reactions, the point is considered as:

- ***Mobile blue*** if the point reacts to **blue 44** during automatic respiration and then switches to **orange 21** during apnoea. Treating this type of point is liable to produce the most favourable result.

- ***Fixed blue*** if the point reacts to **blue 44** on both respiration modes, thus not switching from one mode to the other. Such a point can be considered "second best" to treat.

- ***Mobile orange*** when the point reacts to **orange 21** during automatic respiration and then switches to **blue 44** during apnoea (opposite reaction to mobile blue). Despite its inverted reaction to the two colours, its mobility is considered positive. It is, therefore, possible to treat it but *preferably "on its blue side"*. This can be done by inserting an extemporaneous needle or an ASP during the brief duration of inspiratory apnoea.

- ***Fixed orange*** if the point consistently responds to **orange 21** on both respiratory modes. Treatment of an ear point having this type of reaction should clearly be avoided because the result bears a considerable risk of failure or even aggravation.

All four situations are summarised in **Table 15.1**.

**Table 15.1 Anticipation of the Reactive Quality of an Ear Point before Treatment**

| Automatic respiration sympathetic aspect | Inspiratory apnoea parasympathetic aspect | Formula | Treatment |
|---|---|---|---|
| Blue | Orange | Mobile Blue | Positive |
| Blue | Blue | Fixed blue | Possible |
| Orange | Blue | Mobile orange | Possible, if treated "on the blue side" |
| Orange | Orange | Fixed orange | Avoid treatment |

## 15.4 CONCLUSION

Considering the possible effects of treating a point, the question of knowing whether it should be treated or not can, to a certain extent, be anticipated. This technique may appear complex at first glance, but in fact, takes merely a few seconds. In practice, paying attention to the reactive quality of ear points before treating them may be particularly appropriate when considering patients in poor physical or nervous condition or hypersensitive patients. These situations require caution regarding the *reactive quality* and at the same time a limitation of the *number* of points treated at each session.

## REFERENCES

1. Nogier, Paul. Biotic points and antibiotic points, *Revue Auriculomédecine* 8, 1977, 15
2. Rouxeville, Yves. *Index of Dr. Paul* Nogier's *lectures*: February, March, and September 1983

# CHAPTER 16

# Pulse Reactions to Mechanical Pressure Applied to the Skin

**Anthony de Sousa**

## 16.1 INTRODUCTION

In addition to exposure to light at a short distance from the skin (using lamps, test rings, and detectors), it is also possible to trigger a vascular response through direct mechanical contact with the skin.

The response to mechanical stimulation involves pressure-sensitive sensors located within the skin, probably so-called tonic receptors such as the superficial Merkel discs (**Figure 5.12**). These sensors are characterized by slow adaptation, meaning that the delay between stimulus and response is slow, but the response is maintained throughout the duration of the stimulus.

When he began studying mechanical stimulation of the skin, Paul Nogier observed a curious and unexpected pulse reaction. Among the various pressures exerted, some could trigger RAC responses consisting of *rhythmic patterns*, depending on the intensity of pressure. As a result, he ended up describing **three skin "levels": superficial level, medium level, and deep level**, thereby designating the functional link between three separate degrees of pressure onto the skin and the specific responses these pressures triggered on the pulse (**Figure 16.1**).

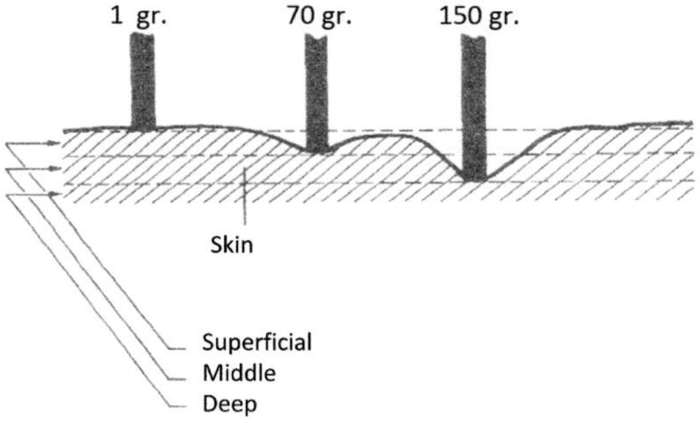


**Figure 16.1** The three pressure levels on the skin: superficial, middle, and deep levels.

DOI: 10.1201/9781003753629-16

Initially, Paul Nogier named these types of reactions the "*three tissues*". But later on, to avoid confusion with the histological structure of the skin, he came on to prefer the term **level** (or **layer**), in agreement with a suggestion made by Yves Rouxeville, an experienced colleague from Northern France.

One can reasonably assume that the patterns obtained on the pulse represent three modalities of sympathetic responses to minor stresses of mechanical nature.

## 16.2 THE SUPERFICIAL LEVEL

This level refers to the RAC obtained when applying a pressure of approximately *1 gram per* $mm^2$ to the skin, normally resulting in *1–3 positive RACs*. This, of course, is a standard RAC response and is not rhythmic.

Applied to the **ear**, **the** pressure of this order is mostly of experimental interest, using an instrument seldom used today, called a *needle probe*, consisting of a small bundle of metallic needles mounted on a spring-loaded rod.

By contrast, the superficial level is currently tested on the **soma**, mainly for diagnosis of **pathological skin scars** and **dental foci**. These two situations have already been discussed in Chapter 10. We will briefly summarize them here, insofar as their diagnosis partly implies the superficial level:

### 16.2.1 Pathological or Toxic Scars

The **aspect** of a pathological scar may or may not be swollen, red, or keloid (N.B. keloid scars are not as harmful as their aspect might sometimes suggest).

**Subjectively**, touching a toxic scar can be *felt* by the patient as either unpleasant, painful, or insensitive ("like cardboard"). A notable example is the navel, a scar that everybody has, and which fairly frequently turns out to be pathological.

**Testing a scar with the pulse** can be done in two different ways:

> The **first** technique consists of *scanning over the scar* at a small distance (1 cm) with a black test ring or black rod. This will result in a positive RAC if the scar is pathological (normally, no RAC is expected).
>
> The **second** technique involves stimulating the superficial level by applying light touch to the scar with a finger, cotton wool, or an eraser and slowly moving along the length of the scar. If the scar is pathological, it will respond with a **negative RAC** (except in case of RAC exhaustion, a negative RAC may then be too weak to be felt;

see Chapter 10). At the same time, the patient will be experiencing this touch as either unpleasant or insensitive, as mentioned above. The scar may be pathological over its entire length or only over a restricted segment, often at one extremity. Counting the number of RACs is important because it provides an indication of the degree of pathology. The scar can then be treated *on the ear*, generally on the border locations indicated in **Figure 10.10**.

It is recommended to apply both these techniques using the pulse, one confirming the other.

### 16.2.2 Dental Foci

As opposed to pathological scars, extra-oral diagnosis and location of a dental focus **in situ** (over the maxillary or mandibular skin of the jaw) can only be done using the pulse, using two techniques, similar to those described for testing scars:

The **first** technique involves scanning the soma at a distance of approximately 1 cm over the skin, covering the maxillary and mandibular arcades, using *the tip of a black rod*. If a dental focus is present, a ***positive RAC*** will appear when the black rod reaches the location of the root of the affected tooth.

The **second** technique is once again based on the properties of the ***superficial level***. In this case, one applies *light stationary pressure* with a finger through the skin of the jaw over the root of **each tooth**, one after the other. Pressing on a normal tooth will result in no more than one or two faintly positive RACs. On a dental focus tooth, the same pressure will result in a sharper ***positive RAC***, lasting between 2 and 9 cycles, depending on the importance of the dental focus. In some cases, however, a ***negative RAC*** may appear (except in case of RAC exhaustion, as mentioned earlier). If there is more than one focus, *counting the number of RACs on each one* makes it possible to compare their importance.

To treat the dental focus, we then turn to the opposite ear, specifically the rear border of the lobule (**Figure 10.3**), using two different methods. First, by scanning a ***black rod*** at a distance of 1 cm over the rear border of the lobule, searching for a point reacting by with a **positive RAC**. Then, secondly, by exerting light pressure on the edge of the lobule between the thumb and index finger, thus stimulating the *superficial level*. The reactive point (**positive** or **negative RAC**) corresponding to the dental focus will generally be that representing the second branch of the trigeminal nerve V2 for a focus located on the maxillary arcade and the third branch V3 for a mandibular arcade focus.

**Table 16.1** sums up the reactions obtained when testing a pathological scar and a dental focus with the pulse. In both cases, the responses to light touch are an example of triggering the superficial level.

**Table 16.1 Testing Pathological Scars and Dental Foci with the Pulse**

| | Scanning with black rod | Light touch (superficial level) |
|---|---|---|
| Pathological scar | RAC + | RAC -- |
| Dental focus (in situ) | RAC + | RAC + or RAC -- |
| Dental focus (representation on the ear) | RAC + | RAC + or RAC -- |

*Note*: In both cases, testing using a light touch (Red) is a typical example of superficial-level reactions.

## 16.3 THE MIDDLE LEVEL

We will now describe the **middle and deep levels**. In contrast to the superficial level, both levels have the surprising property of producing rhythmic *pulse patterns*. They can be triggered *on the ear* (not on the soma), using a *black pressure probe* (**Figure 16.2**). This instrument consists of a metal rod with a blunt tip, mounted on a spring. Only the middle level is currently used for clinical purposes. The deep layer has more of an experimental interest (see below).

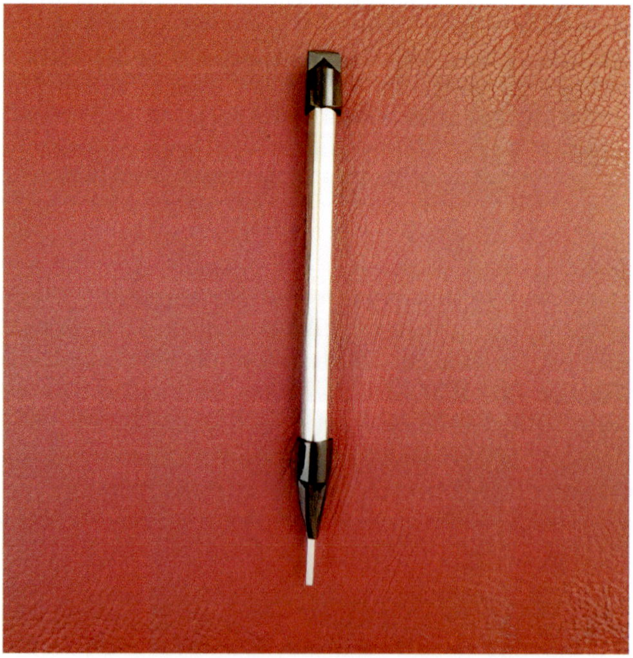

**Figure 16.2** Black pressure probe.

The *middle level* responds to mechanical stimulation of the ear when the black probe is pressed halfway, delivering a continuous *pressure of approximately 70 g/mm²*.

The *normal pulse reaction* of the middle level will consist of a *rhythmic sequence* of *four positive RACs followed by four negative RACs*, alternating as long as the stimulation lasts. To be precise, however, the number of positive and negative RACs is not always strictly limited to four and can often reach five or six pulses.

Under normal conditions, this rhythm is regular, symmetrical, and inexhaustible. It is known as the ***middle-level beat***:

| |
|---|
| *Middle-level beat*: **+ 4/– 4/+ 4/– 4 …** |

One exception should be mentioned: applying the same pressure onto an *ear border* (**Figure 17.4**) will normally cause the pulse to react in a reversed manner, beginning with four negative RACs followed by four positive RACs, and so on:

| |
|---|
| *Normal response of the middle level on an ear boundary*: **– 4/+ 4/– 4/+ 4 …** |

As for the **pathological reactions of the** middle level, they are of two kinds:

1. If the rhythmic pulse pattern does not appear, the middle level is said to be ***flat***. This situation is frequent and indicates hyporeactivity of the sympathetic system, vagotonia, a drop in vitality, or a state of pathological fatigue of functional or organic origin:

| |
|---|
| *Middle-level hyporeactivity*: ***(lack of response)*** |

2. If, on the other hand, the rhythmic sequence disappears in favour of a ***sharp***, ***uninterrupted positive RAC***, this indicates a state of sympathetic hyperreactivity, possibly in a context of allergy: the middle level is said to be ***blocked***.

| |
|---|
| *Middle-level hyperreactivity*: **+ + + + + + + *(uninterrupted positive RAC)*** |

During examination, the black pressure probe (pressed halfway) is applied successively to different parts of the ear, as the middle-level beat may be normal in certain areas of the ear and altered in others, depending on the origin of the disorder.

The observation of a middle-level beat abnormality provides information not only on the general reactivity of the subject (fatigue, hyperreactivity, etc.), but also on the cause of the pathology, for example, ecto, meso, or endo-dermal origin, depending on the area, or embryologic territory, on which the middle level has been found to be altered.

One can then scan this same area with an ear point detector (white rod or Heine's lamp) to identify an ear point related to the problem. Once this point has been detected, located, and tested for middle-level beat, there are two possibilities.

The first is to treat it directly, either with a needle or preferably with a *bipolar north-south magnetic rod* (Sedatelec). This involves exposing the point alternately to each of the two magnetic poles (1–2 mm above the point or in contact) at a rate of once per second for approximately a minute. Such a procedure normally restores the middle-level beat on the point.

The second possibility involves analysing the point using another pulse-related technique, such as frequency responses (see Chapters 20 and 21), and then verifying whether the middle-level beat has been restored. The middle-level reaction on this point then takes on the significance of a *control parameter.*

## 16.4 THE DEEP LEVEL

The deep level is mainly of experimental interest. It responds to mechanical stimulation of approximately *150–160 g/mm² applied anywhere on the ear or at a detected point using the black probe, which is* pressed fully and continuously.

Under **normal conditions,** this rhythm is *asymmetrical.* On a constant total of **20** to **21 RACs**, the first ones are **positive**, and the following ones are **negative**, however, ***in varying proportions:***

- Depending on individual reactivity, Paul Nogier described three types of normal responses, which he called *rapid, intermediate, or slow*, depending on when the RAC switches from positive to negative. Thus, on a total of 20 to 21 RACs:

*A* ***rapid*** *reaction includes:*

***2 to 3 positive RACs, followed by 18 to 19 negative RACs***
**+++/– – – – – – – – – – – – – – – – – – –**

*An* ***intermediate*** *reaction includes:*

***6-7 positive RACs followed by 14-15 negative RACs***
**+++++++/– – – – – – – – – – – – – –**

*A* ***slow*** *reaction includes:*

***18 to 19 positive RACs, followed by 2 to 3 negative RACs***
**+++++++++++++++++++/– – –**

- In **pathological reactions** at the deep level, the switch from positive to negative RACs disappears. The rhythmicity is lost in favour of a fixity of positive or negative RACs. Fixity is known to be pathological:

A negative RAC maintained throughout the duration of the stimulation indicates *a lack of sympathetic response:*

**RAC**

A positive RAC maintained throughout the duration of the stimulation indicates *a difficulty in mobilising the sympathetic response:*

**RAC +++++++++++**

Comparing this to a car engine, the first case (constant negative RAC) would be comparable to an engine that has lost its power, whereas in the second case (constant positive RAC), the power of the engine is unaltered but cannot be transmitted to the wheels because of a clutch failure.

At the time, Paul Nogier commented on the pathological aspects of the deep level; he spoke of energy deficiency and inhibition in mobilising *energy reserves*. Today, these notions lack clarity, which is why we prefer to describe the phenomenon in terms of neurovegetative responses.

Deep-level reactions are sometimes considered more challenging to observe than those of the other two levels and are not often included in clinical protocols. Treating a point related to deep-level disturbances is theoretically possible, e.g. with a needle. However, as for the middle level, it may be preferable to consider the reactions of the deep level as a *control parameter*, which can be checked after the use of other techniques.

## 16.5 CONCLUSION

Summarising these considerations on mechanical stimulation, the superficial level is primarily applied to the soma for diagnosing pathological scars and dental foci, whereas the *middle* and *deep levels* are limited to the ear. The *middle level* is a useful clinical parameter for assessing the general reactivity of the organism. The *deep level* can be considered more like an experimental technique for observing the neuro-vegetative system's rhythmic "echo" response to mechanical micro-stress applied to the skin.

## BIBLIOGRAPHY

1. Nogier Paul. *From auriculotherapy to auriculomedicine* (Maisonneuve) 1981, 115–122
2. Rouxeville Yves. *Auricular Acupuncture* (Sauramps médical) 2000, 91–99

# CHAPTER 17

# Transfers of Information and Ear Borders

**Anthony de Sousa**

## 17.1 INTRODUCTION

Every living organism can be imagined as like an enormous anthill, involved in constant and countless exchanges of information. This has been known for a very long time as a fundamental property of life. What is more recent is the fact that the arterial reflex (RAC) provides us with an original tool for observing this circulating activity and for helping to influence it when impaired.

Classically, we know of many different pathways devoted to the transport and exchange of information: depolarisation waves along nerve fibres, humoral and chemical messengers, hormones and neurotransmitters, probably also to a lesser extent blood cells and various other tissues. From a methodological point of view however, studying circulation of information by way of the RAC gives access to an original and somewhat different viewpoint than that of classical physiology, and for which Paul Nogier introduced a new notion that he named ***transfers of information*** (**Figure 17.1**). This represents a more synthetic concept, adapted to the auricle, regardless of the anatomical pathway. Transfers of information can also be tested on the body, but as such are of lesser importance.

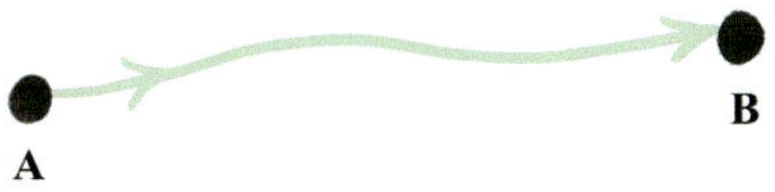


**Figure 17.1** Transfer of information from point A to point B.

The RAC allows us to measure whether transfers on the auricle are normal or pathological. In the latter case, they are described as being *impaired*, *reduced*, or *blocked*. There are many possible causes of impaired transfers. For example, they may reflect acute or chronic damage to the central or peripheral nervous system. Or they may be due to chemical products, infectious disease, pathological scars, or dental foci, or stress. In 1998, Dr Yves Rouxeville made an interesting observation [1] showing a link between reduced transfers and hyperreactivity to $Na+$, $K+$, or $Ca++$ ions (each placed in a test ring and producing at least five RACs when brought into contact with the ear). The role of these ions in nerve transmission is well known.

DOI: 10.1201/9781003753629-17

From a therapeutic point of view, we know that the results obtained by auriculotherapy depend, among other things, on the quality of information transfers. Paul Nogier often insisted on the importance of checking this. For this purpose, he developed an elegant method, called the *double-impact* technique, based on the concepts of *image* and *counter-image*, known in optical physiology.

## 17.2 THE DOUBLE IMPACT TECHNIQUE

A punctual stimulation is briefly applied to the skin surface, for example, with a white light (Heine lamp), a coloured lamp, a white or black rod, or simply by touch. This stimulation is called the **image** (**Figure 17.2**). It will induce a local reaction inside the skin called the **counter-image**, propagating concentrically, like a circular wave triggered by a pebble thrown into a pond. Let us suppose that the speed of propagation of the counter-image depends on the speed of the nerve impulse that carries it.

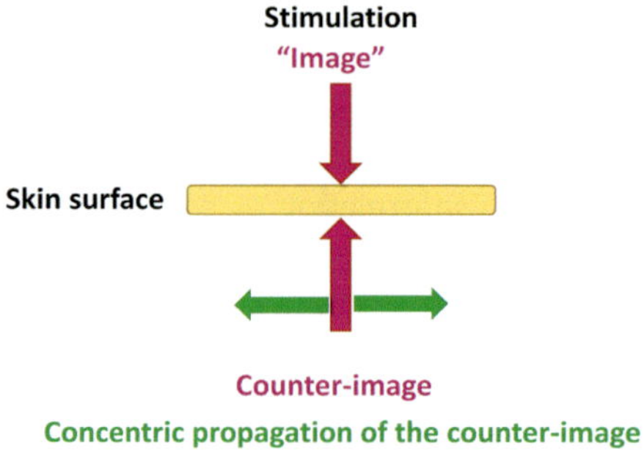


**Figure 17.2** Counter-image induced by punctual stimulation of the skin.

The **double-impact** technique (**Figure 17.3**) consists of a double stimulation. At time **T1**, a brief initial stimulation S1 applied at point A triggers a counter-image (in green on the diagram), which will propagate. At time **T2**, there follows a second stimulation **S2** at point **B**, located a few centimetres away from point **A**, which will induce the propagation of a second counter-image.

The two stimuli must be given with a time lag of approximately a quarter of a second between the two stimulations, **S1** and **S2**, to the effect that the counter-image triggered by **S1** will collide with the counter-image initiated by **S2**, *before the time at which the counter-image triggered by **S1** would have reached point **B***. The idea of a brief time interval is to bring the two counter-images *to* collide. *This collision will cause a strong, single RAC* called a ***rebound***. If the time interval between S1 and S2 is too long, the second impact **S2** at point **B** will occur after the first counter-image has already overtaken point **B**. In this case, there will be no collision of counter-images and no rebound pulse response.

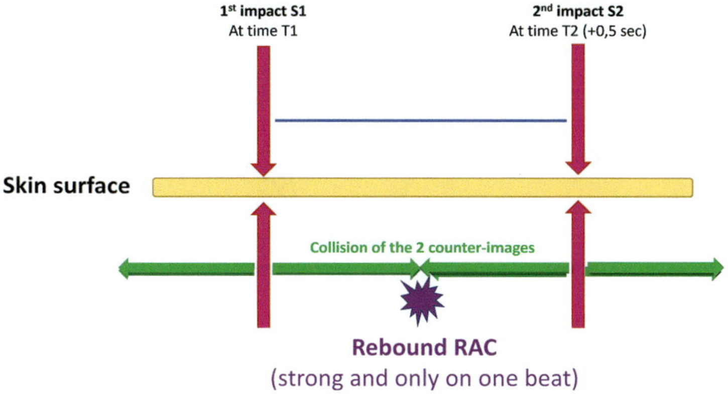


**Figure 17.3** Rebound caused by the collision between two counter-images.

Thus, the *normal* reaction to a double impact is limited to one strong rebound. If the rebound is weak or absent, this will indicate *reduced* or *blocked* information transfers between points A and B. Usually, the rebound reaction is immediate, but it may sometimes occur after two or three beats, especially if the patient is exhausted or even just tired.

Because it carries a somatotopic representation of the whole body, the auricle is a privileged location for checking the quality of transfers and correcting them when disturbed. Theoretically, a double impact can be applied to any part of the ear. However, we will now see that transfers are, to a large extent, related to the notion of ***ear borders***.

## 17.3 EAR BORDERS

Borders are mostly located on linear regions of the ear, defined by anatomical reliefs that mark a morphological separation between two regions. Paul Nogier described several borders, the most important of which are the following (**Figure 17.4**):

- *The helix's root and ascending branch* divide the auricle into upper and lower halves.

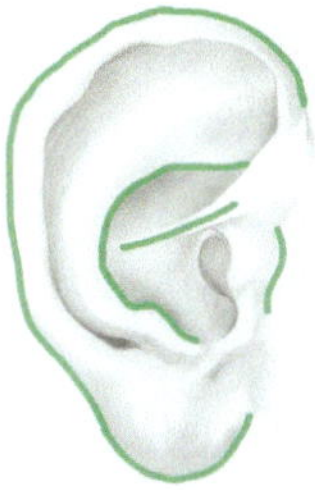

**Figure 17.4** General view of the main borders on the auricle.

- *The rim of the helix* defines the border separating the external and mastoid aspects of the ear as a whole.
- *The anthelical parapet* can be compared to the top of a cliff and marks the limit between the anthelix surface on the upper side and the vertical part known as the wall, leading to the concha on the lower side.
- The external aspect of the tragus is separated (*a*) from its internal aspect by the well-defined *posterior rim* (not marked on the figure) and (b) anteriorly from the pre-tragal region and the cheek by *an anterior groove,* sometimes not very clearly defined.

Functionally, borders have the property of *influencing the passage of transfers that cross them* by enhancing or impairing them. Thus:

- Transfers *between the upper and lower parts of the auricle* (on the external or mastoid aspects of the auricle) depend on the border located on the root and ascending branch of the helix (**Figure 17.5**).

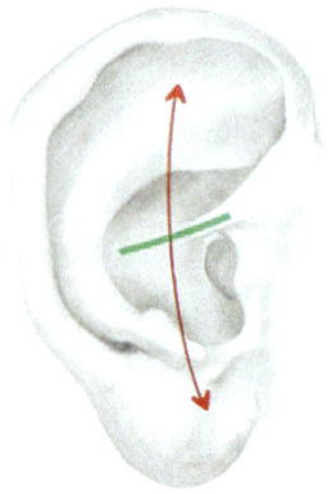

**Figure 17.5** Border between the upper and lower parts of the ear.

- *Transfers between the external and mastoid aspects of the ear* depend on the border of the helix (**Figure 17.6**).

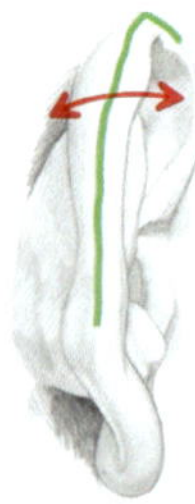

**Figure 17.6** Border between external and mastoid aspects of the auricle.

- *Transfers between anthelix and concha* depend on the border situated on the anthelical parapet (**Figure 17.7**).

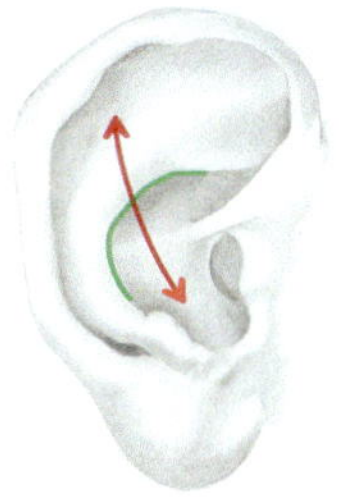

**Figure 17.7** Border between anthelix and concha.

- *Transfers between the concha and the pre-tragal* region depend on the border located on the anterior limit of the external tragus (**Figure 17.8**).

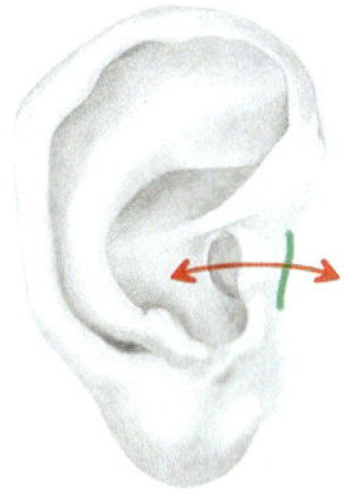

**Figure 17.8** Border between concha and the pre-tragal region.

## 17.4 TREATMENT OF A BLOCKED EAR TRANSFER

The functional properties of borders can offer a therapeutic lever for restoring impaired transfers. When a rebound is not obtained following a double impact, one can proceed by searching with a *black rod* for a "black point" located on the corresponding border, particularly at both ends. Incidentally, an epiphysis point (pineal gland) may also influence an impaired transfer, and so be detected. These so-called "black" points can either be treated directly with an extemporaneous needle or be the subject of further analysis with other techniques.

## 17.5 TRANSFERS BETWEEN THE EAR AND THE SOMA

These transfers involve the *periauricular border* (**Figure 17.9**), which limits the auricle as a whole from the neighbouring regions (cheek, skull). If a particular area of the auricle does not respond to centripetal (from cheek to ear) and centrifugal (from ear to cheek) double impacts, this region is referred to as an "**excluded zone**".

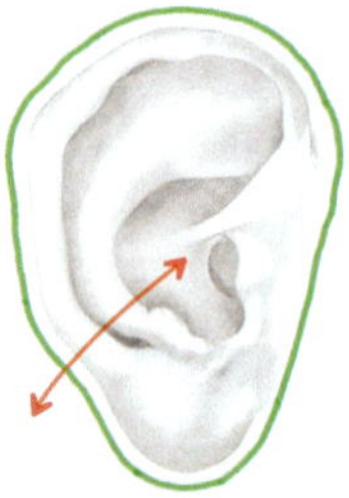

**Figure 17.9** Periauricular border, separating ear, and soma.

Such pathological areas can be examined and treated on the ear with appropriate techniques, generally colours and frequencies (see Chapters 18, 20, and 21).

Double impacts across the periauricular border, comparing between centrifugal transfers and centripetal transfers, can also be applied to a somewhat more whimsical type of test: when a centrifugal double impact produces a rebound stronger than the centripetal double impact, this can indicate that the patient has an outgoing type of temperament, whereas the opposite is rather suggestive of an introverted character.

## 17.6 PERIPHERAL TRANSFERS

Finally, transfers can also be tested between two regions of the body. They do not concern the auricle nor imply a notion of borders. They are of lesser importance than transfers on the ear. Referred to as peripheral transfers, they are mainly used for testing chemical substances:

- In the case of a *pharmaceutical drug*, a double impact with a test ring containing the drug can be applied, for example, from arm to forearm. The quality or intensity of the resulting rebound will indicate whether the chemical information conveyed by the drug is satisfactorily distributed throughout the organism. This test can be used in addition to the classical technique for testing drugs, described in Chapter 23.

Similarly, a double impact can be elicited on the forehead, from one side to the other, with a test ring containing a *neurotransmitter*. The resulting rebound may contribute to assessing the dynamics of the neurotransmitter within the central nervous system in relation to a clinical situation.

## 17.7 CONCLUSION

Among many other factors, the state of good health of a living organism depends on the integrity of the countless networks of exchanges of information that are active within. Pathological conditions are often accompanied by impairments within these systems. Thus, the RAC provides a possibility to globally assess such disorders on the auricle and improve them when they are disturbed.

## PROTOCOL 1: RAC CALIBRATION AND BASIC TECHNIQUES

*To summarize the description of signal medicine techniques, we include a few simple protocols in some of the following chapters, for the purpose of assisting the examiner in the practical application and integration of these techniques. This is the first.*

### Preliminaries

- Standard clinical examination (Chapter 13.1)
- Adequate positioning of patient and examiner (Chapter 4.1)

### Evaluation of the quality of the RAC

- Evaluation of **the resting pulse** (Chapter 13.1). Compare left and right radial pulses (**Figure 9.6**)
- Evaluation **of the RAC** (Sections 13.1–13.3). Triggering a RAC can be done (Section 13.2):
    - ***Either*** by placing a double polaroid test ring on the patient's chest.
    - ***Or*** by approaching a white test ring in line with the ear and measuring the reactive distance.

Normal distance: 8–10 cm. The white test ring technique gives the possibility of (Section 13.5):

1. **Calibrating** the RAC
2. Assessing the patient's **general state of vitality**
3. Assessing the patient's **capacity to cope with an overload** (of stress)
4. Detecting **oscillations**: if the distance varies. If present, treat by solar plexus point bilaterally (needle or cryotherapy)

**Basic techniques** – to give an initial idea of the patient's vitality and general reactivity:

- Check for **RAC exhaustion** and if present, search for pathological scars/dental foci (Chapter 10).
- Check the **neurovegetative formula** (Section 13.6). If necessary, correct it.
- Evaluate **transfers of information** on the auricle (Chapter 17).
- Check the **middle-level beat** (Section 16.3). If weak, no direct treatment. Check again after having treated other parameters.

Search for a **detectable point(s) on the auricle** (Chapter 14) and measure its quality (Chapter 15). Depending on the clinical conditions, ***either*** *treat directly* with needle (extemporary or semi-permanent) or cryotherapy, ***or*** *proceed with further analysis* of the point, e.g. with colour or frequential techniques.

## BIBLIOGRAPHY

1. Nogier Paul. *From* Auriculotherapy *to Auriculomedicine* (Maisonneuve) 1981, 165
2. Rouxeville Yves. *Personalized Auricular Acupuncture* (Sauramps Médical) 2000, 158

CHAPTER 18

# Techniques Using Colour Stimuli

**Anthony de Sousa**

## 18.1 INTRODUCTION

Stimulation of the skin with colours, using filters and lamps, is an important part of pulse-assisted auriculotherapy. It is one of many possibilities of interacting with the body by way of the skin to measure the patient's reactivity and pathological features.

The instrumental aspect has been introduced in Chapter 12. Research with coloured gelatines had shown, according to Paul Nogier, that "not only does the skin perceive colours, but it can, in certain cases, analyse their spectral components" [3]. Coloured gelatines induce a pulse reaction according to their resonance with a function, organ, or system. When the skin is exposed to a colour filter (**Figure 18.1**), it induces *photo-emission*, whereas the same colour projected using a colour lamp (**Figure 18.2**) is more powerful and gives rise to *photoreception*. In this regard, it should be noted that a colour will not necessarily produce the same pulse reaction, depending on whether it is incorporated into a filter or a lamp, even though it has a similar significance in both cases.

To the naked eye, it may sometimes appear that two gelatines are virtually identical in colour, even though their absorption spectra and pulse resonances may be very different.

We can assume that the action of a coloured gelatine on the skin involves two different mechanisms [1, 2]. In the case of a coloured filter, some of the photons emitted by the skin will cross the filter barrier and move away, while others, not unlike a radar, will be reflected back to the skin, which will also be the case for the opaque type of test rings. In the case of a lamp on the other hand, the photons projected by the lamp will pass through the gelatine in the reverse direction and be absorbed by the skin.

Some filters are designed to contain several colours, either superimposed or juxtaposed, and are named *composite* filters. An example is the *seven colours* filter, also called the *colour programme*, visible in the central part of **Figure 18.1**.

## 18.2 THE MOST OFTEN USED COLOURS AND THEIR INTERPRETATION

The colours in *filters* and *lamps* offer a wide range of resonance categories. Discovered on an empirical basis, these categories include a variety of systems,

DOI: 10.1201/9781003753629-18

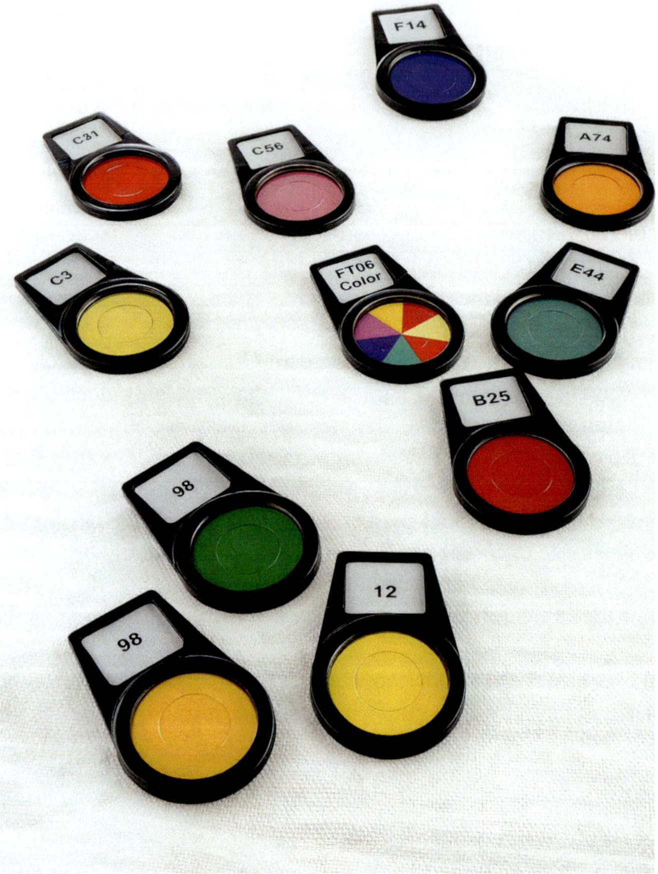


**Figure 18.1** Colour filters.

organs, functions, and pathologies. Colours can help detect an ear point, assess the appropriateness of treating it, or measure the beneficial or toxic nature of a chemical substance. Examples of the most widely used resonance categories are listed below.

The ***seven colours of the colour programme (CP)*** (**Figure 18.1**) are named, respectively, A, B, C, D, E, F, and G, similarly to the designation of fundamental frequencies (Chapters 20 and 21) with which they share the main significances. The colour programme includes the following filters:

**Colour A (Wratten Kodak orange 22 or 21)** has a general significance of toxicity or what is undesirable for the organism. Paul Nogier used to

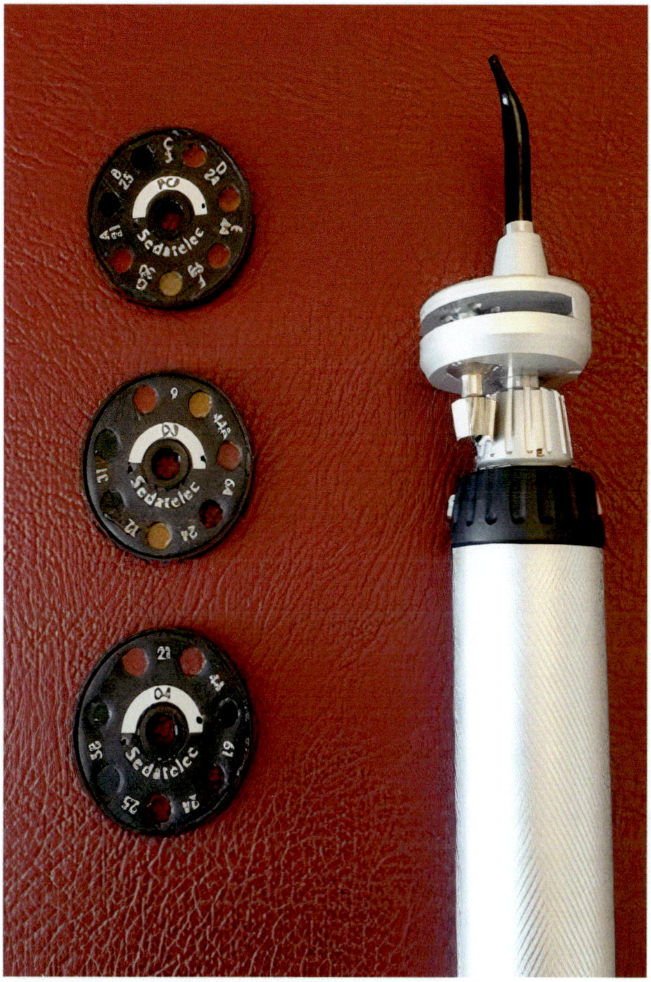


**Figure 18.2** Colour lamp.

describe this as *anti-biotic*. Amongst others, this property is used to evaluate a substance, medicine or drug (see Chapter 23).

**Colour B (WK red 25)** resonates with organs or functions of *endodermal origin*, especially the digestive and respiratory systems, mostly located in both sections of the concha. It resonates with the *parasympathetic* system and is also one of the two colours expressing *phase 1* (Chapter 19), the other being **red 29**.

**Colour C (WK yellow 4)** is related to structures of *mesodermal* origin, i.e. musculoskeletal, which are mainly located on the *anthelix*. It also resonates with *organs* of mesodermal origin, i.e. the circulatory and renal systems.

**Colour D (WK red 23A)** is related to symmetry, commissural structures, and interhemispheric communication. It also refers to movement with displacement.

**Colour E(WK blue 44)** is related to longitudinal nerve structures (spinal cord, peripheral nerves). It is also used to evaluate a substance, signifying a beneficial effect, designated by Paul Nogier as *biotic* (as opposed to colour **Orange 21/22**—see Chapter 23). In addition, this colour expresses *phase 3* (Chapter 19).

**Colour F (WK blue-violet 98)** resonates with diencephalic subcortical structures, the limbic system, emotions and personal interactions.

**Colour G (WK red 30)** evokes the cortico-frontal regions, the higher cortical functions, conscious and unconscious, and the endocrine system.

The **Star** filter, or **CP filter** (at the centre of **Figure 18.1**), combines all the individual gelatines of the colour programme. The juxtaposition of these seven specific colours has a particular significance, having the property of "summing up" the activity of the organism as a whole. Therefore, imposing it on the skin surface of the anterior chest has the effect of stressing the organism (in terms of micro-information) by creating an overload, to which the organism is forced to adapt. In practice, this makes it possible to assess the organism's ability to absorb an overload (see Chapter 13).

## 18.3 VARIOUS OTHER COLOURS

### 18.3.1 Colours Related to the Autonomous System

**WK red 24** is frequently used in disorders of the autonomic system. For example, if filter **red 24** induces a reaction when approaching the axis of the ear, only on one side and not on the other, this may suggest a neuro-vegetative *inversion* (**Figure 13.5**), a blockage on the sympathetic ganglion chain (mainly implying the sympathetic master point, the marvellous point, the stellar ganglion point, the cosmonaut point, an osteopathic blockage of the first rib or a disorder related to the perivisceral plexi.

**WK cyan Blue 65A** is less commonly used; it reacts to a neurovegetative *dissociation*, an abnormally high reaction of the number of RACs to **noradrenaline** placed on the arm (4–5 RACs or more), accompanied by an equally high number of RACs to **acetylcholine** placed on the chest. Paul Nogier suspected this as entailing a suspicion of a cancerous condition.

### 18.3.2 Colours Related to the Cerebrospinal Nervous System

**WK green 58** reacts in a variety of situations involving structures or functions of the central nervous system, particularly in connection with brain asymmetry and laterality and also to functions of the endocrine system. This colour was not originally a part of the colour programme but has been added more recently since it is related to the auricular area responding to the L territory, located just in front of the D territory on the anterior part of the tragus (**Figures 26.11** and **26.12**). Furthermore, Green 58 is the expression of phase 2 (Chapter 19).

**WK yellow 9** is often involved with hyperreactivity of the central nervous system, accompanied by a lowering of the response threshold, either of endogenous or circumstantial origin. Often associated with what the French call a state of spasmophilia-tetany, in fact, this colour expresses nervous hypersensitivities in a more general way, whatever the anatomical structure(s) involved. When treating these hypersensitivity situations, one should be cautious by limiting the number of points treated to avoid a significant aggravation.

**WK yellow 12** reacts to situations of hypersensitivity towards pain or depressive states, generally implying detection of a thalamus point on the antitragal wall. It is also used to select one of the three phases in the ear (Chapter 19).

**WK yellow 15** is usually associated with rhythmic or periodic phenomena (normal or pathological) and often leads to detection of an epiphysis point.

**WK blue 99**, either single or as part of a composite filter **red 31** / **green 58** / **blue 99**, is used in many rhythmical problems, especially in sleep disorders. Imposing these colours induces a sleep-like state (not clinically but in micro-information), which is useful for detecting the appropriate points.

In this respect, mention can also be made of **WK blue 44A**, related to slow-wave sleep phases, and **WK blue 49B**, associated with REM phases.

## 18.4 MEASUREMENT AND PROCESSING TECHNIQUES USING COLOURS

### 18.4.1 Basic Technique Using a Colour Filter

Handling an individual colour filter at the ear is a simple, standard technique consisting of the following stages:

1. ***Approach the filter*** from 10 to 12 cm in line towards the ear (**Figure 12.13**). First, at approximately 6-8 cm, but mainly when the filter ***touches*** the ear by double contact, the normal reaction should not exceed one or two RACs (See "Assessing a TR on the Ear: Three Basic Techniques" in Chapter 12). Three or more RACs indicate a pathological reaction to the element represented by the colour. The number of RACs indicates the importance of the pathology.

2. Impose the filter: If the pulse response is normal, the filter need not be tested further. If, on the other hand, the ***reaction*** exceeds 2 RACs, then proceed to impose the filter by placing it (at inspiration) on the chest if the filter belongs to the colour programme, or on the arm for any other colour filter (see Protocol 2 in Chapter 18, Section 18.6).

   ***Notes***:
   - *As far as the seven filters of the colour programme are concerned, and only these, the rule for imposing them on the arm or the thorax is reversed: to enhance a filter's expression, it must be placed not on the arm but on the thorax, and if on the contrary one wishes to slow down or inhibit its expression, the filter must be placed on the arm.*
   - *Generally speaking, however, a more dynamic way of selecting whether to impose a filter on the arm or chest consists of testing the filter by briefly (for a half second) placing it first on the arm and then on the thorax and comparing the two resulting RAC responses. The filter will then be imposed at the site (arm or chest) where it has induced the strongest RAC (qualitatively, i.e. it is not necessary to count the RACs.*
   - *Testing* a filter, as described above, by *approach and touch* naturally *requires a RAC response.* On the other hand, *imposing* the filter on the arm or chest merely implies selecting a piece of specific information and *does not involve a vascular response.* It should also be remembered here that after approximately one minute, the information disappears, so the filter must be re-imposed.

3. ***Scan the ear***: in the presence of the filter which has been imposed, scan through the ***entire*** ear (**Figures 14.1–14.3**), either with a white tip or more specifically with a colour lamp bearing the same colour as the imposed filter, at a distance of about one centimetre. Search for a point induced by the imposed filter, meaning that the point would not have been detectable when scanning on an "empty ear", i.e. without any filter imposition.
4. ***Treat the point***: Once identified, the ear point can be treated directly, by needling, by cryotherapy or by massaging the point with a special glass rod.
5. ***Check*** that the filter's ***reaction*** at the ear has disappeared after treating the point. If this is not the case, the filter can be reimposed to find a second ear point.

The filter to be tested is often *chosen* by the practitioner for its likely relationship with the clinical aspects (e.g. choosing colour filter **C4** in the presence of osteo-arthritic problems to select ear points more specifically related to this type of pathology).

### 18.4.2 Sequential Techniques

In our practices, however, a high proportion of patients who wish to be treated by techniques such as signal medicine suffer from chronic pathologies. These are often complex, characterised by a combination of multiple causes and effects that have added up over a lifetime and compensate each other to ensure adaptation and homeostasis. While exploring these pathological networks with the pulse, Paul Nogier developed a category of techniques called *sequential*. Three examples will be described here: the *random sequence*, the **red 24** *sequence*, and the *colour programme sequence*.

#### *18.4.2.1 The Random Sequence*

Regardless of the clinical picture, the filter may simply be one of several filters chosen randomly for screening. The filter producing the strongest response with the RAC (the highest number of RACs) will then be imposed to detect one or more ear points related to the imposed filter.

After treating these points, test the remaining filters, select the most reactive one, impose it, treat the corresponding ear points, and so on at each level, until all the filters have been tested.

#### *18.4.2.2 The Red 24 Sequence*

As we have seen, the colour filter Wratten Kodak **red 24** is linked to disorders of the neurovegetative system that frequently occur. For this reason, it can be used according to a repetitive sequential technique, using the same filter at each level. To do this, using both the filter **24** and the red colour lamp **24**, we will proceed as follows:

**First level**: The **red 24** filter is tested using the above standard technique. If the colour does not react beyond one to two RACs, there will be no sequence. If, on the other hand, three or more RACs occur, then the filter **red 24** will be imposed (at inspiration) on the patient's arm to detect the *first point* related to the colour. The point will then be treated, preferably by an extemporaneous needle or by massaging with a glass rod. The duration of insertion of an extemporaneous (traditional needle used, e.g. in Chinese acupuncture) can vary from the remainder of the treatment session down to taking it out immediately upon insertion. Paul Nogier taught that it is also possible to do it while having the patient hold his breath, which makes the needle action more powerful.

**Second level:** treating the first point will induce another point reacting to the same colour, **red 24**. So, one will test the same filter **red 24** once again on the ear, and if it reacts, impose it again on the arm, looking for a *second point*, which will be treated in the same way.

**Following levels:** This same sequence will continue until double contact of the **red 24** on the ear no longer gives a reaction. In most cases, two to four successive levels can be found before reaching this last point, considered the "*causal point*". It can be treated with a semi-permanent needle. Thus, this point is reached when the last and all previous levels have been treated, using the selected set of filters.

## 18.5 EXAMPLE OF RED 24 SEQUENCE IN A FUNCTIONAL DISORDER

A 62-year-old female patient in satisfactory general health was suffering from nausea and irritability, with a feeling of pain in her stomach and oppression in the chest. She was exposed to intense professional stress.

Classical examination shows nothing. Nor does an "empty" scan of the ear (without the imposition of a test ring), but a reaction of six RACs appears on testing the filter **red 24** at the ear (approach and touch) (**Figure 18.3**). When imposed on the arm, this filter then reveals a *liver–gallbladder poin*t on the right ear, probably in connection with nausea (first level). After treating this point using an extemporaneous needle, filter **red 24** reacts again at the ear, and its imposition on the arm induces a *solar plexus* point (second level), possibly in connection with the sensation of stomach pain and thoracic oppression. In the same way, an *aggressivity point* appears (third level), corresponding to irritability. This point can be considered as the causal element of an episode of somatisation because after treatment of this point, filter **red 24** no longer reacts at the ear, and the patient feels more relaxed.

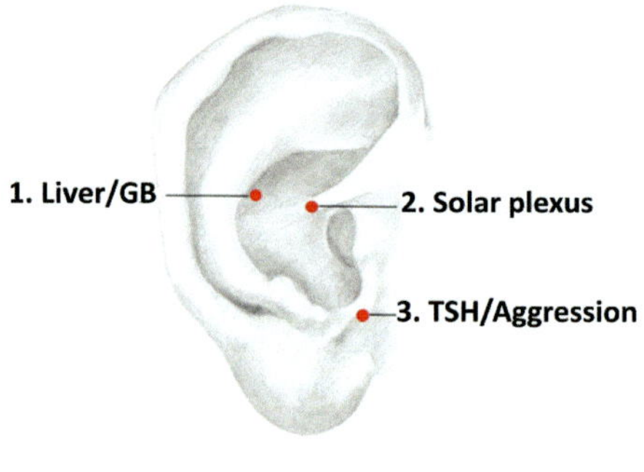


**Figure 18.3** Example of a three-level red 24 sequence.

### 18.5.1 The Colour Programme (CP) Sequence

Whereas the **red 24** sequence tests the same colour at each stage, the **colour programme** sequence involves all seven colours of the CP. One proceeds as follows:

- **First level**: Each of the seven filters of the CP is tested by approaching and double contact on the ear, in random order, to select the colour that reacts with the highest number of RACs.

  This colour filter is then ***imposed*** (at inspiration) on the chest to scan both ears with the white rod or Heine's lamp in search of a reactive point. This first point can be ***treated*** either with an extemporaneous needle or by massage with a glass rod. Then, the imposed colour filter should be tested again on the ear to ensure it no longer reacts. If, however, it still reacts, then another point should be searched for. If it no longer responds, one can proceed to the second level.

- **Second level**: the remaining six filters will all be tested on the ear in the same way, to select the filter causing the most reactive RAC, impose it on the chest, and look for a *second level point* by scanning both ears. This point will also be treated with an extemporaneous needle or by massage with the glass rod.

The **following intermediary levels** will be explored similarly, trying out the remaining filters. Each level appears after having treated the previous level. The process is repeated until the last colour tested at the ear has led to detection of what is referred to as the "**endpoint**" or "**causal point**". Considered the most important, this last point will be able to produce a therapeutic impact on all the preceding points. It is therefore treated either by a semi-permanent needle, cryotherapy or, more specifically, by a sequence of seven fundamental frequencies at "therapeutic" intensity (as provided on the frequency generators described in Chapter 12). In most cases, a sequence will show between two and four levels. The sequence can be interpreted as "witnessing" the series of adaptations the organism has faced over the period a chronic disease or impairment has lasted.

## 18.6 EXAMPLE OF A COLOUR PROGRAMME SEQUENCE

Three weeks prior to consultation, a 53-year-old female patient had undergone the last of three surgical interventions for perforated colonic diverticulitis. The operations had proved difficult due to complications with bleeding and resistant abdominal pain. On the day of the consultation, the pain was improving, but she reported feeling exhausted and depressed.

Testing the seven-colour programme (CP) filters at the ear (approaching and double contact), came out with four levels (**Figure 18.4**):

- ***First level***: reaction at the ear, with Wratten Kodak **G 30 red filter,** which, after being imposed on the chest, produces an **ACTH point** at the ear, probably due to the intense stress experienced by the patient during this period. The point is treated with an extemporaneous needle.
- ***Second level***: consists of a reaction at the ear of **B 25 red filter**. Imposing it on the chest reveals a bilateral ***sensory colon point***, probably related to the abdominal pain.
- ***Third level***: reaction to **D 23A red filter**, which induces an ear point on the pre-tragal region, representing the **anterior white commissure**, which

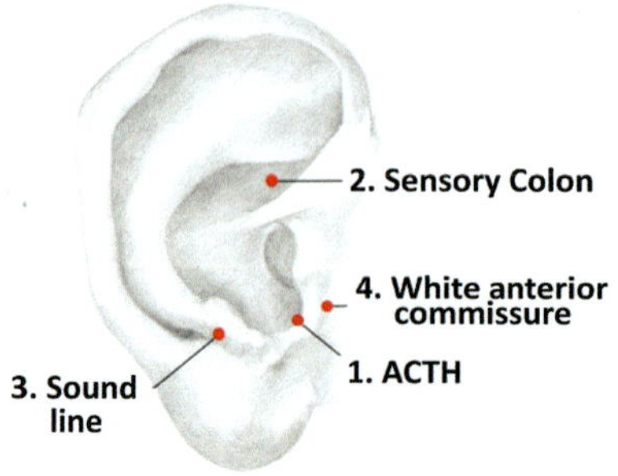


**Figure 18.4** Example of a four-level colour programme sequence.

connects the right and left parts of the limbic system and is involved in deep emotional reactions.

- ***Fourth level***: reaction to **F 98 purple filter**, which reveals a point on the **sound line**. As no other CP filter reacts, this point is considered the **endpoint**.

*Interpretation*: Whereas the first two levels were related to the aspects of stress and pain due to the diverticulitis and the surgery, the last two levels can be seen as a psychosomatic participation concerning a difficult spouse relationship, which the patient had experienced during several years with grief and feelings of abandonment.

## 18.7 TECHNIQUE FOR COUPLING BETWEEN EAR AND PERIPHERY

When a filter belonging to the colour programme reacts at the ear, i.e. produces more than 2 RACs (normally, a colour filter should not cause a reaction on approaching and contact at the ear), the same colour filter can then be scanned over a peripheral region chosen according to the clinical problem and the significance of that colour.

For example, in the case of a digestive disorder, if a reaction with the **red 25** filter (a colour known to resonate with the digestive system) is obtained on approach and contact with the ear, it is then possible to scan this **red 25** filter over the abdomen at a distance of approximately one centimetre. This will probably produce a reaction over the skin projection of a diseased organ. Conversely, imposing the **red 25** filter on the reactive part of the abdomen will likely facilitate detection (with the white rod or the **red 25** lamp) of an ear point related to the clinical problem, which can then be treated.

## 18.8 COMMENTS

- Whereas it may be interesting to know the meaning of each intermediate point found during the course of a sequence, this is by no means compulsory. It is sufficient to simply follow the dynamics of the functional and organic disorders accumulated with time, and having led to the endpoint, the identity of which is more important to discover.
- The term "causal" is not to be interpreted in a strictly mechanistic sense. The elements of these sequences should rather be understood as a biological link between a wide scope of adaptive responses throughout time.
- A general remark concerning examination using the vascular signal: after a sequence has been treated, it can be of interest to return to some of the "witness" parameters measured at the beginning of the examination, such as the reactive distance at the ear, the resistance to overload (Chapter 13), or the middle-level beat (Chapter 16). If they initially were pathological, it is helpful to determine whether these control parameters have recovered due to the sequential treatment. It will often be the case.
- By and large, sequential techniques with colour filters provide a simple and elegant method for "untangling" the web of disorders that have accumulated over time and influence each other within an organism that is constantly seeking to adapt.
- **Nota Bene**: Colour filters were first manufactured by **Wratten Kodak** (WK) Company, for the use of photography and theatre lighting. A completely different use arose by chance, when Paul Nogier discovered that, analysed with RAC techniques, many of these colour filters unexpectedly demonstrated resonating properties with biological functions or parameters. For example, filter WK red 25 has resonating properties with endodermic organs and tissues.
- Unfortunately, Wratten Kokak has drastically slowed down or stopped its production of colour filters, because of lack of demand for its initial applications. The Sedatelec company in Lyon, France, still provides colour filters, but they are obliged to find them with a different manufacturer, called **Lee**.
- **Lee** uses another nomenclature (e.g. Lee 204) and the filters are not produced with the same exact spectrum but for all filters mentioned in the book there are corresponding Lee filters. Since the original research was made using the WK filters, we use WK filter numbers in the book.
- Information can be obtained from Sedatelec, as to the latest updated correspondences between Wratten Kodak and Lee filters, from the point of view of their significances when using the arterial reflex.

## PROTOCOL 2: COLOUR FILTERS

*The content of the techniques and tests, and the order in which they are applied, is suggested as a guideline and can be adapted to each clinical situation.*

*The term "control parameters" refers to elements that are not subject to direct treatment or correction. Their evolution is to be reassessed after treatment with other techniques.*

### Preliminaries

- Positioning of a finger over the pulse and assessment of the resting pulse
- **RAC calibration** (see Chapter 13)
- **Searching for RAC exhaustion** (see Chapter 10)
- Checking the **neurovegetative formula** (see "The Two Territories for Imposition of test rings: The Neurovegetative Formula" in Chapter 13)
- Assessment of the **middle-level beat** (see Chapter 16)
- **Scan the entire ear** without any imposition using a white rod or Heine's lamp. Note the detected points without treating them directly, so that they can be compared with points revealed later by imposing colour filters

### Diagnosis and Treatment Using Colour Filters

Review the set of colour filters chosen to be tested using **on approach and double ear contact** and note those that respond with 3 or more positive RACs.

- If the clinical problem is simple, choose an appropriate colour filter, impose it and then search for an ear point that was not there when scanning without any imposition. Consider testing the "quality" of the detected point to evaluate whether or not it is favourable to be treated (see **Table 15.1**).

- If the problem is more complex or chronic, choose a sequential technique:

  - **Red 24 -sequence**
  - **Colour programme sequence**

- Possibly apply an ear–periphery **coupling** technique (see Section 18.7 above).

## BIBLIOGRAPHY

1. Ackermann John. Human biophoton emission and VAS. Annals of GLEM 2006–2007
2. Bourdiol René. L'Auriculo-somatologie (Maisonneuve) 1981; 155–160
3. Nogier Paul. From Auriculotherapy to Auriculomedicine, (Maisonneuve) 1981, 133–182
4. Nogier Paul. Utilisation des couleurs en auriculomédecine, Revue Auriculomédecine (Maisonneuve) 1977, 41–43
5. Rouxeville Yves. L'acupuncture auriculaire personnalisée (Sauramps médical), 2000, 111–118

CHAPTER 19

# Overview of the Concept of Phases

**Anthony de Sousa**

Phases are a complex subject, the many aspects of which witness the evolution auriculotherapy has undergone from the early days of the discovery of ear mapping to the gradual build-up of signal medicine that we know of today and the possibility of measuring parameters with the RAC.

## 19.1 PHASES AS RELATED TO MAPPING VARIANTS

Shortly after his discovery of auricular mapping in 1951, we know that Paul Nogier was puzzled when faced with certain inconsistencies between the original maps he had found and other mapping systems that had been elaborated after him by other researchers, particularly the Chinese. Eventually, he thought of a hypothesis based on the embryological origins of each organ or function. He imagined that the ear could be capable of displaying not only one, but in fact, three distinct mapping systems, which he named phase 1, phase 2 and phase 3. Nogier divided the auricle into three territories (basically anthelix, concha, and lobule) with their respective innervations (the third branch of the trigeminal nerve, vagus nerve, and C2). Each localisation was "placed" within one of the three territories according to its embryological origin, and with a dynamic permutation mechanism in which each of the three ecto-, meso-, and endo-leaflets would shift to a different territory within each one of the three phases (**Figure 19.1**).

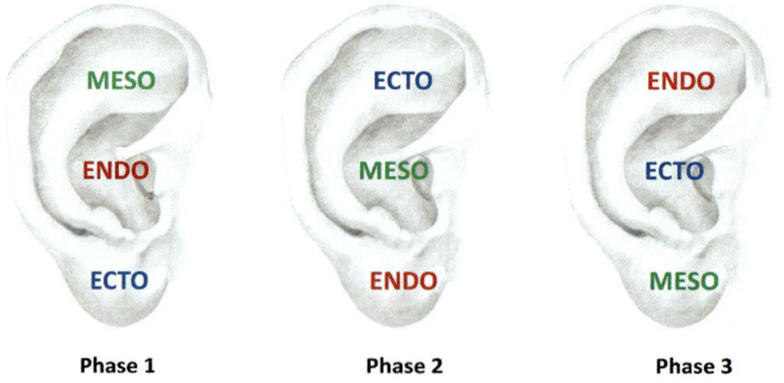


**Figure 19.1** The three phases: distribution of locations in the three territories, according to their embryological origin.


DOI: 10.1201/9781003753629-19

This concept had two logical implications [5]. First, an ear point would bear a correspondence with three distinct organs, each one having a different embryological origin. Second, any somatic structure could potentially have three representations on the ear, one in each territory.

### 19.1.1 Interpretation

The notion of phases is in accordance with the findings that the ear-mapping is not only engraved in the histological architecture of the skin. The auricle can also be considered like a computer screen, capable of virtually displaying different mapping systems, depending on the levels of integration of information reaching the central nervous system. In 2002, phases were defined by a working group [1] *as transient neurological representations of the body on the ear, resulting from the integrative response of the brain to information, both environmental and due to physiological or pathological conditions.*

Within approximately 85% of healthy individuals, *mapping in the central nervous system functions according to the S1 somatotopic* representation, equivalent to Penfield's homunculus. On the auricle, this configuration appears as ***phase 1***. It is the most important among the different mapping systems and prevails in normal conditions. The other two phases are examples of brain *plasticity*, capable of adapting to a functional or organic disturbance of the paths leading from the periphery to the nerve centres [2]. Thus, in the event of damage to the *thalamus*, the level of integration of information reaching the CNS would lead to displaying ***phase 2*** on the ear, whereas in the case of *medullary* disturbances, the level of integration would have ***phase 3*** appear on the auricle.

From an experimental point of view, it is of great interest to recall that Michel Marignan and William Bismuth conducted a study between 1995 and 1997 at the CNRS (French National Centre for Scientific Research) on thermography applied to the auricle. They showed that the occurrence of peripheral pain induced not only one but, in fact, three different thermographic responses located in three different territories of the auricle [4].

## 19.2 REACTIVE PROPERTIES OF PHASES

After having discovered the vascular signal, Paul Nogier extended the notion of phases, showing that, in addition to the mapping aspects, each phase was characterised by specific reactive properties which were measurable with the RAC [6]. However, as these aspects are sometimes excessively complex, we will limit our description here to an overview of the relationships between phases and colours and between phases and fundamental frequencies.

### 19.2.1 Phases and Colours

Apart from the variations in mapping, Paul Nogier empirically found that each phase had a link with a specific colour and could therefore be "identified" by its reaction to this colour. Hence:

**Phase 1** reacts to **red 25** (or to **red 29**, as shown by Bernard Julienne and Alain Mallard, close research collaborators to Paul Nogier). Phase 1 (and therefore phase 1 mapping) can be actively selected at the ear by imposing either a **red 25** or **29** filter or a **yellow 12** filter *on the arm.*

**Phase 2** reacts to **green 58**, and phase 2 mapping can be actively selected by placing either a **green 58** filter *on the arm* or a **yellow 12** filter *on the chest.*

**Phase 3** responds to **blue 44**, so phase 3 mapping can be actively selected by imposing either a **blue 44** filter on the arm, or **yellow 12** filters on both the arm and the chest. Spontaneous display of this phase does not normally appear on the ear. However, like the two other phases, it can be actively selected by placing either a **blue 44** filter on the arm or by placing two **yellow 12** filters, one on the arm and a second **yellow 12** filter on the chest.

From a theoretical standpoint, Nogier is not known to have precisely defined the physical nature of these links. Nevertheless, when using the pulse reaction, one can *identify* what phase the (left or right) **auricle** spontaneously expresses. Nogier had the view that under normal conditions, the **right ear** preferentially displays **phase 2** (and therefore phase 2 mapping) and that the **left ear** preferentially expresses **phase 1** (and therefore phase 1 mapping). This observation is mainly of experimental interest.

From a practical point of view however, depending on the clinical aspects, it may indeed be useful to actively *select* a specific phase on both the **auricles**, as previously described.

To identify the phase spontaneously expressed on each ***auricle***, one can *either* test the three phase colour **filters** one after the other, first approaching, and then touching the ear, to evaluate which one produces the greater number of RACS (3 or more), *or* project one after the other the three phase colours with a colour **lamp** on any part of the auricle.

1. Paul Nogier observed that normally the left ear spontaneously reacts to **phase 1**. In addition to the phase spontaneously expressed, the auricles can be actively selected to express a specific phase, either by imposing one of the phase filters, **25**, **29**, **58**, or **44**, on the arm or by imposing a **yellow 12** filter on the arm and/or on the chest.
2. To understand *the significance* of an ear point, it is useful to find out to which phase it belongs. This can be easily done using a colour **lamp** and projecting onto the point the three phase colours **red 25** (or **red 29**), **green 58**, and **blue 44** one after the other, and estimating which of the three colours produce the greatest number of RACs.

**Table 19.1** summarises these properties.

**Table 19.1 Colours Used for Diagnosis and Selection of the Three Phases**

| Phase | Phase colour | Imposing the phase |
|---|---|---|
| 1 | Red 25 or 29 | Red 25 or red 29 or Yellow 12 **imposed on the arm** |
| 2 | Green 58 | Green 58 **imposed on the arm** or Yellow 12 **on the chest** |
| 3 | Blue 44 | Blue 44 **imposed on the arm,** or Yellow 12 **on the arm and chest** |

A phase is considered **pathological** when more than three to four positive RACs are produced by a filter *approaching at 5–6 cm* or ear *contact* of the phase corresponding colour (**25**, **58**, or **44**). If this is the case, one can impose the filter(s) according to **Table 19.1** and search for a point on the ear to treat the pathological phase.

### 19.2.2 Phases and Frequency Sequences

Amongst various properties attributed to phases, Paul Nogier observed that *phase 1* and *phase 2 both* expressed *different frequency sequences* (*see* Chapter 21). Hence, the ***left ear*** reacts to phase 1 and to the *direct frequency sequence*, whilst the ***right ear*** responds to *phase 2 and to an indirect (or inverted) frequency sequence.*

As for *phase 3*, it does not react in the same way. When phase 3 is selected (by imposing either a **Blue 44** filter on the arm or **Yellow 12** filters on both the arm and thorax), the different areas will no longer respond to a specific sequence of frequencies. Instead, all the areas on both ears react to one specific frequency, the deviated **A+10%** (321 Hertz). It should be noted that this frequency is not pathologic. It is, in fact, the normal frequency of the middle level (see Chapter 16).

Note that when a phase is imposed, either with its own colour filter or with **Yellow 12** filter(s), then both ears will react according to the selected phase and the corresponding frequency sequence. However, the observations described in this sub-chapter are not often applied in clinical situations and are mainly of theoretical interest.

### 19.2.3 Phase Tonality

Even though each phase contains most (but not necessarily all) of the body's localisations, Paul Nogier has shown that each phase has a particular "vocation", i.e. a predominance of physiological and pathological expressions, as well as a privileged relationship with one of the three embryological layers [6]. Hence, we can speak of the tonality or vocation of a phase:

- **Phase 1** is mainly *neurovegetative* and *endodermal*
- **Phase 2** mainly expresses *cerebrospinal* and *ectodermal* aspects
- **Phase 3** is mainly *neuroendocrine* and *mesodermal*

## 19.3 CLINICAL USE OF PHASES

Let us describe two typical situations, the first related to mapping and the second to reactive properties of phases.

### 19.3.1 Determining the Phase(s) to Which a Point Belongs

As mentioned earlier, it may be of interest to find out which phase a point detected on the auricle belongs to and at the same time, its embryological origin. For this purpose, a *colour lamp* will expose the ear point successively to the three phase colours **red 25**, **green 58**, and **blue 44**, and observe which of the three colours induces the strongest RAC reaction (according to the intensity and number of RACs). Furthermore, the phase to which a point belongs gives an idea of the clinical *tonality* of the problem expressed by the point (according to Section 19.2.3, above)

In the event of a point reacting to *two or even three phases at the same time,* this single point will naturally be a clinical expression of a multiple problem, each one related to a phase and to one of the three embryological layers. Although such associations are not always significant, some of them correspond to a group of symptoms, which Paul Nogier used to call a **syndrome**. In this case, treating the point will act on all the symptoms.

**Example**

Nogier often used to mention a point located on the anterior part of the superior hemiconcha, corresponding respectively to the colon in phase 1, the shoulder in phase 2, and the prefrontal cortex in phase 3 (**Figure 19.2**). Such a point may indeed be effective against a relatively common triad consisting of irritable bowel, shoulder pain, and anxiety.

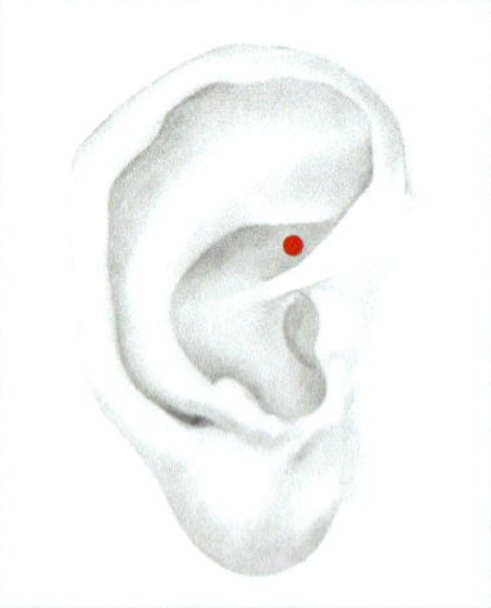

**Figure 19.2** "Syndrome" point expressing a triple clinical problem, according to the significance of the point in the three different phases, respectively.

### 19.3.2 Determining Whether One or Several Phases Are Pathological

This consists of individually testing each one of the three phase colour filters, first by approaching and then double contact touch at the ear to determine if one or several of these filters react with 3 RACs or more.

The technique for **treating a pathological phase** is simple. It consists of imposing the filter corresponding to the impaired phase on the arm (at inspiration) and then scanning the auricle with the colour lamp bearing the same colour as that of the pathological phase. This point can then be treated with an acupuncture needle or by cryotherapy. If other phase colours are found to be impaired, the same procedure will have to be applied again before checking that all the impaired phase colours have been corrected.

## 19.4 CONCLUSION

Theoretically, the meaning of concepts such as phases and localisations is probably not yet fully understood. Even at the brain level, the notion of mapping and localisations has become more relative, implying less fixity and more plasticity and consisting of loosely interconnected networks [3]. It would, therefore, hardly be surprising if the notion of auricular mapping were also to progress towards greater diversity and if the discovery of phases could contribute to opening the way towards a more dynamic understanding than the merely static representation of organs. During his research, Paul Nogier had already envisaged the possibility of making a distinction, for example, between points related to organs and others to functions, wakefulness and sleep, and between day and night. So, in the future, the concept of phases could perhaps be of use in the evolution of mapping.

## BIBLIOGRAPHY

1. Ackermann John, Franck Bryan, Marignan Michel, Nogier Raphaël. *Working group on the definition of phases*, International Symposium on Auriculotherapy, Puerto Rico, 2002
2. Alimi David. Auriculotherapy course, CMU Geneva 2005
3. Duffau Hugues. *L'erreur de Broca* (Ed. Michel Lafon) 2016
4. Marignan Michel. *Introduction to the founding principles of auricular mapping*, International Symposium on Auriculotherapy, Lyon 2021
5. Nogier Paul. *Complements of the auricular reflex points* (Maisonneuve) 1989
6. Nogier Paul. *From Auriculotherapy to Auriculomedicine* (Maisonneuve) 1981
7. VIgneron Jean-Luc. *Phases: myth or reality?* Annales du Glem, Lyon 2010–2011

## PROTOCOL 3: WORKING WITH PHASES

*The content of pulse measurements, as well as the order in which they are carried out are proposed as a guideline which is to be adapted to each clinical situation.*

### Preliminary Measures

- Positioning and assessment of **resting pulse**
- RAC **calibration** and checking for RAC **depletion**

### Use of the Mapping Aspects of Phases

- Find out to **which phase an ear point belongs** (Section 19.3.1)**, and if it turns out to be more than one phase**, **see whether the clinical situation suggests a phase syndrome**
- **Possibly assess which seems the most effective phase** for a given clinical problem in relation to phase tonality (Section 19.2.3)

### Use of the Reactive Aspects of Phases

- Search for a **pathological phase** (see Section 19.3.2 above).
- Approaching and touching the auricle with each of the colour filters corresponding to the three phases. One or several phases are pathological if they react with 3 or more RACs.

### *Comments on the use of phases:*

Diagnosing a clinical "syndrome", i.e. one ear point being active on more than one symptom, can be useful in view of limiting the number of points treated.

Using different mapping aspects of phases can provide alternatives for treatment in difficult cases.

Testing the reactive aspects of phases can give access to the patient's personal reactivity, independently of the clinical picture.

CHAPTER 20

# Introduction to Fundamental Frequencies

Anthony de Sousa

## 20.1 HISTORICAL BACKGROUND

During the seventies and eighties, continuing his work on skin *photoemission* induced by colour filters, Paul Nogier studied the vascular reactions (RAC) resulting from more powerful skin stimulation using a wide-beam lamp, thus inducing *photoreception*. From then on, he had the idea of working with *intermittent* light sources, also known as pulsed or *frequency stimulations*, using a diode connected to a frequency generator.

In the process, Nogier discovered that intermittent light stimulation of the ear could induce a vascular response, particularly when projected onto a well-defined region of the ear, which he first called a reflex area and which he defined as "*a portion of the dermis having a reactive identity to a well-defined stimulus*". The first thing he observed was that the projection of a frequency of approximately 5 Hertz onto the ear produced a RAC, the intensity of which was represented by a bell-shaped curve with a maximum amplitude appearing at 5 Hertz (**Figure 20.1**) only when the stimulation was directed onto the concha (**Figure 20.2**). When projected onto other areas of the ear, the same frequency did not produce a vascular response.

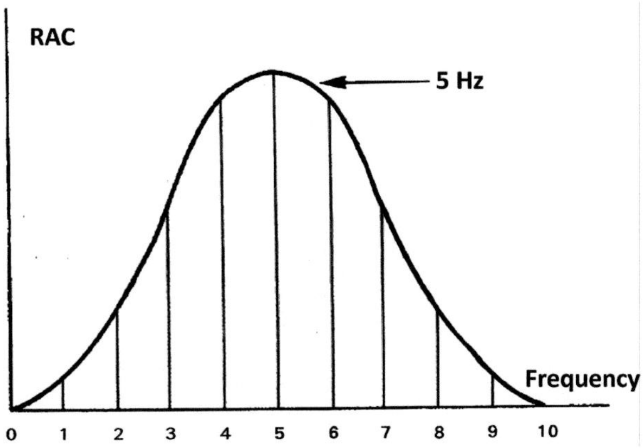


**Figure 20.1** Bell curve showing pulse resonance after stimulation of the concha with a frequency of 5 Hertz. (Copyright Raphaël Nogier.)

DOI: 10.1201/9781003753629-20

To avoid any confusion, let us remind here that an area, e.g. the whole concha (see **Figure 20.2**), is of course much larger than a single point, the diameter of which does not exceed a fraction of a millimetre.

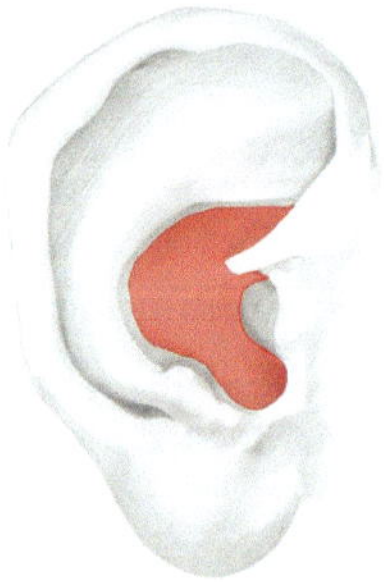

**Figure 20.2** The concha area responds to a frequency of 5 Hertz.

Nogier observed that exposure of the auricle to a continuous narrow light beam did not produce any noticeable pulse response. In contrast, the pulse reactions resulting from narrow intermittent, frequency-modulated light beams revealed homogeneous and well-defined territories (areas). According to this principle, Nogier identified at first six, then seven different frequencies capable of producing a pulse reaction when projected onto the ear, each frequency reacting on a different area. These frequencies were called *fundamental frequencies*, or *Nogier frequencies,* and each of them was identified with the same code as that of the area in which it produced a pulse response: **A**, **B**, **C**, **D**, **E**, **F**, and **G**. These seven areas are represented on **Figures 21.4–21.11**.

## 20.2 PROPERTIES AND DEFINITIONS

While studying the relationships between these different frequencies, Nogier described several aspects

- **Frequency sequence**: (not to be confused with the notion of sequential deparasitation, described in Sections 21.6.1 and 21.6.2): the fundamental frequencies form a well-defined sequence, in which each frequency has twice the value (in Hertz) of the preceding frequency and half the value of the following one. Physically, this constitutes a harmonic series. The term *frequency sequence* refers to the order in which the areas of the ear respond to the fundamental frequencies. Under normal conditions, this order can be either *basic or inverse.* If each frequency occupies the area designated by the same letter, it is said to be a *basic frequency sequence.* When this order is inverse, it is called an *inverse* or *indirect frequency sequence* (frequency-A occupies area G, frequency-B is located in area F, and so on).

- Nogier also observed that under normal conditions, a right-handed person's *left* ear showed a *basic* sequence, whereas the *right* ear had an *inverse* sequence. The therapeutic relevance has not been established, so we can simply consider that each area may normally display one of two frequencies corresponding to the basic or inverse sequences.
- **Natural frequency**: the two frequencies normally liable to react in a given ear area are called natural frequencies. Generally, an ear point will resonate preferentially with the two natural frequencies of its area.
- **Parasite frequency**: designates any frequency to which a point is liable to react other than the two natural frequencies of the area in which the point is located. This implies that the point will express the pathological significance linked to the parasite frequency. For example, a *stomach* point (situated on the left ear) will normally be expected to react with either **B**- or **F**-frequencies, the natural frequencies of the concha. If, in addition, it also reacts to **D**-frequency, this frequency is pathological and will represent a parasite frequency.
- Note that an ear point does not necessarily have to respond to a parasite frequency. Conversely, it may possibly react to several parasite frequencies at the same time.
- Parasite frequency is a widely used notion. It is as if the natural frequency were to "migrate" from its own territory to another area to which it does not usually belong, leading to a frequency parasitisation of any point located within this area. From a diagnostic point of view, we will later be describing a process called ***deparasitation***, by which it is possible to trace back to the origin of this "migration", thus being able to better understand a possible etiological relationship between different symptoms and pathologies.

### Example of a Parasite Frequency

A sore throat in children, apart from the infectious context, may at the same time be the expression of anxiety (note that the terms *anxiety* and *angina* both have the same linguistic origin) due, for example, to stress before an examination or to family tensions. When examining the ear, a throat point will generally be easy to locate (at the upper part of the inferior hemi-concha, close to the superior part of the ear duct). Using a frequency generator (**Figure 20.3**), it is possible to analyse the frequencies to which the point responds. Considering the clinical picture, it will not be surprising if, besides the natural frequencies of the concha area (either **B or F**), the point responds to a parasite G frequency, for instance. One can then trace this G-frequency back to its own specific area

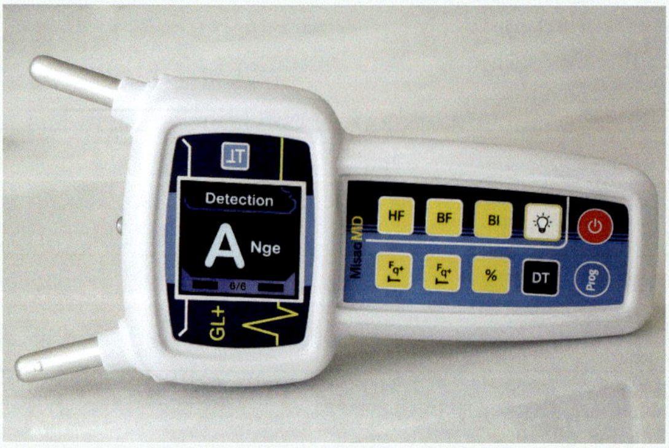


**Figure 20.3** Micropad GL+ frequency generator.

(prefrontal) and detect a relevant point in this area, responding to this same G frequency. The point expresses the etiological impact of the emotional problem. This "endpoint" will then be treated, with or without the original throat point.

- **Direct and complementary frequencies**: as described above, the fundamental frequencies form a sequence, in which each frequency has twice the value (in Hertz) of the preceding frequency, and half the value of the following one. For this reason, the seven fundamental frequencies can be represented as if they formed a symmetrical candlestick bearing seven candles. Each of the first three, referred to as the **direct** frequency, is symmetrically linked to one of the last three, called its complementary frequency:

  The complementary frequency of A is G, and vice versa
  The complementary frequency of B is F, and vice versa
  The complementary frequency of C is E, and vice versa

The **D**-frequency has no complementary frequency, being located "at the centre of the candlestick".

Direct and complementary frequencies are notions mainly used when treating an ear point with frequencies. Treatment using the complementary frequency is sometimes considered more efficient than using the direct one, whether natural or parasite.

## 20.3 PRACTICAL USE OF A FREQUENCY GENERATOR

A commonly used generator is shown in **Figure 20.3**. Micropad's GL+ is a frequency generator, allowing the selection of a light beam intensity for either diagnosis or treatment.

Whether they operate with visible, infrared, or laser light, frequency generators can emit at two different intensities. Low intensity is used for *detection*, referred to as "**diagnostic mode**", and high intensity is applied to *treatment*, called "**therapeutic mode**".

**In diagnostic mode**, there are two distinct types of use:

- **Scanning the ear surface with one selected frequency** at a distance of about one centimetre from the skin, searching for a point responding to this frequency by an RAC.
- **Examination of a point which has already been located to** determine the frequency to which this point reacts. Practically, the tip of the generator is placed in contact with the point, exposing it to all seven frequencies one after the other (scrolling) and finding which one produces a RAC. The point is said to "respond" to one or several frequencies.

In both cases, the response is based on the qualitative intensity of the vascular response (RAC) but can be more accurately measured by counting the number of RACs. A reaction is considered significant if at least 3–4 RACs are produced.

## BIBLIOGRAPHY

1. Nogier Paul. *From Auriculotherapy to Auriculomedicine* (Maisonneuve) 1981; 155–165
2. Rouxeville Yves. *Auricular acupuncture* (Sauramps Médical) 2000; 119–143

CHAPTER 21

# Areas of the Ear and Fundamental Frequencies

**Anthony de Sousa**

## 21.1 INTRODUCTION

From the notions we have of general auriculotherapy (without using the pulse), we are already familiar with the fact that the ear can be divided into different territories, representing at the same time the *innervations* of the ear and the *embryological origins* of the structures and organs represented.

As described in the previous chapter, the research undertaken by Paul Nogier on stimulation of the ear by intermittent or pulsating light sources (loosely referred to as "frequencies"), led him to discover a remarkable fact, that specific areas of the ear responded (by a RAC reaction) to each of these different *frequencies*, and according to the same distribution as that representing the different *embryological origins and innervations* of the ear.

After initially describing six fundamental frequencies and areas, Nogier eventually defined seven and the same number of areas. More recently, however, Raphaël Nogier has shown that there are, in fact, *eight areas and eight fundamental frequencies*. Each area and its corresponding frequency are designated by the same letter of the alphabet: **A**, **B**, **C**, **D**, **E**, **F**, **G**, and **L**. They will be described individually hereafter.

Furthermore, considering the law of somatotopic representation, Paul Nogier observed that each area of the ear also had a correspondence with a *peripheral skin territory* on the body (soma), insofar as both reacted to the same frequency. The *concha*, for example, is innervated by the vagus nerve and represents structures of endodermic origin. However, the concha also has a link with a peripheral area, i.e. the skin of the front wall of the chest and abdomen, situated between the clavicles and the lower limit of the T12 dermatome, in that both areas, auricular and somatic, have in common that they will respond by a RAC when exposed to a frequency of 5 Hertz (**Figure 21.1**).

As a result, the sum of peripheral territories added to areas of the ears covers the entire skin surface (**Figure 21.2**). It should be noted, however, that in a healthy individual, the reactions to the projection of a frequency on the somatic territories are tenuous and considerably more difficult to observe than on the ear.


DOI: 10.1201/9781003753629-21

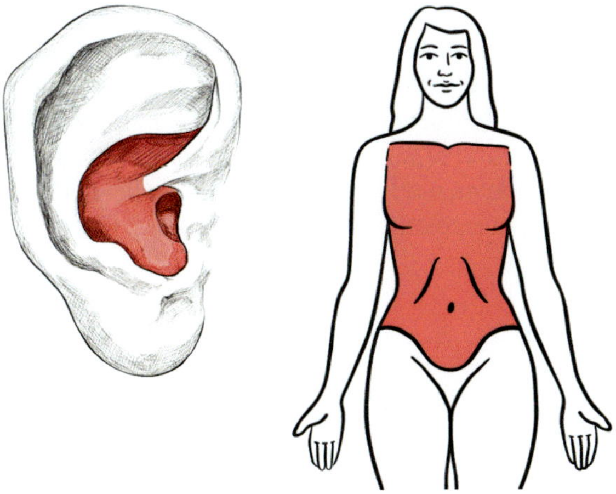

**Figure 21.1** The concha and the anterior aspect of the thorax and abdomen: both respond by a positive RAC to the projection of a frequency of 5 Hertz.

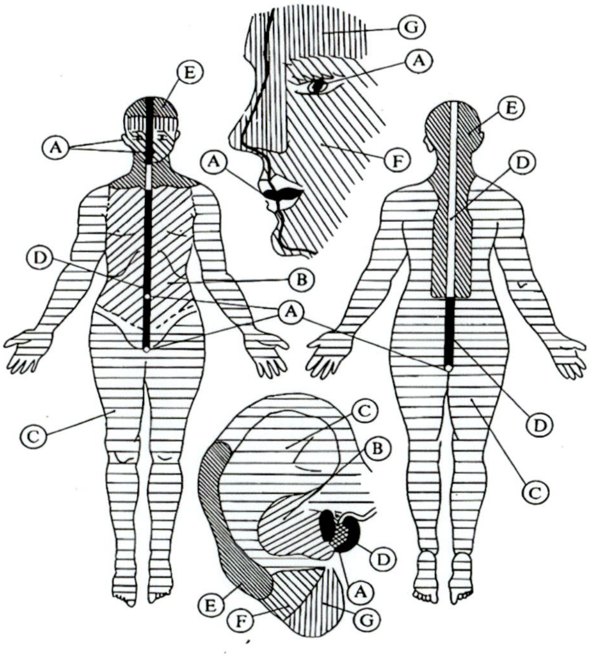


**Figure 21.2** Correspondences between auricular areas and peripheral skin territories, when considering their reactions to the projection of intermittent light. (Copyright Raphaël Nogier.)

In pathological situations, however, whether functional or organic, the somatic RAC responses stand out more clearly than in normal conditions and can be used in a clinical context. In a case of digestive tract disturbance, for example, scanning the abdominal wall with a **B**-frequency while taking the pulse will be likely to define with some clarity the outline of an underlying pathological organ (**Figure 21.3**). It follows that this diagnostic method may be of use in the field of internal medicine as well as in pulse-assisted auriculotherapy.

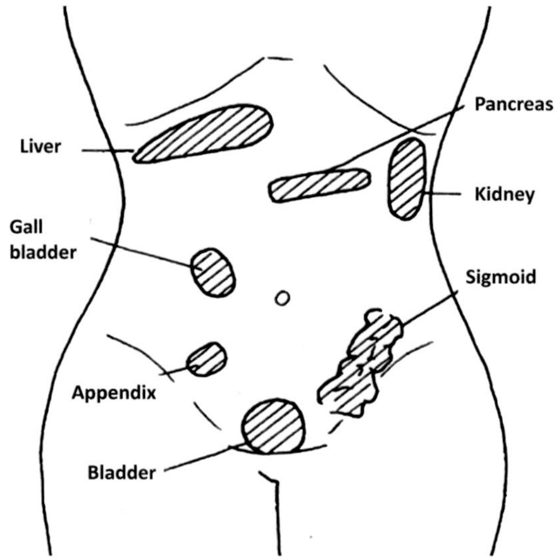


**Figure 21.3** Projection zones of disturbed abdominal organs onto the abdominal wall, as they can be identified by a RAC reaction when scanning the abdomen with a B-frequency.

## 21.2 INTERPRETATION

Reactions of the sympathetic system (RAC) to specific frequency stimulations suggest the existence of a virtual but coherent micro-organisation of the skin, upon which we can rightly speculate on its finality and significance. It appears that, in addition to the many basic properties we are already familiar with in the field of dermatology, the skin is sensitive to a complex environment of electromagnetic fields and radiation originating from the environment, be it close or distant. The skin, therefore, functions as an *interface*, capable of subtle exchanges between the body and its electromagnetic environment.

Although we have not yet identified any receptors to that effect, we can assume that the various territories of the skin (whether auricular or somatic) are distributed according to their individual reactivity to a specific variety of electromagnetic fields to "supply" information to different systems in the body according to their needs.

Specific couplings may even exist between frequential fields and neurotransmitters, as suggested by *experiments carried out on rabbits* (Chapter 8.2).

## 21.3 GENERAL ATTRIBUTES OF AURICULAR AREAS

With these considerations in mind, we will now present a detailed review of the eight auricular areas as they can be represented today: their localisation on the ear and on the body, the frequency to which the pulse respond, their normal and pathological significance, as well as their innervation and the embryological origin of the structures they represent (Chapter 8). We will then introduce a few preliminary considerations on symmetry and laterality, and finally describe the various techniques for diagnosis and treatment based on these properties.

***Area A***

***Ear location***: interior aspect of the tragus (**Figure 21.4**) area A

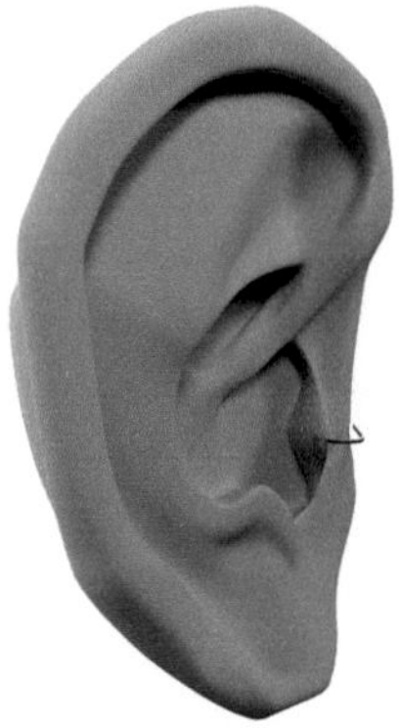

**Figure 21.4** Area A.

***Peripheral location***: *natural orifices*: eyes, mouth, nostrils, vagina, urethral meatus, anus, umbilicus (**Figure 21.2**). Also included are *scars,* healthy, or pathological

***Frequency-A***: 2.28 Hertz

***Biological functions***: anabolism

***Pathological significance***: toxicity, cellular disorganisation, inflammation, allergies, tumours, trauma, pathological scars

***Auricular innervation***: VII bis (Wrisberg's intermediate nerve)

***Embryological origin*** *of the structures implied:* ectoderm

***Area B***

***Ear location***: concha (**Figure 21.5**) area B

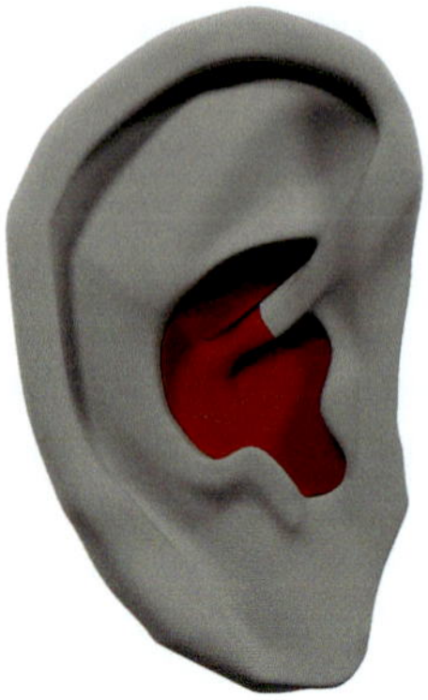

**Figure 21.5** Area B.

***Peripheral location***: anterior aspect of chest and abdomen (except the sagittal line), between the clavicle and the lower limit of dermatome T12 (**Figures 21.1** and **21.2**)

***Frequency***: 4.56 Hertz

***Biological functions***: nutrition, digestion, assimilation, respiration, parasympathetic reactions

***Pathological significance***: digestive and nutritional disorders, including oral and dental, respiratory problems, osteoarthritic disorders, because of impaired nutrition of cartilage

***Auricular innervation***: Vagus nerve (X)

***Embryological origin*** *of organs implied*: endoderm

### *Area C*

***Ear location***: area C anthelix, upper part of helix until the Darwin level, scaphoid groove, ending at the antitragus. This is the largest area (**Figure 21.6**)

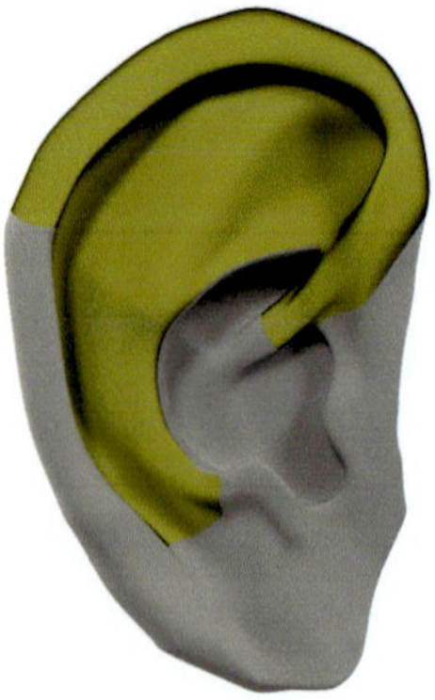

**Figure 21.6** Area C.

***Peripheral location***: dorso-lumbar region of the back (except sagittal line); the four limbs (**Figure 21.2**)

***Frequency***: 9.12 Hertz

***Biological structures and functions***: musculoskeletal structures involved in locomotion, smooth and striated muscles; movement without displacement; cardio-circulatory and renal systems

***Pathological significance***: locomotor and musculoskeletal disorders, vertebral (osteopathic) blockages; cardio-circulatory and renal disorders

***Auricular innervation***: 3rd branch of trigeminal nerve (V3), auriculotemporal nerve

***Embryological origin*** *of organs implied:* mesoderm

### *Area D*

***Ear location***: area D external aspect of tragus (**Figure 21.7**)

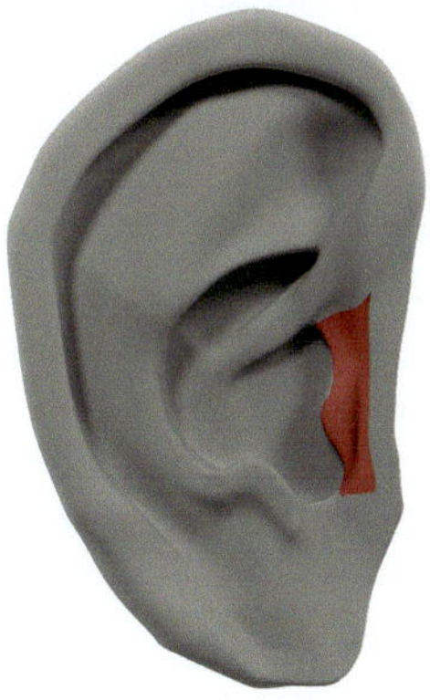

**Figure 21.7** Area D.

***Peripheral location***: median sagittal line starting from the pubis anteriorly up to the skull and then posteriorly down the middle of the back to the anal region (**Figure 21.2**)

***Frequency***: 18.25 Hertz

***Biological structures and functions***: cerebral commissures, interhemispheric communications, symmetry, movement implying displacement; regulation of muscle tone (NB: not relevant for laterality disorders)

***Pathological significance***: commissural and inter-hemispheric disorders; pathologies implying symmetry disorders: hemiplegia, unilateral pain; psychological symptoms implying hesitation and indecision.

***Auricular innervation***: 3rd branch of trigeminal (V3), with occasional resurgences of nerves IX and III

***Embryological origin*** *of structures implied*: ectoderm

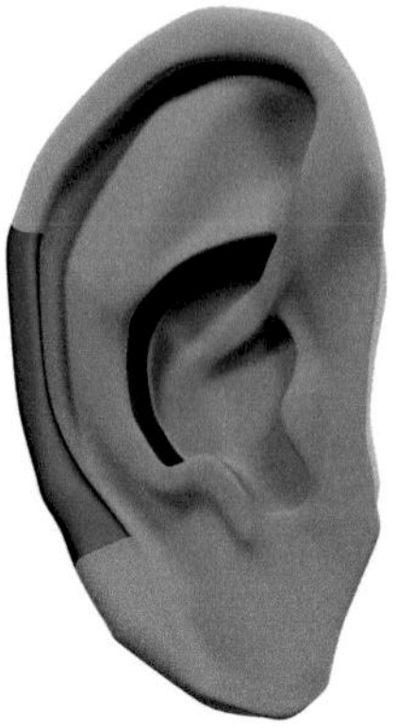

**Figure 21.8** Area E.

### *Area E*

***Ear location***: area E the main location is the tail of the helix from the Darwin level downwards until the helico-lobular incisura. A second location consists of a resurgence on the wall, starting at its upper end at the level of the superior hemi-concha, and continuing down until its termination at the level of the post-antitragal groove (**Figure 21.8**)

***Peripheral location***: neck, anterior and posterior aspects except the midline; scalp, except the midline, with its anterior aspect descending until the eyebrows, and posterior aspect descending until T12 on either side of the dorsal midline (D territory), between this midline and the C territory (**Figure 21.2**)

***Frequency***: 36.5 Hertz

***Biological structures and functions***: spinal cord, longitudinal nerve communication (as opposed to transverse communication); sympathetic system; peripheral nervous system

***Pathological significance***: spinal cord, radicular and PNS disorders, vegetative nervous disorders, pain

***Innervation at the ear***: superficial cervical plexus, probably C3

***Embryological origin of the structures shown***: ectoderm

### *Area F*

***Ear location***: area F posterior-superior part of the lobule, extending upwards, and then vertically downwards to the foot of the antitragal wall (**Figure 21.9**)

***Peripheral location***: face (**Figure 21.2**)

***Frequency***: 73 Hertz

***Biological structures and functions***: diencephalon and subcortical regions, limbic system, thalamus; emotions, instinctive behaviours, interpersonal and emotional relationships

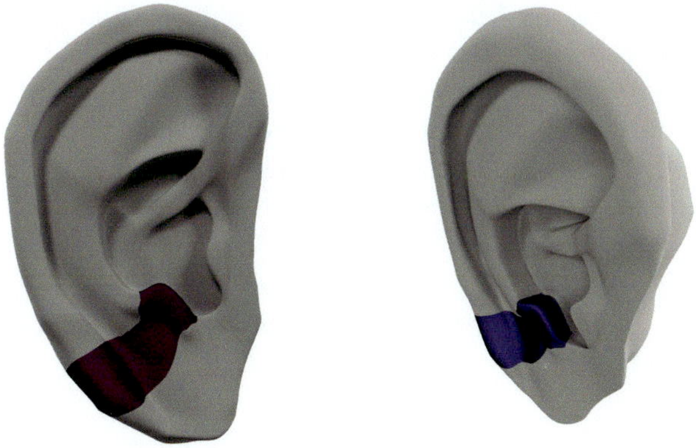

**Figure 21.9** Area F.

***Pathological significance***: fragility of the limbic system, relational disorders (sound line). On the organic level, the F-frequency is that of ulcers, scars, and bone calluses (relationship between the two edges of a tissue rupture)

***Innervation at the ear***: superficial cervical plexus, probably C2

***Embryological origin*** *of the structures shown:* ectoderm

### *Area G*

***Ear location:*** area G antero-inferior part of the lobule, extending upwards and then vertically downwards to the foot of the wall of the intertragal incisura (**Figure 21.10**)

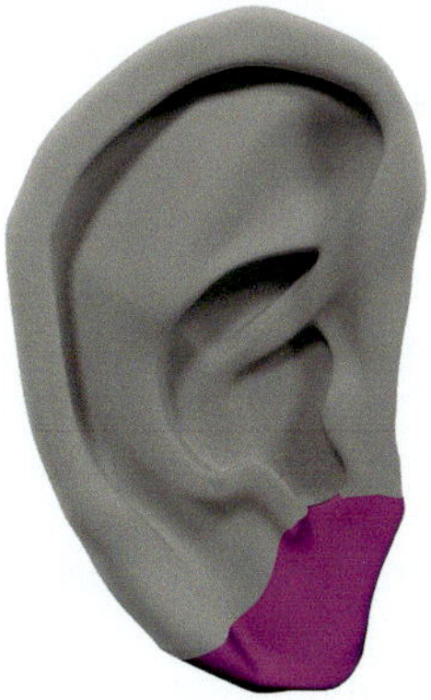

**Figure 21.10** Area G.

***Peripheral location***: frontal and nasal regions, except midline (**Figure 21.2**)

***Frequency***: 146 Hertz

***Biological structures and functions***: cortex, higher mental functions, conscious and unconscious, rationality; endocrine system
***Pathological significance***: cortical and mental overload, anxiety; endocrine disorders, olfactory and visual pathologies
***Innervation at the ear***: superficial cervical plexus, probably C1
***Embryological origin*** *of the structures shown*: ectoderm

*Area L*

***Ear location***: area pre-tragal region, anterior to the external tragus (**Figure 21.11**)

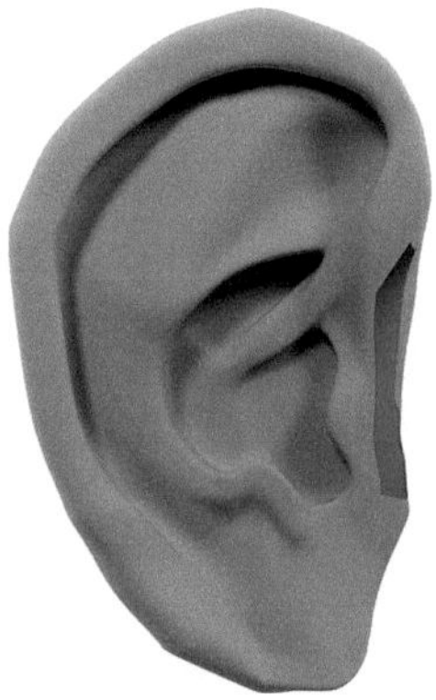

**Figure 21.11** Area L.

***Peripheral location***: *middle line of the skull, beginning on the upper limit of the forehead*, behind the **D** line, and continuing towards the base of the occipital region **Figure 26.5**
***Frequency***: 276 Hertz
***Biological functions***: reinforcement of brain dominance, management of laterality
***Pathological significance***: laterality disorders
***Innervation at the ear***: third trigeminal branch V3 (same as the D range)
***Embryological origin*** *of the structures implied:* ectoderm

### 21.3.1 Overview of the Distribution of Auricular Areas

After having described each area individually, a general view of the ***eight auricular areas*** is presented in **Figure 21.12 (a)**, with a comparative reminder of the original seven areas described by Paul Nogier in **Figure 21.12 (b)**.

Apart from the presence of the eighth area **L**, the main difference between the two lies in the aspect of the **F** area and its border with the **C** area. Furthermore, the

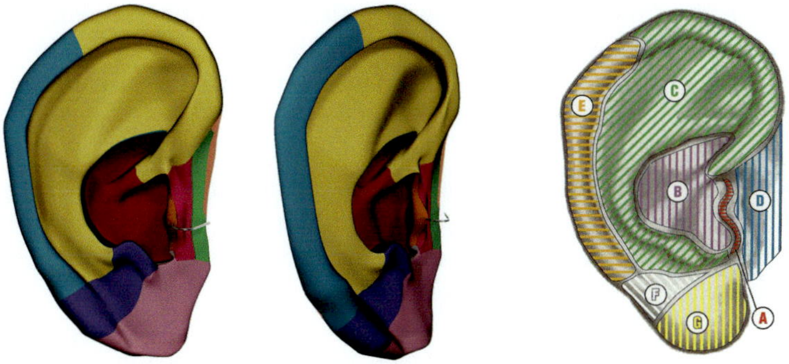


(a) (b)

**Figure 21.12** (a) The eight areas (A area turned). (b) The original seven areas.

wall is not clearly shown in either of these illustrations. This is mainly because the ear is drawn as if it were a flat surface, thus overlooking its vertical aspects.

## 21.3.2 Comments on the Wall and the F Area

The wall can be described as a kind of vertical "cliff", the aspects of which are detailed on the 3D model represented in **Figure 21.13**. The wall is divided into two parts. First, the **longer**, **upper** portion of the wall (which, incidentally, forms the inner part of the two **E** areas, represented in visible in *blue* on **Figure 21.8**). At its upper border, it is longitudinally connected with the **C** area on the anthelix (*yellow*), just below the representation of the spine. At its lowest border, i.e., the foot of the cliff, rests on the floor of the concha, which is the **B** area (*red*).

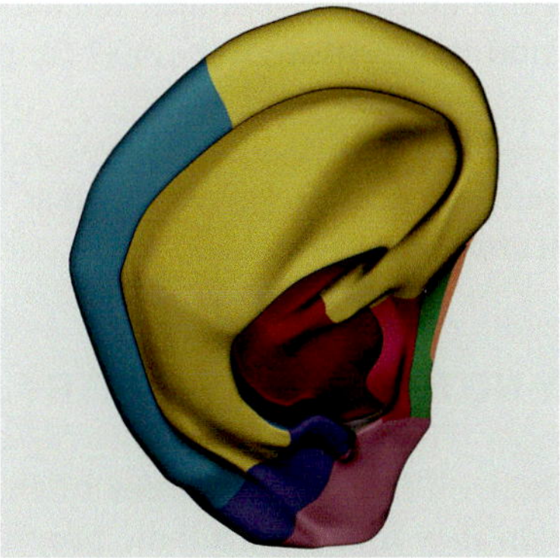

**Figure 21.13** The vertical aspects, i.e. the two different segments of the wall, on a 3D ear model.

The second part of the wall is the lower **antitragal** portion vertically connected to the longer **E** portion at the level of C1, which is represented in purple in **Figure 21.13**. At its front end, the antitragal wall extends to the incisura, whereas its upper border joins the external aspects of the lobule.

Whereas the antitragal part of the wall is well defined anatomically, there is some doubt as to which frequency it responds to. Paul Nogier is not known to have defined it precisely, and to our knowledge, no research has since been undertaken, so the question can currently be considered open.

As for the anterior end of the antitragal wall, near the antitragal notch, indicated by the tip of the arrow on **Figure 21.13**, it is not yet certain whether it should normally respond to F- or G-frequency

However, we will formulate a simple hypothesis based on the principle that the areas of the auricle and their frequencies are related explicitly to the type of anatomical structures that their mapping represents, which gives an indication of the frequency of the area. For example, area **B** bears structures of endodermic origin, such as respiratory and digestive organs. Similarly, we know that a major part of structures located on the antitragal part of the wall, which is situated in the continuity of the **F** zone at the external rear part of the lobule, represents structures belonging to the CNS. Hence, we may reasonably suppose that the frequency resonating on the antitragal part of the wall is the same as that of the external rear part of the lobule, that is, **F**-frequency, and not **C**-frequency as implied on **Figure 21.12 (b)**.

Finally, we have reason to believe that both aspects of the antitragal region, the lobular external part as well as the antitragal wall, can be defined as the F area, as suggested on **Figure 21.13**.

As for the anterior end of the antitragal wall, near the antitragal notch, it is not yet certain whether it should normally respond to **F**- or **G**-frequency.

These considerations still require confirmation. However, it does not contradict our own experience, and despite its uncertainty, we feel that it temporarily makes the best allowance for clinical application.

## 21.4 PRELIMINARY NOTIONS ON SYMMETRY AND LATERALITY

Frequential responses obtained in different areas of the ear have very special characteristics. Not only do they form a harmonic progression from the physical point of view, but they can also be said to witness increasing evolutionary stages, biologically speaking. In this respect, our knowledge of their significance has evolved somewhat since Paul Nogier first started research on the subject. This is particularly the case of **D**-frequency (18.25 Hertz), related, as we have seen, to inter-hemispheric and commissural functions and to the notion of right-left *symmetry*.

Initially, however, it was thought that this **D**-frequency was at the same time dedicated to *laterality*, a brain characteristic that emerged with the human species and which, in fact, results in a different functional tone for each hemisphere. Human thought, language, and writing do not require *symmetry* of the hemispheres but are indeed dependent on ***a**symmetry* and the dominance of one over the other. Laterality, therefore, necessarily implies a notion of asymmetry. At this point, it must be admitted that there is a contradiction: it makes no sense to consider that the same frequency **D** can simultaneously be an expression of both *symmetrical* and *asymmetrical* functions.

The credit for raising this objection goes to Raphaël Nogier. He had noticed that using **D**-frequency in therapeutic mode on points representing the brain commissures localised on the tragus for treating *laterality disorders* (e.g. left-handedness, language disorders, enuresis) was not very effective. This reinforced the idea that **D**-frequency was, in fact, not involved in these types of *asymmetrical* brain disorders and led Raphaël Nogier to search for a new frequency specifically related to laterality and its disorders. He eventually found it to be 276 Hertz and named it the **L-frequency** (**L** for laterality). This frequency elicits a pulse response when projected on the ear, onto a new area located just *in front of the **D** area*, between the tragus and the rear part of the jaw. The corresponding colour filter is *green 58,* and the related *somatic* area is located *on the middle line of the skull, beginning on the upper limit of the forehead*, behind the **D** line and continuing towards the base of the occipital region (see ). So finally, due to recent progress, eight areas can now be identified on the ear, reacting to eight frequencies. These notions are developed in greater detail in Chapter 26.

Another important corollary should be mentioned regarding the **D**-frequency. Whereas it can no longer be considered related to laterality and its disorders, the significance of **D**-frequency should include the notion of *movement* previously attributed to the **C**-frequency.

Although organs devoted to locomotion, such as bones, muscles, and joints, are basically related to the **C**-frequency and are located on the mesodermal territories of the ear (in phase 1), the notion of *movement with displacement* should be introduced as a function of its own. Raphaël Nogier has shown that *movement with displacement* (as opposed to movement without displacement, e.g. activity of the bowel) implies the notion of *symmetry*, as much so in living beings as in machines designed for movement, such as automobiles, airplanes, etc. Thus, it follows that *pathologies implying movement and asymmetry induced by pathological situations* (e.g. hemiplegia) also imply **D**-frequency and not **C**-frequency, as previously assumed.

## 21.5 RELATIONSHIPS BETWEEN COLOUR PROGRAMME, AURICULAR AREAS, AND FUNDAMENTAL FREQUENCIES

Looking back briefly to the filters of the colour programme (Chapter 18), let us remind that Paul Nogier had initially described *areas* of the ear as being closely correlated with these *colours* and with the seven fundamental *frequencies*. In line with this, René Bourdiol, a neuroanatomist close to Paul Nogier, used to speak of "*frequency colours*" [1]. It also followed that colours, areas, and frequencies were considered a unity, all of which were named with the same letters **A**, **B**, **C**, **D**, **E**, **F**, and **G**.

This is certainly true to some extent. From the physics point of view, however, admittedly, we do not know of any common denominator between the absorption spectrum of a colour filter and the frequency emitted by a generator. Hence, the question remains as to what could form the basis of such correspondences between colours, frequencies, and areas. Whereas it seems clear that each area of the ear will react selectively to one of the fundamental frequencies, this can hardly be said of colours: first because the projection of a colour with a lamp will tend to be too powerful and have the ear surface react as a whole (this was already mentioned when discussing phases in Chapter 19). And when it comes to colour *filters*, their sheer size makes them technically inappropriate for testing on such small surfaces as the auricular area.

Nevertheless, experience still leads us to believe that areas, colours, and frequencies have something in common, especially from a clinical point of view. First, they have similar reactions when tested with the RAC. Secondly, the *interpretations* attributed to areas, colours, and frequencies, respectively (**Figures 21.5–21.12**) are, for the most part, close or identical. For example, *colour **B*** (**red 25**) and *frequency-**B*** (*4.56 Hertz*) are known to react with organs and functions of *endodermal origin* and are all located in the concha area. Nevertheless, even if such connections can be taken into consideration on empirical grounds, it must be kept in mind that the notion of a precise correspondence between colours and frequencies lacks a physical basis and, therefore, can be misleading. Practically speaking, this entails that colours and frequencies often have a close significance but are not always interchangeable.

## 21.6 DIAGNOSTIC TECHNIQUES USING FUNDAMENTAL FREQUENCIES

### 21.6.1 Auricular Diagnosis

In general, the following two steps should be carried out. First, scan through the whole auricle with a white tip or Heine's lamp in search of a point that appears "on an empty ear" (i.e. without imposing any information). This point generally expresses one of the aspects of the clinical picture. If several points are detected, the rule is to select the one that reacts with the greatest number of RACS.

The second step then involves **analysing** the detected point using a frequency generator. The tip of the generator is placed in contact with the point. By scrolling through the eight frequencies in diagnostic mode (i.e., with low intensity exposing the point to the eight frequencies one after the other), the frequency that causes the largest number of RACS is selected.

Usually, the point will predominantly react either to the *natural frequency* of the area in which the point is located, to the *complementary frequency,* or both. This is a normal reaction. The question is then whether the point also reacts to a *parasite* frequency, that is, a frequency that is neither the natural nor the complementary frequency of the area in which the point is located.

If the point reacts solely to the *natural frequency of the area* or *to its complementary frequency,* it can be assumed that the pathology expressed by this point remains relatively mild and is not correlated with other pathological aspects. For instance, this could be the case of a minor injury or an acute inflammation. If, on the other hand, the point does react to a *parasite* frequency, it can be assumed that the problem is more complex and could be influenced by another pathology *located in the area from which the parasite frequency originates*, thus possibly suggesting a causal link between the two pathologies.

### 21.6.2 Somatic Diagnosis

Frequency resonance can also be applied for diagnosis directly onto a *somatic* localisation without necessarily using the ear, as illustrated by the following situation:

- In the event of acute abdominal pain in the left iliac fossa, solving a differential diagnosis between colonic diverticulitis and ureteral lithiasis can be facilitated by projecting fundamental frequencies onto the painful area using a frequency generator. This technique is possible if the two possible pathologies are known to respond to different frequencies. If the problem is due to a colonic disease, a RAC will clearly appear on a projection of **B**-frequency, known to resonate with endodermic structures. If, on the contrary, the pain originates in the urinary tract, the pulse will respond to the projection of **C**-frequency, which has a connection with mesoderm structures. Optionally, confirmation can be obtained by searching for related ear points, their location, and the frequency to which they react.

## 21.7 OPTIONS FOR TREATMENT

Following the detection of an ear point and analysis of what frequency this point responds, the question of which treatment to apply will mainly depend on the problem's complexity level.

### 21.7.1 Treatment by the Natural or the Complementary Frequency

If the point reacts to the natural or complementary frequency of the area in which the point is located, the problem can be treated *directly*, either with a ***needle*** or by the ***natural frequency*** or by *the **complementary frequency (using*** strong intensity, i.e. "therapeutic mode").

**This choice depends** on the "reactive quality" of the point (see Section 15.2). If the point responds as "mobile blue", treating it with the complementary frequency may prove more efficient than treating it with the direct frequency. This rests on the assumption that if the point is "mobile", it means that the body's reaction will be capable of actively reversing the complementary frequency into the direct frequency, which is considered more powerful therapeutically than injecting the direct frequency. If, however, the ear point responds as "fixed blue" (**Table 15.1**), this means that it reacts passively, i.e. the body will not be capable of actively reversing the frequency and should, therefore, be treated by the direct frequency. The duration of the frequency injection should be approximately 30 seconds or until the extinction of the RAC.

### 21.7.2 Treatment by Simple Deparasitation

If, when tested, the point additionally responds to a parasite frequency, one can break the causal link of this frequency belonging to a different area. This is called *deparasitation* and consists of treating the point (here again in "therapeutic" mode, and until the extinction of the RAC) either by the complementary frequency if the point is *reactive*, that is, *"mobile blue"*, or by the parasite frequency itself, if the point is *passive,* that is *fixed blue.*

Parasitation of a point means that this point is somehow influenced by some deeper pathology, often preceding in time and originating in some other auricular area. The process of deparasitation can be seen as somewhat "forcing" the parasite frequency back to the auricular area from where it originated.

### 21.7.3 Treatment by Sequential Deparasitation

An initial deparasitation may well result in one or more additional parasite frequencies appearing one after the other on the same point. This will require a ***sequential deparasitation***. Much like *sequence 24* and the *colour programme sequence* (both described in Chapter 18), sequential deparasitation, also known as a *frequency sequence*, is a step-by-step approach consisting of several successive deparasitations.

The notion of sequence is an interesting process. It offers the possibility of analysing how different pathological elements have cumulated over time and compensated one another to induce multiple causalities. The various levels of a sequence can also contribute to bringing forward an element of the patient's history that had not been mentioned (see example below).

Practically speaking, the sequence involves a combination of (1) scanning the surface of an auricular area using one selected frequency in search of a reactive point and (2) scrolling through all the different frequencies on one individual point to find out which frequency this point reacts the most to.

It can be carried out as follows:

***First level***: one searches for a point by *scanning* the whole ear with a white tip or Heine's lamp. If several points appear, select the one producing the greatest number of RACs. If it bears a parasite frequency, then deparasitise it as mentioned above.

***Second level***: the auricular area from which the first parasite frequency originates is scanned with the natural frequency of this area in diagnostic mode (this time not with a white tip) in search of a second point. We then assess whether this point also bears a parasite frequency. If so, we **deparasitise** it by projecting the parasite frequency (or its complementary frequency) in therapeutic (strong) mode.

***Following levels***: these are dealt with similarly until an auricular area with a **terminal** or **causal** point is found. The terminal point can be recognised by the fact that it reacts either to *all eight fundamental frequencies (maybe one or two could be missing)* or only *to the frequency of the area in which the point is located.* As a rule, one may usually find between one and four different levels, rarely more.

***Final level***: **treating the terminal point** can be done in several ways: with the frequency generator in therapeutic (strong) mode and successively *projecting the eight frequencies one after the other at approximately one per second (this rhythm is usually programmed in the generator). The process could be described as "therapeutic scrolling". Alternatively, one can treat* with a semi-permanent needle (ASP) or by its equivalent: cryotherapy (injecting a point with nitrogen at −40 degrees for half a second). But whatever the type of treatment, *the remarkable aspect of this sequencing technique is that only the terminal point needs to be treated because all the points related to the previous intermediary levels will have de facto been automatically treated during the process.*

### 21.7.4 Example of a Frequency Sequence

A 48-year-old patient goes to see her physician because of recurrent throat infections over the past two months, with pain when swallowing and moderate fever. She is in her pre-menopausal period, so family and professional tensions make her feel even more irritable, but otherwise, she has no serious medical problems.

Analysing the frequency sequence, we come across four successive levels (**Figure 21.14**):

1. ***First level***: by scanning both auricles with a white tip, the first point appears on both ears, located on the posterior border just above the helical-lobular angle. It can be interpreted as representing the ***glossopharyngeal***

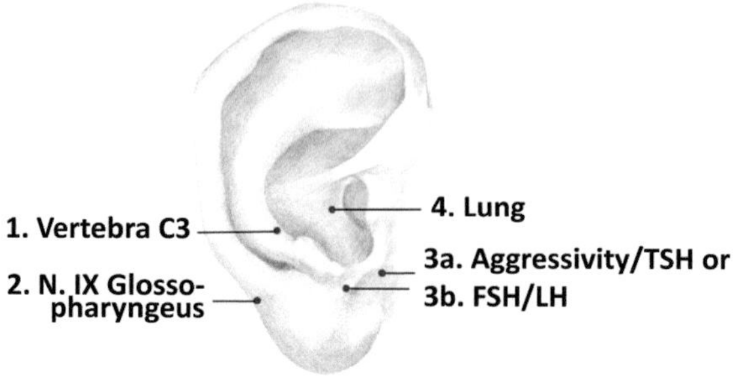


**Figure 21.14** Example of a frequency sequence.

***nerve IX***, which transmits pain signals from the throat and, therefore, can be considered related to the main symptom. The point is located at the limit between the ***E*** and ***F*** areas**,** but by scrolling through the frequencies (in diagnostic mode), we find that this point is ***parasitised by the C-frequency***. Consequently, we deparasitise this point by removing the parasite frequency, injecting the same C-frequency into the point (in therapeutic mode) to "push it back into its own **C** area".

2. ***Second level***: we then scan through the C area (which supposedly exerts a pathological influence on the glossopharyngeal nerve) with C frequency and find a second point representing the ***C3 cervical vertebra.*** This is hardly surprising considering that, clinically, vertebral blockages in the cervical region are prone to induce pharyngeal inflammatory disturbances. We then scroll through all the frequencies (in diagnostic mode) on the C3 vertebral point and find it is parasitised by the ***G frequency.***
3. ***Third level***: following the same progression, we scan the **G area** with **G frequency** (in diagnostic mode). This time, two points are found: ***an FSH/LH point and an aggressivity (TSH) point***. While the former suggests a possible vulnerability induced by the pre-menopausal phase, the aggression point can be related to the irritability described by the patient. The point reacting with the highest number of RACs is the FSH/LH point, so we select this point to scroll through the series of frequencies (in diagnostic mode) and find that the point reacts to a ***parasite B frequency***.
4. ***Fourth (and final) level***: scanning (in diagnostic mode) through the **B area** with **B-frequency** reveals a fifth point located on the left ear, in the central part of the lower hemi-concha, which can be identified as a lung point. This point responds to all eight frequencies and is therefore ***considered*** the ***causal or terminal point***.

When questioned once again on her medical history, the patient informs us that she had suffered from pulmonary tuberculosis at the age of 25! ***N.B. The fact that the lung point has appeared on the left ear of a right-handed patient can be understood as referring to a medical event that occurred in the past and not in the present.***

***Treatment:*** This terminal point was treated with a semi-permanent needle, which entails clearing all the previous points that have appeared throughout the sequence. Clinically, a treatment by auriculotherapy proved satisfactory, without antibiotics.

## 21.8 CONCLUSION

The techniques involving fundamental frequencies devised by Paul Nogier provide an elegant and relatively simple approach to understanding and solving the complexity of disorders that tend to accumulate over time within an organism in perpetual quest for adaptation.

### PROTOCOL 4: TECHNIQUES USING FUNDAMENTAL FREQUENCIES

*The content of measurements and techniques and the order in which they are carried out are proposed as a guideline to be adapted to each clinical situation.*

#### Preliminaries

- Positioning of patient and practitioner
- Assessment of resting pulse
- RAC calibration
- Searching for **RAC exhaustion**
- Checking the neurovegetative formula
- Possibly include other optional parameters from previous protocols

#### Diagnosis and Treatment Using Fundamental Frequencies

- Searching for an ear point with a white tip or Heine's lamp
- **Frequency analysis** of the detected point
  If the point only reacts to the natural frequency of the area:
  - **treat it directly with this frequency** (in therapeutic mode) or the **complementary frequency**, or with an **extemporaneous needle**

  If the point is parasited by another frequency, then treat this point by:
  - **simple deparasitation** (one level), or
  - **sequential deparasitation** (several levels)

## BIBLIOGRAPHY


1. Bourdiol René. *L'Auriculo-somatologie* (Maisonneuve) 1981; 97–151
2. Nogier Paul. *From Auriculotherapy to Auriculomedicine* (Maisonneuve) 1981; 155–165
3. Nogier Paul. *Advanced Course in Auriculomedicine*, Lyon 1981–1994
4. Rouxeville Yves. *Personalized Auricular Acupuncture* (Sauramps Médical) 2000; 119–133

CHAPTER 22

# Other Techniques Based on Fundamental Frequencies

**Anthony de Sousa and Jean-Luc Vigneron**

The deparasitation and frequency sequence techniques described in the previous chapter are certainly among the most used. In addition, the following techniques can provide valuable complementary information:

- The central reaction test
- Deviated fundamental frequencies
- The passing band

## 22.1 THE CENTRAL REACTION TEST

Paul Nogier developed the central reaction test in the mid-1980s. The test enables us to diagnose a pathological frequency. In the previous chapter, we began by identifying an ear point and then analysing and treating it based on its frequency characteristics. We will now show that it is also possible to proceed the other way around, i.e. to start by identifying a disturbed frequency and then find a point that can correct that frequency.

The principle of the test is based on the following two characteristics:

1. Suppose a given frequency is injected for about 10 seconds at high intensity ("therapeutic" mode) onto a random somatic spot on the forehead (marked with a small circle), the frequency will be absorbed, causing a reaction within the skin. If the same frequency is injected immediately after, at the same spot, but this time, with low intensity ("diagnostic" mode), this second injection results in an RAC response, clearly stronger than if one had not applied the first injection. This response is called an echo.

   To put it another way, the first frequency injection at high intensity is sometimes referred to as the image, while the echo response obtained when the frequency is injected a second time at low intensity is called the counter-image, or echo.

DOI: 10.1201/9781003753629-22

Note that the central reaction test is conducted on the forehead and not on the auricle since it does not involve mapping. The forehead, being the part of the soma anatomically closest to the brain, makes it an ideal spot for the test.

2. Since fundamental frequencies are separated by equal harmonic intervals, the lowest frequency A can be seen as summarising or virtually containing all the other harmonic frequencies.

The central response test combines the two properties. Frequency **A** is injected at high intensity ("therapeutic mode") onto any random (but marked) spot on the forehead. This image will produce an echo or counter-image. And, since frequency **A** virtually contains all the other harmonics, re-injection (at low intensity) will produce an echo not only of frequency **A** but also of all its harmonics, i.e. all the fundamental frequencies. Normally, all the fundamental harmonics should respond with a positive RAC.

However, it can happen that one or more of the frequencies are missing and produce no RAC or only a small RAC response. This is called a **frequency gap** and is a sign of a pathological frequency.

In practice, the technique consists of four steps.

### 22.1.1 Searching for a Frequency Gap on the Forehead

The **A** frequency is injected for 10 seconds at high intensity (therapeutic mode) into a randomly selected point on the forehead (previously marked with a circle).

Then, at low intensity (diagnostic mode), all the fundamental frequencies are successively scrolled through the same point on the forehead, collecting the echo of a positive RAC (qualitatively and quantitatively) for each of them.

If one or several of the frequencies injected turn out to be unresponsive (or weakly responsive), this shows a **frequency gap**, or **missing frequency**, indicating that there is something to be corrected in the field of that frequency.

### 22.1.2 Searching for a Correction Point on the Auricle

Returning to the auricle, one then scans the ear (in diagnostic or low-intensity mode) with the missing frequency in search of a point responding to that frequency. As a rule, one should scan the whole ear surface, although the point will most likely be found within the area where the missing frequency belongs.

### 22.1.3 Determining Whether the Subject Reacts Actively or Passively

To implement the most adequate correction of the diagnosed point, we take the organism's reactionary mode into account, remembering that to any stimulation, whether diagnostic or therapeutic, the organism responds by seeking to re-establish the best possible homeostasis. So, taking into consideration the patient's *constitutional mode of reaction*, being either **active** or **passive**, we proceed as follows:

We again inject an **image** of the **A** frequency on the forehead (at therapeutic, or strong intensity) for 10 seconds. We then compare the intensity of the **echo** response (in diagnostic or low intensity) *between the two frequencies*, **A**, *and its complementary frequency*, **G**.

- If the **G** frequency echo is more intense than the **A** frequency echo, the organism is reacting in an **active** mode, thus adapting by *reversing* the initial **A** stimulation into its complementary **G** frequency.
- If, on the other hand, the echo simply reproduces the **A** frequency without reversing it, this indicates a **passive** reaction mode. The body undergoes the stimulation without trying to adapt.

### 22.1.4 Treatment of the Detected Point by Complementary Frequency

Paul Nogier considered that the power of the treatment could be enhanced if it were carried out using the *complementary* frequency. Hence:

- If the subject's reactivity mode is active, the point will be treated in similarity using the direct frequency, because an active organism will invert the injected frequency by itself.
    - For example, with a **B** frequency gap in active mode, the **B** frequency in therapeutic (strong) intensity is injected since the organism, in active mode, will spontaneously reverse this stimulation by itself.
- If, on the other hand, the subject's reactivity is passive, the point is treated by the complementary frequency to compensate for the organism's lack of reactivity.
    - In the example of a **B** frequency gap, one injects the complementary **F** frequency since the organism will not actively reverse the injected frequency by itself.

## PROTOCOL 5: THE CENTRAL REACTION

### Diagnosis of a Pathological Frequency, by Searching for a Frequency Gap

Inject frequency **A** at high intensity for 10 seconds at any point on the forehead (marked by a circle).

- Search for an echo on all the frequencies. If one of them does not respond, it corresponds to a **frequency gap** or **pathological frequency**
- Search for a point at the ear by scanning the pathological frequency

### Determining the Subject's Reactive Mode

At a point on the forehead, inject **A** at high intensity for 10 seconds.

Compare the RAC echoes produced between **A** and **G** in low intensity:

- **If A** prevails: **Passive** mode
- **If G** prevails: **Active** mode

### Treatment

If the reaction mode is **passive**, treat the point with the **complementary gap frequency**.

If the reactive mode is **active**, treat the point in ***similarity*** with the **direct gap frequency**.

*Repeat the test to determine if another frequency must be corrected.*

## 22.2 DEVIATED OR ALTERED FREQUENCIES

The fundamental frequencies (so-called Nogier frequencies) discussed until now are most often characterized by precise values (in Hertz); we, therefore, call them **pure** frequencies. However, one may also encounter minor variations in Hertz values within a range of **–30%** to **+30%** of the pure frequency. These are referred to as **deviated** or **altered** frequencies. Most generators we work with are designed to produce the following (discrete) variations: **–30%, –20%, –10%, +10%, +20%,** and **+30%**, in both weak ("diagnostic") and strong ("therapeutic") intensities. Variations exceeding **30%** are not taken into consideration as they no longer correspond to the notion of harmonics.

The fundamental frequencies are referred to by their letter, for instance, "C", whereas altered frequencies will be referred to by their letter and the deviation, for example, "**C+30**" or "**C−10**", and so on.

For any detected ear point, the RAC can be used to determine which fundamental frequency, pure or deviated, this point resonates with.

### 22.2.1 Predetermined Deviated Frequencies

Note that several pathological situations are known to respond *a priori* to a particular deviated frequency. For example, **minor intervertebral disorders (MIDs)** are known to resonate with frequency **A+30**. This makes it possible to perform a low-intensity **A+30** scan of the spinal region from top to bottom on both sides of the spine to locate the MID level.

Similarly, a region of the body suffering from **intense pain** will likely respond to a frequency of **G+30**. Hence, from a *diagnostic* point of view, it is possible to locate the painful area by scanning the region with **G+30** (at low, "diagnostic" intensity). The same frequency can also be applied for treatment (at strong, "therapeutic" intensity), either by direct contact in *loco dolendi*, on a corresponding ear point, or both.

### 22.2.2 The Case of +10% Frequencies

Pure frequencies are the closest to normality. But Paul Nogier's research led him to the opinion that frequencies deviated by **+10%** are ***not** pathological* but may indeed represent a sign of the **best possible degree of vitality** for the point or region that carries them, even more so than the pure frequency. Therefore, treating a frequency deviated by +10% will not be necessary. This is consistent with the fact that biological norms are often not rigid but are characterised by slight intervals of physiological *oscillations*.

### 22.2.3 Detection and Treatment of a Deviated Frequency

This technique is applied to points detected on the ear as opposed to the forehead, as was the case with the central reaction. First, the tip of a frequency generator is placed in contact with the ear point, and without displacing the tip, one reviews all the fundamental (pure) frequencies one after the other to find out to which of these frequencies the point reacts the most. Secondly, while maintaining the same frequency, one reviews all possible deviations, starting from + or - 30% (except for +10%, which we have seen, is not pathological), to determine which deviation the examined point reacts to. Combining the two, we may, for example, determine that the point resonates with **B+20**.

We then proceed to treat this deviation. For this purpose, it is once again necessary to know whether the subject under examination reacts in an **active** or **passive** mode, which is measurable by a test called the *central reaction to the deviated frequency*.

Let's say that the point reacts to **B+20**. We then inject the same deviated frequency into the point on the ear for 10 seconds in therapeutic mode and observe the **echo**. If it reacts with the **direct frequency B+20**, the reaction is **passive**. Conversely, the reaction is considered **active** if the echo reacts with the complementary frequency **F+20**.

*Important note: It should be emphasised that the inversion only concerns the letter, which refers to the fundamental frequency. The deviation itself is not reversed. Thus, B+20 becomes F+20 and not B−20 or F−20.*

If the reaction is **passive**, the point will be treated in *compensation* mode, by **F+20**. If, on the other hand, the reaction is **active**, the point will be processed in *similarity* mode, by **B+20**.

### 22.2.4 Significance Attributed to Altered or Deviated Frequency (Text by Jean-Luc Vigneron)

The meaning or interpretation that can be attributed to a frequency deviation deserves further detail. This chapter, therefore, includes a text describing the personal experience of Dr Jean-Luc Vigneron, a senior colleague in charge of research at GLEM.

As described in Chapter 20, the Nogier frequency system is articulated symmetrically around frequency **D** so that frequency **A** is complementary to **G**, **B** is complementary to F, and **C** to **E**. Whereas, D has no complementary because it is the centre of symmetry. By contrast, the deviated frequencies are complementary at the same level of deviation: for example, **G+10** is complementary to **A+10**, or **G−30** is complementary to **A–30**, etc. However, for **D,** we can consider that **D+10** is complementary to **D−10**, etc.

An ear point reacting to an altered or deviated frequency has a pathological significance. To interpret the meaning of this "parasite" frequency, we must consider the location on the ear and the corresponding area. For example, a **C−30** frequency will not have the same meaning if found in area B as in area **C**. The list below reflects my experience:

**Frequency A**

- **A−30**: cellular alteration pathology related to an infection, a scar, a cellular lesion, etc.
- **A−20**: a scar that requires stimulation.
- **A+10**: see below Section 22.2.5.
- **A+20**: an allergic and inflammatory type reaction.
- **A+30**: osteoarticular blockage.

**Frequency B**

- In my view, any deviation of this frequency is related to metabolic suffering or some digestive pathology. It should be considered according to the location of the point and requires checking for food intolerance or allergy (see Chapter 27).

**Frequency C**

- **C−** deviations: degenerative pathology concerning mesodermal organs: bones, joints, muscles, etc.
- **C+** deviations: inflammatory pathology of the same elements.

**Frequency D**

- **D+ or −** deviations: disorders of left-right coordination.

**Frequency E**

- **E + or −** deviations: neuralgic pain, or degeneration of the reflex loop (example: neurological complications of diabetes).

**Frequency F**

- **F + or −** deviations: loss of control of subcortical functions, interpreted according to the localisation.

**Frequency G**

- **G−30**: suggests disorders of the psyche, especially towards depression
- **G+30**: like above, with a tendency towards vehemence.

**Example**

A liver point, in phase one, is detected in the concha. The pathological significance depends on what frequency the point reacts to:

- **A−30**: The liver cell has been organically *injured*, for instance, by hepatitis A, B, or C, by an Epstein–Barr virus, by medication, or by a toxic substance.
- **B−30**: Indicates dysfunction: Is there a food intolerance (see Chapter 27)?
- **C+/−30**: The liver pathology has an impact on the muscles and the vessels. (NB: In Chinese medicine, the muscles, tendons, and veins are related to the liver.)
- **E−30**: Involves degenerative and possibly painful phenomena of the nerve endings.
- **F−30**: In our experience, this suggests intoxication by an aggressive substance or by medication. In this case, we will also find **F−30** on points connected to the mesonephros.
- **G−30**: Very frequent. The patient feels irritated or angry because of some unpleasant situation.
- **G+30**: Like the above, but with additional virulence.

Of course, this list is not exhaustive and can be enriched by the experience of each practitioner using the pulse.

### 22.2.5 The A+10 Frequency

In a physiologically well-balanced individual, **A+10** frequency elicits 7–8 RAC reactions when the tip of a frequency generator is placed at 1.5 cm above any part of the external aspect of the auricles and tragus (not necessarily on an ear point). No RAC is produced on the ear's mastoid aspect (back side) with **A+10**, except over the representations of the heart and lungs.

The **A+10** frequency has been associated with what has been described in Chapter 16 as the *middle level* and is often referred to as "the middle-level frequency". The *middle level* acts as a link between the *deep and superficial levels*, exerting as if it were an active pump-like mechanism between the two.

Referring to the symmetrical structure of the **ABCDEFG** frequency system, as described in Chapter 20, It should be kept in mind that each fundamental frequency (except **D**) has a *complementary*, or *opposite* frequency in relation to the "central" frequency **D**. This implies that an ear point bearing an altered (deviated) frequency can be treated by the opposite frequency, but with the *same deviation*. For example, a point reacting to **A–30** can be treated by **G–30**, except in the case of reactive exhaustion.

### 22.2.6 The G+10 Frequency

In this respect, the **G+10** frequency is "opposite" or "complementary" to the **A+10** frequency.

In the event of **A+10** not reacting over the ear, a point reacting to its complementary frequency **G+10** should be found and, in this case, treated by this same frequency **G+10**, which in turn can be expected to restore the normal reaction to **A+10** over the ear.

**A+10** and its *complementary* frequency **G+10** both play a particular role in relation to the fundamental frequencies **ABCDEFG** and their deviations. They have the property of being able to *support and improve* the fundamental frequencies **of ABCDEFG in their actions at the cellular level by** boosting them or slowing them down, according to what is necessary.

**Example**

A knee point is found in the triangular fossa of the external ear. It reacts to **C–30**. Provided it is a *mobile* point (see Chapter 15), it is possible to treat such a point with the same frequency and the same deviation **C–30**. In addition, we will test the point's reaction to frequency A+10 to assess its supportive action on the C−30 frequency active on the knee point. At 1 or 2 cm from the point, **A+10** should produce 7 or 8 RACs.

If the response is up to 10 or even 20 RACs, this means that the influence of **A+10** is **excessive**. It will be necessary to reduce its influence by treating the knee point with **A+10**.

If, on the contrary, the response is merely 1 or 2 RACs, this means that the influence of **A+10** is **insufficient** and will need to be enhanced using **G+10**.

## PROTOCOL 6: DEVIATED FREQUENCIES

Here we work on the **ear** and not on the forehead.

1. **Given a point on the ear**, determine to which **fundamental frequency** this point reacts. Then find the **maximum deviation** that still gives a response.

   **Determine the active or passive reactive mode of** the point, using the central reaction to the deviated frequency: inject the frequency and its deviation (e.g. **B+20**) in therapeutic mode. If the echo is **B+20**, the reaction is **passive**. If the echo is **F+20**, the reaction is **active**.

2. **Treatment**
   - In case of a passive reaction, the compensation is treated with **F+20**.
   - In case of an active reaction, the treatment is similar but with **B+20**.

     N.B. Remember that the deviation does not change when dealing with complementary frequencies.

3. **Consider** the significance of the deviation observed (see text in Section 22.2.4).

4. **Examine the reactions to A+10** (in view of its supportive action on the fundamental frequencies): with the tip of the frequency generator at a distance of 1.5 cm from the ear, test reactions to **A+10** over the whole ear and/or over a point which has been detected: this should normally produce 7–8 RACs
   - If there is no reaction, or if only 1–2 RACs, then treat the point with the complementary frequency G+10 to compensate for a ***lack*** and *restore* the normal response to **A+10** (7–8 RACs).
   - If 10–20 RACs, treat the point with **A+10** to reduce ***excess***.

## 22.3 MEASURING THE BANDWIDTH

(*Text by A. de Sousa*)

In addition to the possibility of measuring a frequency deviation and including this deviation in the treatment, it can also be of interest to evaluate *to what degree of deviation* the brain is still capable of recognising and integrating a frequency. In other words, how "wide" is the brain's capacity to recognise a deviated frequency?

To illustrate this, we may compare it to the old-time mid-twentieth-century radio receiver systems that functioned in analogue mode. The "tuner" button on the condenser made it possible to select a radio station, not in a discontinuous digital mode as today, but in a progressive discrete mode. The sound varied gradually in the form of a bell-shaped reception curve. At the top of the curve, reception quality was at its highest, and then gradually decreased on either side of the curve until it was lost. Radio stations varied according to how "wide" the reception curve was.

Similarly, to describe the brain's capacity to recognise deviated frequencies, Paul Nogier used the term **bandwidth**. This parameter can influence the efficiency of some of the communication channels within the organism.

**Technique for measuring the bandwidth**: For this particular purpose, **D** frequency is the most appropriate because it can *deviate* but has no *complementary* frequency other than itself, so injecting **D** frequency can only produce an echo on the same **D** frequency, whether the subject reacts actively or passively.

The technique is conducted as follows: Frequency **D–0** (**D zero** or just **D**) is injected for ten seconds on any point of the forehead, in therapeutic mode (high intensity).

1. *The degree of deviation* for **D** is then assessed at the same point on the forehead, in diagnostic mode (low intensity). We start with the highest deviations, **D+30** and **D–30**. If the echo is still felt under these conditions, it shows that the brain has a *wide* bandwidth. If the echo does not appear in **+/–30**, then **D+20** and **D–20** are tested, and if this produces an echo, the bandwidth is considered *medium*. Finally, if there is no echo, **D–10** is tested (but not **D+10** as it is a sign of vitality and not pathology), and if necessary, **D–0**. If the echo only occurs with **D–10** or **D–0**, this indicates a *narrow* bandwidth.

### 22.3.1 Treatment

If the bandwidth turns out to be *narrow*, the objective is to *"widen the channel"* so that the brain can still understand a frequency deviated up to **+/–30%**. For this purpose, we will use frequency **A** because of its ability to sum up all the other frequencies. Scan the auricle in search of a point capable of reacting to both **A+30** and **G–30%** in diagnostic mode and then inject this same point in therapeutic (strong) mode, first with frequency **A+30** and then with **A−30**, for 30 seconds or until extinction of the RAC. This should broaden the bandwidth for all frequencies and can be verified by re-testing with frequency **D** on the forehead, as described above.

### PROTOCOL 7: MEASURING THE BANDWIDTH

1. **Objective**: Assess the brain's ability to understand deviated frequency information.
2. **Diagnosis**: Inject **D−0** in therapeutic (strong) mode, onto a point on the forehead.
   Search for an echo in diagnostic mode, with all the deviations of **D** frequency starting with **D+30** and **D−30**, to determine how far the echo still occurs.
3. **Treatment**: Scan the ear for a point that responds to both **A+30** and **A−30**, then treat the point with **A+30** and **A−30** in therapeutic (strong) mode. This should have the effect of broadening the bandwidth for all the frequencies.
4. **Check** that this is the case by repeating the initial measurement with **D** on the forehead.

## 22.4 CONCLUSION

Frequent stimulations constitute a very important field. The responses to these stimulations reflect the state of health or pathology of the organism. This led René Bourdiol (well-known neuroanatomist and auriculotherapist who worked with Paul Nogier for years) to name the frequency system "the royal road" among our techniques.

Furthermore, let us mention that we also work with a separate frequency system developed by Paul Nogier, called **beat frequencies**. They will be discussed in the fifth part of this book (Chapter 26).

From the therapeutic point of view, we can influence disorders of these frequency systems through fine adjustments, which can lead to powerful resonance effects. Of course, this also implies acting on these systems with caution.

## BIBLIOGRAPHY

1. Bourdiol René. *L'Auriculo-somatologie* (Maisonneuve) 1981; 97–15
2. Rouxeville Yves. *Personalized Auricular Acupuncture* (Sauramps médical) 2000; 130–141
3. Rouxeville Yves. *Les fréquences +20 et −20*, Revue Auriculomédecine 22 (1981); 31–32

## CHAPTER 23

# Evaluation of a Drug Substance

**Anthony de Sousa**

## 23.1 INTRODUCTION

Empirical evidence with the vascular reflex shows that the can react not only to colours or frequential stimulations but also to substances, whether natural, synthetic, medicinal or food. We do not know precisely by what analytical mechanisms or if the skin harbours specific micro-receptors; however, this certainly represents another example of photoreception on the skin surface.

It is well known that pharmaceutical companies have devoted considerable research resources over several years to determine a drug's therapeutic properties and adverse effects before introducing it to the market. This research is largely based on statistical evaluation methods, which form the basis of pharmacological knowledge of a drug. However, once the clinical indications of a drug have been defined, there remains considerable uncertainty as to how an individual patient may react to it.

Among the predictive methods that are beginning to be explored to answer this question, the vascular response, using the RAC, can be very effective, particularly when having to choose between different drugs for a given problem. It can help us determine, *in an individual patient*, if the substance is likely to have a positive effect and to what extent the undesirable effects are likely to be an obstacle. Paul Nogier used to say: "Checking the effect of drugs on human beings *by means of micro-information is a medical act of the utmost importance*" [1].

## 23.2 TECHNIQUES

To examine a drug using RAC, the drug is placed between the two transparent polycarbonate plates of an **empty test ring** (**Figure 12.6**). The substance to be tested can be a liquid, powder, a crushed tablet, or the content of a capsule. If the substance is liquid, a small round blotter will be soaked with the substance before placing it between the two polycarbonate plates but this is not compulsory. When several substances are placed in separate test rings for comparison, great care can be taken with handling to avoid contamination of one substance by another. The same precautions should, of course, be taken when a tablet or

 DOI: 10.1201/9781003753629-23

capsule is picked up with bare fingers for testing without using a test ring (this should be avoided).

Two different methods can be used to assess a drug, one using the test ring alone, the other using the test ring coupled with a colour filter.

### 23.2.1 Method Using the Drug Test Ring Alone

This method consists of the following three stages:

1. **Measure the distance at which a RAC occurs** by **approaching the** test ring on the axis of the ear. Start at a moderate speed from approximately 50–60 cm from the ear. The number of RACs, usually 3 or more, is unimportant for this technique.
   - The measurement can be repeated to confirm it, but also to determine if there are oscillations (at each approach, the pulse reacts at a different distance) and to correct them if necessary (see Chapter 13).
   - A RAC occurring about 6 to 8 cm from the auricle merely indicates that the organism recognises the substance and can, therefore, be considered normal. A RAC triggered *between 40 and 10 cm indicates **hyperreactivity***, the importance of which will be proportional to the distance measured. Clinically, this is equivalent to the non-desirability of the substance and may express either a possibility of side effects or intolerance to the substance.
2. **Contact of** the test ring on the auricle provides a second way of detecting ***hyperreactivity***. It involves one **first contact stage, this time** counting the resulting number of RACs. The contact should be maintained during the count.
   - **In a second stage**, the contact is repeated three to four times in rapid succession. Contact is then maintained whilst the number of RACs is once again counted.
   - The purpose of these two successive stages is to measure the difference *between the number of RACs* produced in both situations. *If the number of RACs produced by the second contact exceeds that produced by the first contact*, it indicates *hyperreactivity*. As with the approach manoeuvre described above, this may inform of possible side effects, but does not necessarily eliminate the prescription of the drug, except if the difference is very large, as this could be a sign of intolerance to the product.
3. **Rapid withdrawal of the test ring from the ear**, following the previous two stages, will now measure the ***desirability of the substance***.

The test ring is held against the auricle for one or two seconds and then abruptly "pulled" away from the ear. If there is no significant response, this indicates that the product is not expected to have a positive effect on the patient. If the substance can be helpful to the patient, this will be expressed by a marked, usually single RAC response (rebound). The process can be imagined as if the pulse reaction were to express a micro-stress of the organism due to suddenly being "deprived" of a substance which could have been capable of producing a positive effect.

The three stages described above should be considered as a unity in their interpretation. Together, they provide the practitioner with a personalised possibility of predicting the advantages and disadvantages of prescribing a particular drug to a given patient. In general, a rebound immediately after rapid withdrawal of the test ring indicates that a predominantly positive effect can be expected, unless there is a very strong response to the two hyperreactivity evaluations *(approach and contact).*

### 23.2.2 Method Using the Drug Test Ring Coupled with a Blue 44 or Orange 21 Colour Filter

Another personalised way of assessing a drug is to couple the test ring containing the drug either with a **Blue 44 filter**, indicating a biotic, i.e. beneficial, aspect of the product, or with an **Orange 21 (or 22) filter**, expressing the non-biotic, undesirable character related to side effects or intolerance.

The colour filter is placed between the drug test ring and the ear. While holding them together, **a single contact is made** against the auricle, and **the resulting number of RACs is counted**. This time, without the use of either approach or rapid withdrawal. The same procedure is then repeated with the drug coupled to the opposite colour filter, **Blue 44**. The order is not important.

Thus:

1. The number of positive RACs obtained by presenting the drug coupled with **Blue 44** is a measure of ***the desirability of*** the drug.
2. The number of positive RACs obtained by presenting the drug coupled with **Orange 21** measures ***the non-desirability of*** the drug.

Comparing the number of RACs obtained with the two colours assesses whether the substance should be prescribed. Intermediate situations are possible, from a reaction only to **Blue 44** (the substance is beneficial) to only to **Orange 21** (not beneficial). Intermediate situations, in which a vascular response to both colours is found, are

**Table 23.1 Summary for the Assessment of a Drug's Desirable and Undesirable Effects**

| | Hyperreactivity or undesirable effect | Desirable effect |
|---|---|---|
| **Drug alone** | RAC on approach (between 10 and 40 cm). Number of RACs at 2nd contact greater than Number of RACs at 1st contact | Strong RAC (rebound) on rapid withdrawal of the test ring from the ear |
| **Drug coupled with colour** | Reaction at contact with **Orange 21** | Reaction at contact with **Blue 44** |

to be considered individually. **Table 23.1** summarises the two techniques, both techniques have their advantages.

The one using the drug alone can provide a rapid first estimation, while using colour filters gives more quantitative accuracy due to counting the number of RACs.

## 23.3 COMMENTS

In various severe clinical situations requiring extensive chemotherapy, it may help to compare the responses (number of RACs) to **Blue 44** and **Orange 21** to choose between several relevant drugs. It may be that the number of RACs to **Blue 44** for a given substance is much higher than for the other substances, thus determining the choice, despite pharmacologically predictable adverse effects and a clear response to **Orange 21**. The best response is, therefore, not necessarily in favour of the drug with the least toxicity or side effects. The body appears to be able to indicate through cutaneous photoreception the drug that is most likely to be effective, regardless of the side effects. These tests, therefore, provide us with an aid for deciding whether to use a drug for a given patient, thus, to some extent, being able to personalise the treatment.

On a more anecdotal level, in general medicine practices where the physician has taken the habit of currently checking on the vascular response when prescribing a drug, the medical assistants who work in the office can often notice a considerable reduction in telephone calls from patients complaining about the adverse effects of their treatments!

## PROTOCOL 8: EVALUATION OF A DRUG

### Instruments

1. The test ring containing the drug to be tested
2. A **Blue 44 filter** and an **Orange 21 filter**

Measurements can be made with the test ring containing the drug either alone or coupled with the colours.

### Preliminary Measures

- RAC calibration

### Criteria for a "Favourable" Drug

#### *Drug Alone*

1. Lack of reaction on approach and contact with the ear
2. Rebound reaction to abrupt withdrawal of the drug from the ear

#### *Drug Coupled with Colours*

1. Contact reaction of the drug with **Blue 44**
2. No or little reaction at contact with the drug, coupled with **Orange 21**

### Criteria for a Drug That Is Toxic or to Which the Patient Is Hypersensitive or Intolerant

#### *Drug Alone*

1. Presence of reaction at a distance and at contact
2. Lack of reaction to rapid withdrawal from the ear

#### *Colour-Coupled Drug*

1. Reaction on contact with **Orange 21**
2. No reaction on contact with **Blue 44**

## BIBLIOGRAPHY

1. Nogier Paul and Raphaël. *L'Homme dans l'Oreille* (Maisonneuve) 1979; 142–144
2. Rouxeville Yves. *Personalized Auricular Acupuncture* (Sauramps Médical) 2000; 15

CHAPTER 24

# The RAC Applied to Smoking Withdrawal

**Anthony de Sousa**

## 24.1 INTRODUCTION

The harmfulness of tobacco dependency is proportional to the difficulty of giving it up. Although it can in many cases be achieved without too much difficulty, as a rule it takes some perseverance, partly because cigarette makers currently use substances to the effect of increasing dependency. As practitioners, we can be of considerable help in reducing the difficulty, provided we obtain the patient's active participation. In this field, it is not possible to overlook the patient's motivation.

In the field of smoking cessation, the vascular response (the RAC) has three main advantages:

1. *The possibility of measuring the degree of dependency*, particularly for comparing dependency before and after treatment.
2. *Personalisation of the points to be treated* for withdrawal.
3. *Anticipation of the pathologies* that would be likely to result from continuing to smoke.

Before going to a medical consultation for withdrawal, the patient is advised to have smoked the last cigarette at least three hours before the interview. Furthermore, the practitioner needs to take sufficient time to get acquainted with the patient, who is often seen for the first time, to understand the historical context and, above all, to assess the motivation and circumstances that led them to this decision. Without a strong demand and efficient cooperation, it is hardly possible to achieve a successful withdrawal.

The intention of cessation for the sake of pleasing another person, for instance a spouse, is almost certainly due to fail. The decision can only be made by oneself. It is also important to ensure that the process of quitting does not coincide with a period of existential difficulties, and to postpone the project if necessary. It can take up to three or four unsuccessful attempts before being able to "measure the obstacle" sufficiently well to get through the process successfully.

## 24.2 MEASURING THE DEGREE OF DEPENDENCY

**A test ring containing tobacco** must be available. Usually, a practitioner has a small collection of these, from which he can choose a tobacco close to that of the patient. If not, he can produce a test ring containing tobacco brought by the patient.

DOI: 10.1201/9781003753629-24

As with the evaluation of a drug discussed in the previous chapter, we can use the tobacco test ring either alone or in combination with the **blue 44** and **orange 21** colour filters.

The technical aspects are the same as with a drug, but their *interpretation is reversed*, since the object is not concerned with finding an adequate therapeutic substance, but with a toxic substance that has already created an addictive process within the brain.

Thus, a strong, unique RAC (rebound, which is not to be counted) on rapid withdrawal from the ear of a tobacco test ring *alone*, as well as a RAC reaction (which can be counted) *to ear contact* when the tobacco test ring is coupled with **blue 44**, does not mean that the substance is beneficial, as would be the case for a drug, but that *the brain "wrongly" considers it desirable.* This is the sign of addiction.

Conversely, a distant reaction to the *approach of tobacco alone*, or a reaction to contact when the tobacco test ring is coupled with the **orange 21**, means that the brain has "recognised" the substance as non-beneficial and is, therefore, to be rejected. This is a sign of an absence or reduced addiction. These data are summarised in the following **Table 24.1**.

**Table 24.1 Measures Indicating Tobacco Dependence and Non-Dependence, Respectively**

| | Addiction (before treatment) | Non-addiction (or after successful treatment) |
|---|---|---|
| Tobacco alone | No reaction on approaching: Rebound on rapid withdrawal | Reaction on approaching: No reaction on rapid withdrawal |
| Tobacco coupled with colours | Reaction on contact with **Blue 44** | Reaction on contact with **Orange 21** |

Prior to treatment, the measurements generally correspond to the situation described under Addiction (left-hand column in the table). The aim of treatment is *to* ***reverse the measurements to non-addiction*** (right-hand column on the table) as thoroughly as possible. If this is not the case, the treatment should be repeated.

## 24.3 DETECTION OF THE MAIN EAR POINTS DETECTED FOR TOBACCO WITHDRAWAL

By imposing the **tobacco test ring on the chest**, *points corresponding to the effects of tobacco deprivation* will appear on the ear. These can be detected by scanning the ear with a white tip or Heine's lamp. This step is essential, as it will define the points to be treated for a personalized treatment. It should be noted that we will often come across points that were already part of the anti-tobacco programmes seen in general auriculotherapy (without the pulse). But working with the pulse allows the treatment to be directed and personalised, often restricting the number of points to those most likely to be active. The points are usually treated with semi-permanent needles or cryotherapy.

Among the points usually detected for RAC-assisted withdrawal under imposition of a tobacco test ring on the chest, the most frequent are illustrated below (**Figure 24.1**).

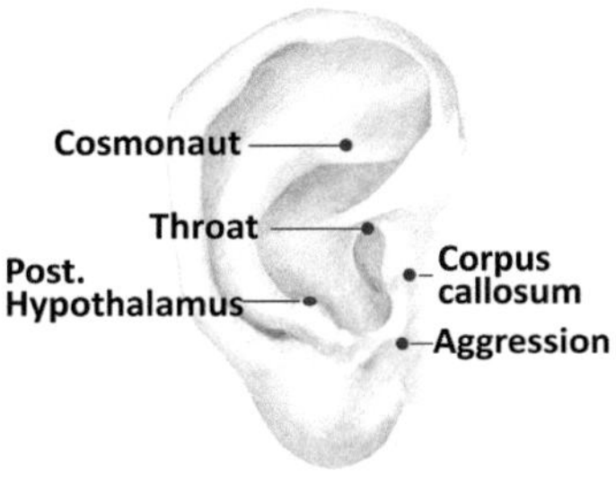


**Figure 24.1** Commonly detected points during tobacco withdrawal.

- *The "cosmonaut" point*, representing the paravertebral sympathetic ganglion D12-L1, is the first to send an electrical signal to the brain in case of stress.
- *The corpus callosum point* involved in interhemispheric communications.
- *The TSH point, the so-called "aggressivity point",* reflects the irritability often associated with withdrawal.
- *The posterior hypothalamus point* may compensate for the vagotonia linked to withdrawal.
- *The throat point is* related to the local sensation of pleasure when smoking.

## 24.4 POSSIBLE ESTIMATION OF ORGANS AFFECTED BY SMOKING

The ear points generated by the stress of withdrawal are one thing. Quite another are the points related to tobacco-induced pathologies. These can be at least partially estimated, even if it makes no sense to treat them. This step is not meant to lead directly to withdrawal but offers the possibility of a valuable discussion for the patient.

Technically, ***by imposing the tobacco test ring on the arm***, one or more ear points corresponding to possible pathological targets already present or likely to appear in the event of continued smoking will be induced and detected by scanning both ears. The most frequently encountered potential targets are, of course, the cardiovascular and respiratory systems. For some patients, providing this kind of prognostic information may reinforce their decision to quit smoking. For others, of course, it would only cause anxiety and would therefore better be avoided. It is up to the physician to adopt the best possible strategy applicable to an individual patient.

## 24.5 CHECKING AFTER TREATMENT

Immediately after auriculotherapy treatment, a new assessment of the degree of addiction should be performed, as described above. At this stage (see **Table 24.1**), the tobacco test ring alone should induce a RAC at approach and not produce a rebound at rapid withdrawal. When coupled to colours, the test ring should no longer react to ear contact when coupled to **blue 44**, but react when coupled to **orange 21**. If this is not the case, or if the addiction is only partially reduced, the ear should be scanned again under imposition of the tobacco test ring on the chest.

## 24.6 CLINICAL EXAMPLE

A 61-year-old male patient with satisfactory general health and an athletic, nervous temperament has been in the habit of smoking approximately 20 cigarettes a day since the age of 18. He has been reluctant to quit for a long time, fearing weight gain.

On pulse-assisted ear examination, the basic parameters are normal.

Examination with the tobacco test ring shows no reaction to an approach in line with the ear but gives a strong response to **rapid withdrawal from the ear**. Coupled with **blue 44**, the test ring induces 12 positive RACs but no reaction when coupled to **orange 21**. These are typical data for an installed addiction.

**Imposing the tobacco test ring on the chest** simulates tobacco deprivation. It allows detection of ear points that will be useful for withdrawal treatment (**Figure 24.2**). In this right-handed patient, three points appear on the right ear: corpus callosum, throat, **and TSH/aggressivity**, and two points on the left ear: **corpus callosum** and

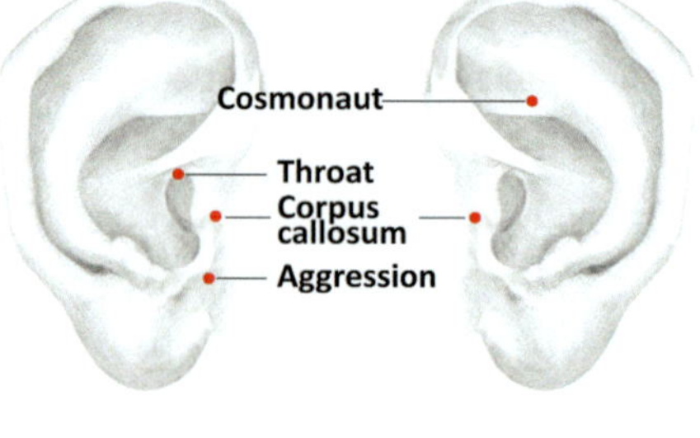


**Figure 24.2** Points detected under smoking deprivation (test ring imposed on the chest).

the so-called **cosmonaut** point. This relatively small number of points proved sufficient to induce a non-addiction formula after treatment. The patient succeeded in stopping smoking.

Finally, imposition of the tobacco test ring on the arm, to anticipate potential pathological targets due to tobacco, reveals on both ears the presence of **lung** points in the lower hemi concha and a **mucosal bladder** point at the base of the wall of the upper hemi concha (**Figure 24.3**). These points, marked in blue in the figure, were not intended to be treated and were only of prognostic interest. Eventually, even though he had managed to stop smoking, the follow-up showed that the patient developed cancer of the bladder two years later.

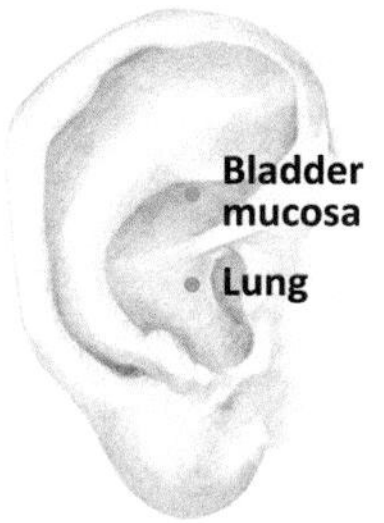


**Figure 24.3** Prognostic points of organs that could be altered in the long run by tobacco.

## 24.7 INSTRUCTIONS AFTER WITHDRAWAL

The instructions to follow after withdrawal, including the frequency of follow-up visits, hydration, and nutrition, remain unchanged from those described in general auriculotherapy.

## PROTOCOL 9: SMOKING WITHDRAWAL

1. ***Instruments to be used***

   - A **tobacco** test ring containing tobacco similar or identical to that of the patient
   - A **blue 44** filter **and** an **orange 21** filter
   - Measurements can be made with tobacco alone or coupled with colours

2. ***Criteria for tobacco dependency***

   **Tobacco alone**
   - Lack of reaction on approach and contact
   - Reaction to rapid withdrawal

   **Tobacco coupled with colours**
   - Reaction to contact with tobacco coupled with **blue 44**
   - No reaction to contact with tobacco coupled with **orange 21**

3. ***Detection of the points to be treated***: under imposition of the tobacco test ring (alone) on the thorax

4. ***Treatment of detected points:*** with the same imposition

5. ***Criteria for successful treatment*** (or non-dependence): formula reversed from **3**

   **Tobacco alone**
   - Presence of reaction to approach and contact
   - Absence of reaction to rapid withdrawal

   **Tobacco coupled with colours**
   - Reaction to contact of tobacco with **orange 21**
   - No reaction to contact of tobacco with **blue 44**

6. ***Possible estimation of the organs that may be affected by tobacco:*** detection under the imposition of the tobacco test ring on the arm

## BIBLIOGRAPHY

1. Nogier Paul. *Les Programmes Delta*, Revue Auriculomédecine No 5: (1976) 46–48
2. Nogier Paul and Raphaël. *L'Homme dans l'Oreille* (Maisonneuve): 1979; 89–94

CHAPTER 25

# The Photogram

Raphaël Nogier

## 25.1 PRINCIPLE

A photogram is a technique that allows us to assess the photoreception of coloured light on the skin. When we carry out a white light test that will trigger RACs, we are unaware of the wavelength(s) of light responsible for inducing the RAC. White light is, in essence, very composite, ranging from 380 to 780 nanometres in wavelength. It is therefore made up of photons of different wavelengths. Any stimulation with light, white or coloured, should trigger a RAC. In pathological situations, however, despite of a normal white light test, there can be a lack of reaction to one or more coloured lights. This is called a *photoreception gap and* may be linked to certain pathologies, which we will deal with specifically.

## 25.2 TECHNIQUE

A photogram requires an adequate lighting system. For many years, we have been using the Theralight, made by Sedatelec. Today, we use the Microlight, an Italian instrument made by Micropad (**Figure 25.1**). This device, which we have contributed to developing, contains a wide lamp, making it possible to project light onto a large surface of the thorax and abdomen. The front panel contains the controls for selecting either white light or one of the 15 pre-programmed colours.

Normally, any coloured light should trigger a RAC over three pulse cycles. If the reactivity index is seven with white light, the reactivity index will be seven for each coloured light.

It is important to wait for the RAC to come to extinction after each colour illumination.

This technique aims to determine if there are any photoreception gaps, i.e. any colour for which there is no reaction.

## 25.3 INTERPRETATION

We believe that each wavelength of light stimulates the production of a particular chemical neuromediator. Yellow light is expected to stimulate dopamine production, while red light stimulates the production of serotonin.

Therefore, a photoreception gap signifies a “deficiency” in producing a particular neuromediator.

DOI: 10.1201/9781003753629-25

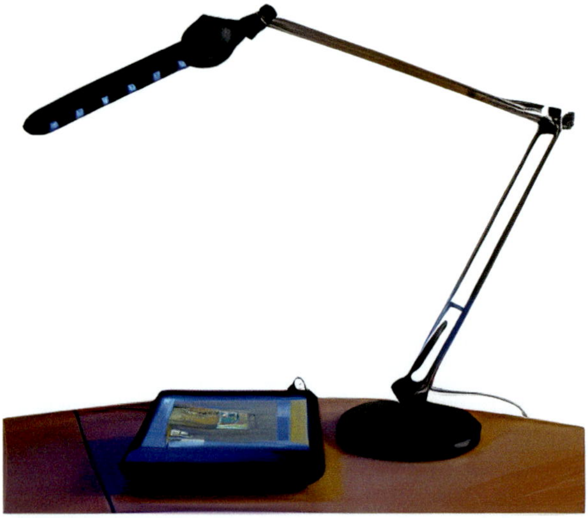

**Figure 25.1** The Microlight, made by Micropad, can illuminate both large areas of the body and ear points.

## 25.4 TREATMENT

Treating a skin photoreception gap implies searching for one or several points on the ear, which produce a RAC when exposed to the colour that fails to produce a RAC when projected on the body. If, for example, there is a photoreception gap with blue light, we will search for the ear points that produce a RAC when exposed to this same blue light. For this, the Micropad is equipped with a special point detector capable of emitting punctual beams of the same colours projected on the body.

**Psoriasis** is a demonstrative example. In this type of disease, the healthy-looking parts of the skin appear free of any lesions. However, they fail to receive blue light. Indeed, projection of blue light on these parts of the skin does not induce a RAC, whereas projection of the same blue light onto the psoriasis lesions does produce a RAC reaction. We then search on the ear for points reacting to blue light and confirm them with an electronic point detector. These points can then be treated, generally with acupuncture needles inserted for approximately 20 minutes.

To study skin photoreception in depth, a photogram must be systematically tested. If there is a defect in the photoreception of coloured light, food tests (RAFT: see Chapter 27) cannot be carried out, because their interpretation is based exclusively on skin photoreception.

## BIBLIOGRAPHY

1. Nogier Raphaël. *Introduction to Auriculomedicine*. Haug 1993

CHAPTER 26

# Symmetry, Laterality, and Tragus
## *The Case of Multiple Sclerosis*

**Raphaël Nogier**

## 26.1 INTRODUCTION

Referring to the fundamental frequency concepts described in Chapter 21, clinical practice reveals that the skin is not receptive to the same frequencies on the right and left sides of the body (hemi-bodies). Paul Nogier had observed with the RAC that there is an asymmetry of photoreception for some frequencies. Knowledge and understanding of this phenomenon enable us to diagnose and treat numerous pathologies such as postural disorders, dyslexia, depression, multiple sclerosis (MS) attacks, and autoimmune disease attacks.

While Chapter 21 established the theoretical framework distinguishing **D** frequency (symmetry) from **L** frequency (laterality), clinical application requires a deeper understanding of these two complementary yet distinct biological functions and their therapeutic implications.

## 26.2 THE BIOLOGICAL FOUNDATIONS OF SYMMETRY AND LATERALITY

### 26.2.1 The Notion of Symmetry

We have two arms, two legs, two eyes, and two ears because, fundamentally, we are built on a principle of symmetry. It is indeed impossible to conceive locomotion in a living being without a symmetry axis, on either side of which two identical parts are designed as in a mirror image. This symmetry exists in all animal species: insects, spiders, reptiles, birds, and mammals. Symmetry is an absolute necessity.

Embryologically, organs derived from the endoderm are single: one oesophagus, one stomach, one intestine, one liver and one pancreas, whereas those derived from the mesoderm are double: two arms, two legs, but also two kidneys, two ovaries, two testicles The mesoderm is the embryological layer from which locomotion originates and thus gives rise to symmetry and to double organs.

Along with the evolution of species, Guy Lazorthes, a French physician and embryologist, reminds us that the mesoderm is the embryological layer that

DOI: 10.1201/9781003753629-26

appears last, after the endoderm and the ectoderm. He clearly associates mesoderm with symmetry:

> *The acquisition of a third cell layer, the mesoderm, will provide the Metazoans, which appeared later and are said to be triploblastic, with extensive potentialities, especially the possibility of developing organs with a specific function, in particular fast-contracting muscles. By becoming triploblastic, animal beings have taken a big step forward. An essential and inexplicable phenomenon is the fact that animals acquire symmetry and an axis with a 'front' and a 'back'* [1].

Although finding a precise finality for Man and life in general is difficult, let us remember that a large part of an animal's nervous system tends towards a single objective: locomotion. Being able to move is indeed vital and is one of the characteristics of the animal world compared to the plant world. To avoid predators, search for food, protect itself from cold and heat, eliminate undesirable animals, and reproduce, it is essential to develop locomotion and, therefore, symmetry. It should be stressed that a large part of the nervous system tends to stimulate movement and locomotion. Sensory systems would not exist if locomotion did not exist. Indeed, most sensations, such as hunger, thirst, cold, heat, or even feelings like fear and jealousy, only make sense if there is a possibility of movement by locomotion. When an animal is hungry, it looks for food; when it is hot, it looks for shade; when it is afraid, it will run away.

The symmetrical aspect of animal architecture must be understood from the point of view of locomotion. Every animal has a tendency towards symmetry, to the extent that we can even speak of symmetry as a function (**Figure 26.1**). This is particularly striking with butterflies.

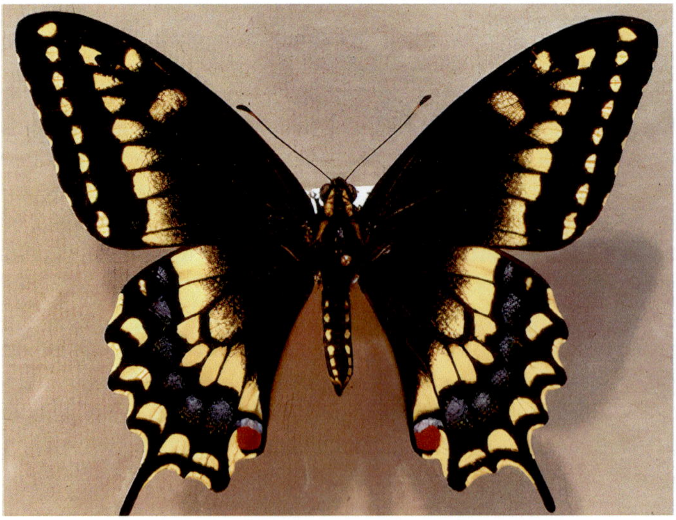

**Figure 26.1** Symmetry can be observed in all animals.

The following law could be stated:

> *Every animal organism has a symmetry function that naturally tends to develop two identical sides with respect to a central axis.*

This function of symmetry, under the control of several nerve centres, is undoubtedly one of the most complex and stable functions in living organisms. It can be observed that congenital malformations in humans do not concern symmetry, which is generally maintained in most cases.

The near-perfect symmetry within animals is indeed astonishing. For example, the wings of a butterfly are identical point by point when looked at with a mirror, as is the feathering of a bird of prey.

The nervous system of all animals is organised around this binarity. The brain comprises two cerebral hemispheres linked together by inter-hemispheric fibres, which promote coordination and exchange of information between the hemispheres. This dual configuration is found in birds, reptiles, and mammals. Each hemisphere controls the motor functions of the opposite hemisphere. No animal can be found in nature with a brain made of one piece. The brain is always split into two parts, regardless of the animal. This rule is absolute.

A functional symmetry accompanies this anatomical and geometrical symmetry. The animal uses one side or the other indifferently. If we consider monkeys tapping a coconut with a stone, 50% of the monkeys use one hand and 50% the other.

An animal is built on an almost perfect symmetry.

### 26.2.2 The Notion of Laterality: When Binarity becomes Duality

Unlike animals, humans will give preference, as far as motricity is concerned, to one side of the body rather than the other, although they are, at birth, geometrically built on both sides of a symmetry axis. This phenomenon, known as laterality, leads to progressive loss of symmetry. It has been found that approximately 90% of human beings write with their right hand, kick a ball with their right foot, and have a directing eye on the right. This preference, called dextrality, is found indifferently north as well as south of the equator and on all continents. It is genetically programmed and leads to a morphological and functional dissymmetry.

We know that, from the moment of birth, a baby will show a preference for one side: 90% of newborns lying on their back turn their head towards the right side, whereas only 10% towards the left. This preference, hardly noticeable at first, will become increasingly evident over the years. As the child grows, they will use one hand more than the other, one foot more than the other, and acquire an increasingly marked motor preference for one side (right or left). This will lead, on the one hand, to anatomical asymmetry (one shoulder higher than the other) and, on the other, to cerebral asymmetry. Furthermore, it is difficult to make the difference between cause and effect: is it because there is a motor laterality that the hemispheres become asymmetrical? Or does motor laterality depend on the fact that the hemispheres are asymmetrical? I think the answer can be argued both ways. From birth, a baby has a natural tendency towards laterality. However, it is by using one side more than the other that the child will really settle into their laterality and will, therefore, stimulate one hemisphere more than the other.

In humans, the two cerebral hemispheres develop different functions. Born with two identical cerebral hemispheres, the left hemisphere, under the influence of education, will gradually acquire capacities that the right hemisphere does not possess.

In the 19th century, Broca was credited with the discovery that 96% of patients suffering from right-sided hemiplegia lose the ability to speak. So, it was Broca who discovered that the left hemisphere is the hemisphere of language. He then spoke of a dominant major hemisphere (the left) and a dominated minor hemisphere (the right). This notion of dominant and dominated hemispheres led to much confusion among neurologists for many years.

It was not until the end of the twentieth century that the function of the hemispheres became clearer. Sperry, Nobel Prize winner in 1981 and neurosurgeon, understood that the two cerebral hemispheres each have their own function.

The right hemisphere is more related to perception.
The left hemisphere is more related to abstraction.

Although examples of very limited functional asymmetry can be found within animals, it can be said that their two hemispheres are almost identical.

The hen, for example, can use the right eye **independently of** the left. Thus, the two eyes can be used for two different tasks simultaneously.

It all starts in the egg. Just before hatching, the chick's head is positioned so that the right eye is pressed against the shell and, thus, perceives light coming from outside the shell.

The left eye, on the other hand, is directed against the body of the chick. If it has not hatched, this eye does not perceive anything.

After hatching, each eye specialises. The right eye serves to find food. Thus, its near vision is better. The left eye is used preferentially for spotting predators. Thus, its distance vision is better.

In birds, song is a function located in the left hemisphere.

However, all these differences are minimal, whereas they are significant in humans.

### 26.2.3 Hemispheric Specialisation in Humans

What will happen if a right-handed patient's right hemisphere is out of order?

This situation can occur in strokes or if a selective unilateral electroshock neutralises the right hemisphere. The patient will function only with their left hemisphere.

The left hemisphere subject will retain certain aptitudes and lose others. Emotionally, he is well-tempered, sociable, and cheerful, and can, if asked, collaborate with those around him to answer questions or participate in tests. Speech, as we have seen, is preserved. The subject will speak normally. Speech is fluid; there is no hesitation in the choice of words. The melody of speech, however, is altered. The tone is monotonous. If asked to perform a complicated calculation, division, or multiplication, his skills are excellent and they are not only preserved but improved. If the subject is made to listen to a famous song—for example of "*The Sound of Silence*"—the left hemisphere subject is unable to recognise the voices of Simon and Garfunkel, or whether it is a man or a woman singing, they will be unable to recognise the melody, let alone sing it. But on the other hand, he will be able to recite the words of the song and understand them. If the subject is shown two similar drawings: in the first, a house with one door and three windows; in the second, a house with two doors, five windows, and two chimneys on the roof, the subject will not be able to see the differences; he will say that the first drawing represents a house and that the second also represents a house. As can be seen, the faculties of perception are diminished, but those of abstraction are preserved or even increased.

What happens if the left hemisphere is artificially neutralized in a right-handed person?

In this situation, the right hemisphere subject will lose speech and become aphasic. He will utter unintelligible gibberish. His mood is affected, and he becomes emotional, pessimistic, and less cooperative. He understands only a small number of words. He cannot say where he is, the date, or the year. If he is made to listen to "*The Sound of Silence*", he will recognise the voices of Simon and Garfunkel and will be able to hum the melody but will have difficulty with the text of the song. His mathematical skills are non-existent. On the other hand, if he is presented with two drawings that look alike, he will recognise the differences at first glance.

To quote once again Guy Lazorthes: "*We can therefore conclude that the left hemisphere governs logical and abstract analytical thinking as used in language and mathematics; the right hemisphere governs concrete thinking and mental imagery as used in artistic creation, for example*".

### 26.2.4 Laterality, Intelligence, and Development

While animals have two almost identical hemispheres, the two hemispheres in humans are functionally different and perfectly complementary. This allows humans to develop exceptional abilities and differentiates them from other animals that do not have a "left hemisphere".

What makes man superior to the great ape is his capacity for abstraction due to the left hemisphere. Socrates' "know thyself" or Descartes' "I think, therefore I am" are thoughts that require exceptional cerebral machinery. The consciousness of being, i.e. the consciousness of oneself, requires a sum of abstractions that only the left hemisphere can produce. This self-awareness is also expressed by being able to recognise oneself in a mirror, something that dogs, cats, and even great apes are incapable of doing.

Another specific human capacity is autonoetic consciousness. It consists of being aware of time and moving freely through this dimension. *Yesterday, I went shopping; tomorrow, I will go to the countryside; next year, I will buy a new car; and in 1066, William the Conqueror won the Battle of Hastings.* Each of us can walk through history by taking reference points. One minute has 60 seconds. Sixty minutes amount to one hour. Twenty-four hours define a day. A year is made of three hundred and sixty-five days. This seems natural to us, normal, and easy. Yet, animals do not seem to be capable of thinking this way. Lucretius reminds us in "*De natura rerum*" that an animal lives in the present. It evidently has a memory due to learning but does not measure time. A cow cannot anticipate the next day and think *tomorrow, I will go and graze in the field out there.*

Perception of time is a very elaborate function. Without a brain, time does not exist, any more than colours could exist without eyes. A child only begins to understand time at a late stage. Whereas it acquires speech very early and can make complex constructions and draw, it takes several years for a child to distinguish between today, yesterday, and tomorrow. Virtually, a child lives in eternity. It is only around the age of six, the age of writing and of reason, that a child leaves the world of eternity to enter the world of finality and, therefore, of death. He then understands that man has an end and that he is mortal. He gradually realises that his days are limited and so are the people he sees every day. His mother and father are not eternal. This is why the child begins to develop metaphysical anxieties at this stage. From a neurological point of view, this perception of time can disappear if a lesion occurs in the left hemisphere.

Finally, man is creative. This makes the most significant difference from animals. He can elaborate very complex abstractions. The fields of mathematics, literature, and music are evidence of this.

Man considers the world in an asymmetrical manner. According to Guy Lazorthes: *"First, the two hemispheres receive together the information that comes from the surrounding world; subsequently, each hemisphere then extracts what is particularly relevant to it, processes it according to its specialisation and then communicates the processed information to the other hemisphere. Each hemisphere has its own memory, its own archives; one hemisphere perceives the world with its richness and its diversity, and the other hemisphere analyses it".*

When I see the world around me, hear the noises around me, and touch the world around me, the information is processed by the right hemisphere.

When I deal with abstractions, when I talk, or when I calculate, I use my left hemisphere. The left hemisphere is a machine for creating abstractions.

The importance of the corpus callosum in these complex mechanisms should be stressed here. This commissure unites the right and left hemispheres and enables communication from one to the other. The corpus callosum consists of over 200 million axons, originating mainly from cells belonging to the cerebral cortex. A surgical removal of the corpus callosum, sometimes necessary, shows to what extent it is essential regarding laterality.

### 26.2.5 The Paradox

Man must face a strange paradox. He must symmetrize himself to run fast and de-symmetrize himself to be intelligent. This is perfectly antinomic and leads us to a burning issue: can one run fast and be intelligent? Here are a few elements to reflect upon.

Intelligence largely depends on the left hemisphere's abilities for abstraction and conceptualisation. Mathematical reasoning, academic music, and mastery of language all require learning specific abstractions. Today, we often speak of different types rather than one single form of intelligence. The term emotional intelligence is frequently used. Nevertheless, the great geniuses of humanity have been known to work with totally abstract concepts. To do so, they must have worked with dissymmetrical brains. This leads us to believe that it seems difficult, if not impossible, to develop symmetry and its opposite simultaneously. Developing intelligence implies decreasing speed! I am aware, of course, that such comments will hardly be acceptable to many readers. However, facts are facts and cannot be ignored.

Does this entail that we should privilege study over speed? I do not think so. The proverb "*mens sana in corpore sano*" reminds us of the importance of a well-balanced life. We could change this proverb by saying: "*develop intelligence harmoniously without hindering symmetry too much*". Some would say that there is a need for balance.

It should be noted that some types of sports requiring speed or coordinated movements, such as running, gymnastics, cycling, or swimming, tend to develop symmetry, while others, like tennis, table tennis, and golf, tend towards asymmetry.

## 26.3 CLINICAL ASSESSMENT METHODS

We have different types of tests: those that evaluate the subject's symmetry, those that will define the subject's laterality (right- or left-handed), and those that assess the quality of work of each hemisphere. These three types of tests will allow us to establish precise diagnoses.

### 26.3.1 Clinical Tests for Detecting Symmetry Disorders (without Using the RAC)

The idea is to measure the difference in height between the shoulders and between the hands while they rest along the body (**Figure 26.2**). The subject should be standing, with shoes and glasses on, looking to the horizon, feet open at 30°, and there should be no dental contact.

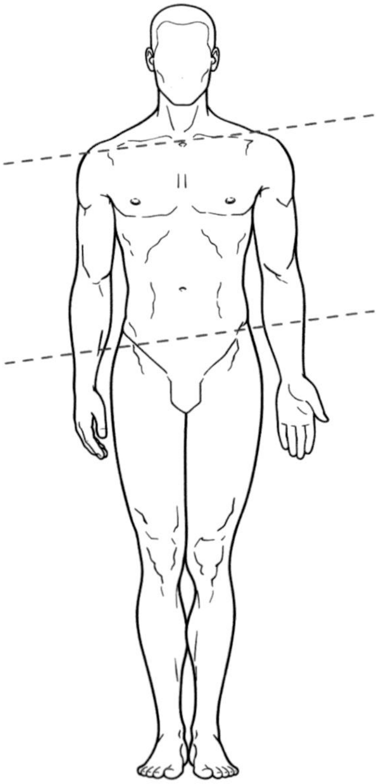

**Figure 26.2** In a right-handed person, the right shoulder is generally lower.

We then observe the shoulder line and the bi-iliac line. A confirmed asymmetry exists when there is a difference of three digits (fingers) between the right and left sides.

### 26.3.2 Clinical Tests to Measure Laterality (without Using the RAC)

How do we determine if a person is right-handed or left-handed?

A right-handed person is defined by the fact that the language centre is in the left hemisphere, whereas a true left-handed person's language centre is in the right hemisphere.

#### *26.3.2.1 Defining the Directing Eye*

To do this, the subject must be asked to look through a monocular microscope or to do as if he were to take a photograph with an ancient type of camera, where one has to look through the viewfinder with only one eye. This test makes it possible to know which eye the subject aims with, which generally coincides with the subject's laterality. However, the test is not valid if the subject suffers from an ocular pathology.

#### *26.3.2.2 Defining the Directing Foot*

The subject stands up in front of the examiner, who gradually pushes them backwards until destabilised. The destabilized subject will move the directing foot towards the rear to prevent falling. It will be the right foot for right-handed people and the left foot for left-handed people.

#### *26.3.2.3 Defining the Directing Hand*

The directing hand is more difficult to define because it is influenced by the "cultural" aspects. Many children have been taught to write with their right hand, whereas they would naturally use their left hand. For ages, society has been conditioned for right-handed people, with left-handed people being considered almost as pathological exceptions. This has forced left-handed people to adapt. To find the directing hand, it is necessary to perform tests in which the cultural aspect is not involved: ball throwing, distributing cards in card playing, slingshot, archery, etc.

Usually, a true right-handed person has a directing eye, a directing foot, and a directing hand all on the right. For the true left-handed person, it is the opposite. The fact is that about 10% of the population is not totally oriented as far as laterality is concerned, and some people write with their right hand but have a directing left eye or a directing left foot. These cases represent a form of dyslaterality, often associated with various disorders.

### 26.3.2.4 Assessing the Activity of the Cerebral Hemispheres: The Eye Deviation Test

The test aims to determine which cerebral hemisphere is predominantly active during "mental imagination activities" or "abstract operations".

When a subject is in a calm, stress-free atmosphere, their eyes deviate to the side opposite to the active hemisphere (**Figure 26.3**). When the right hemisphere is most active, the eyes deviate towards the left. When the left hemisphere is most active, the eyes deviate to the right. This is an easily observable phenomenon because it can be reproduced.

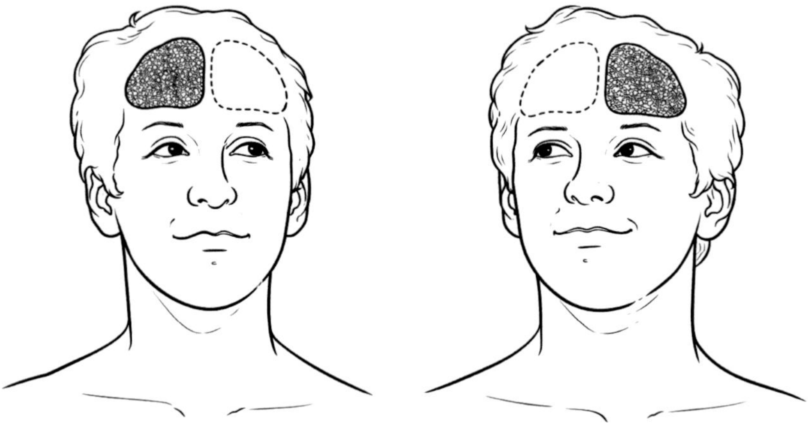

**Figure 26.3** The eyes deviate towards the side opposite to the active hemisphere.

In a well-balanced subject, during a relaxed conversation, for example, the eyes sometimes deviate to the right, sometimes to the left. This shows that the subject will refer to the whole range of information given by his brain: imaginative as well as abstract information.

This deviation of the gaze will be oriented on one side only when the subject must concentrate on a specific situation. The test, therefore, consists of placing the subject in front of a mental situation involving one or the other of the two hemispheres.

If a right-handed subject is presented with a situation that addresses the right hemisphere: "Can you imagine a summer evening on a beach, you hear the sound of waves, the cry of seagulls, a guitar in the distance", the subject will turn their eyes to the left.

Whereas when the subject's left hemisphere is addressed: "How much is thirteen multiplied by seventeen?" the subject will perform a mental calculation, and their eyes will move to the right after a few seconds of concentration.

For this test to be interpretable, it is important that the subject is not familiar with this principle and that the conversation occurs as naturally as possible during a discussion that does not suggest a test. Moreover, the "trick" should not be revealed to the patient after the test so that it can be repeated later.

As we shall see, this test can provide us with valuable information about how our patients function. It will help make diagnoses and monitor the treatments we institute.

### 26.3.3 Testing Symmetry with the RAC

Working with the RAC and with frequencies allows us to obtain a more precise idea of a patient's symmetry function. Using the RAC will help to detect, but above all, to quantify disorders.

**Technique**: we will apply fundamental frequencies and observe the vascular reactions (RAC) obtained when we project each of the frequencies **A, B, C, D, E, F, G,** and **L** onto the **sagittal midline of the forehead** (**Figure 26.4**). Normally, only **frequency D** will produce a RAC response that will last for three pulses. If this is indeed the case, we can deduce that the symmetry function is of good quality. If not, we examine which parasite frequencies produce the RAC and respond instead of **D**. These will indicate which territories on the ear need to be examined and treated to restore the symmetry function.

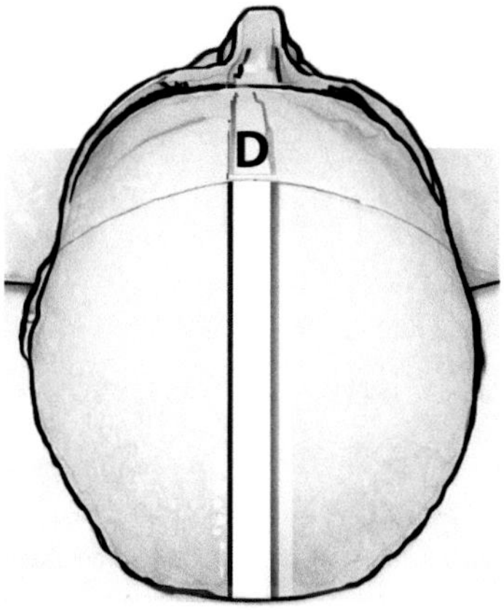


**Figure 26.4** The median sagittal line on the forehead (D line) normally reacts to D frequency.

### 26.3.4 Testing Laterality with the RAC: Two Different Methods

The frequencies we use to measure laterality are of two different kinds: on one side, the **L frequency** (Chapter 21), and on the other, a new type of frequencies called **beat frequencies**.

1. The first method consists of **projecting L frequency** onto the **L line** (**Figure 26.5**). This is a 4 cm wide sagittal midline located on the scalp, under the hair. It follows the **D** line. The **L** line was first described in 2006. Normally, only the **L** frequency triggers a RAC when projected onto the **L** line.
2. The second method for measuring laterality uses a type of **beat frequencies** that Paul Nogier discovered in the early eighties. He described two beat frequencies: the first is called **low frequency** (**BF**), corresponding to **3.75 Hz**[1]. The second is called **high frequency (HF)**, corresponding to **8.74 Hz**. To explore these two frequencies, Nogier developed a specific generator called the **DB 165**. Today, we mainly use the **GL+** by Micropad (**Figure 12.16**), the **Premio 40** by Sedatelec (**Figure 12.17**) or other generators which are capable of delivering both fundamental and beat frequencies.

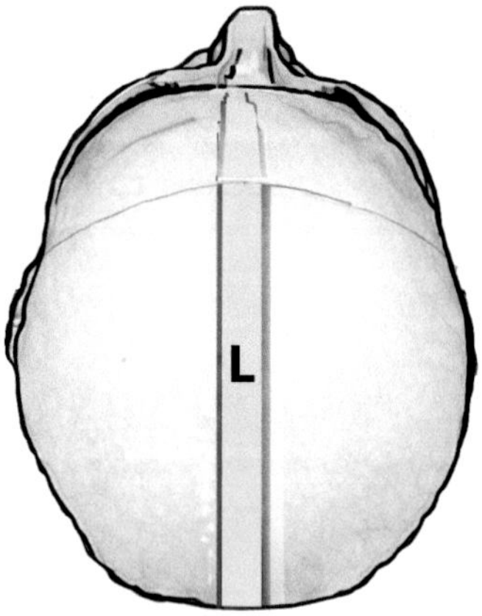


**Figure 26.5** The median sagittal line (L line) on the head normally reacts to the L frequency.

The name "**beat frequencies**" was chosen by analogy with the physics of musical instruments. When two strings of an instrument, say a piano, are tuned to a very close but not strictly identical frequency, the two sounds produced will be only barely different, but in addition will produce a characteristic "beat" sound at regular intervals depending on the (slight) difference between the two frequencies. This can be easily demonstrated on a musical instrument.

The analogy was made when Paul Nogier discovered that these two frequencies, *the harmonics of which were very close*, expressed a difference in "tone" respectively of the right and left hemispheres, and of the opposite sides of the body.

Under normal conditions, the low-frequency **BF** expresses the "tone" of the left forehead (hemisphere) and of the right side of the body. Whereas the high frequency **HF** normally expresses the "tone" of the right forehead (hemisphere) and of the left side of the body. Practically speaking, these reactions can be obtained by projecting the frequency on the left and right foreheads and on the left and right cheeks, to observe where a RAC is produced. The results can be schematically noted on a diagram (**Figure 26.6**) representing four compartments: the right and left hemi-foreheads, and the right and left hemi-bodies.

| | |
|---|---|
| Left body<br>**HF** | Right body<br>**BF** |
| Left forehead<br>**BF** | Right forehead<br>**HF** |

**Figure 26.6** Schematical representation of the normal distribution of beat frequencies between the two foreheads and the two hemi-bodies in a right-handed person. The opposite would be found in a normal left-handed person.

In a right-handed person, the high-frequency **HF**, when projected onto the right hemi-forehead or left hemi-body, will trigger a RAC response during three cycles, whereas if **HF** is projected onto the left hemi-forehead or the right hemi-body, there will be no response. The **HF** frequency has a "right hemisphere" tone (**Figure 26.6**).

The low-frequency **BF**, in a right-handed person, will trigger a RAC response when projected onto the left hemi-forehead and onto the right hemi-body, whereas there will be no response when **BF** is projected onto the right hemi-forehead or the left hemi-body. The low-frequency **BF** has a "left hemisphere" tone. The reverse reactions will prevail for high-frequency **HF** or for low-frequency **BF** in a left-handed subject (**Figures 26.7** and **26.8**).

In short, *beat frequencies* are widely used to explore, determine, and control *frequency disorders* that are linked to various pathological conditions such as autoimmune diseases, which we are about to describe.

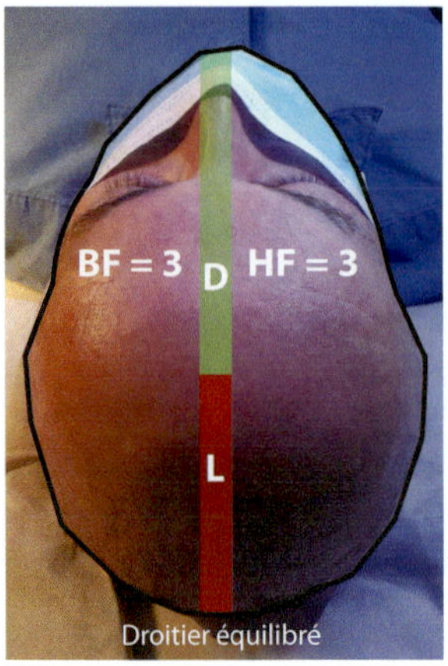


**Figure 26.7** Distribution of beat frequencies HF and BF on the two foreheads of a normal right-handed person.

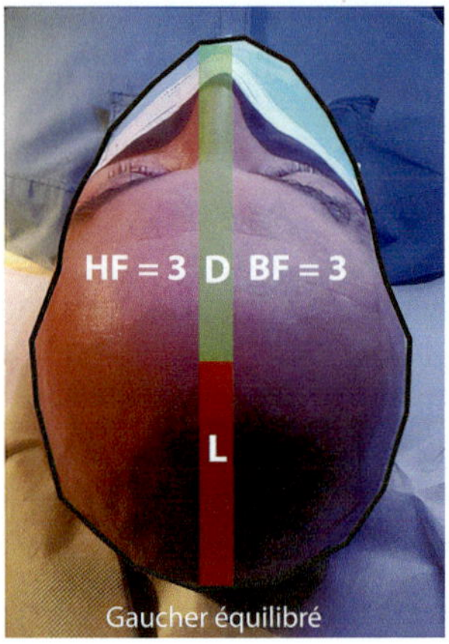


**Figure 26.8** Distribution of beat frequencies HF and BF on the two foreheads of a normal left-handed person.

## 26.4 PATHOLOGICAL CONDITIONS AND THEIR MANAGEMENT

### 26.4.1 Symmetry Disorders

Symmetry and laterality disorders are associated with numerous cases of pain, instability, or vertigo. Eighty percent of low back pain patients have a symmetry disorder, which shows how important it is to reduce asymmetry in patients who require it.

In a study carried out in 2000, Bernard Bricot of Marseille (France) observed that auriculotherapy modified postural tone.

First, we will explore the **D** line on the forehead for parasite frequencies. Identifying these frequencies will inform us which ear zone "contains" the auricular points to be treated. If we find a parasite **A** frequency, we will search for a point on the sub-tragal area. If it is a **B** frequency, we will look for points in the concha. If the parasitic frequency is **C**, we will look for pathological points on the anthelix, etc. It is important to note that, in the case of a **C** parasite frequency, the subject should be examined standing up, as it is known that the points on the ear appear when the subject is put out of balance.

The parasite frequencies liable to be found can also be *deviated*: **A-30%**, A+30%, F–30%, or **F+30%**. Michel Marignan has described these frequencies as being involved in the postural system. According to him, the **A–30** frequency is linked to the postural inputs (eye, foot, inner ear), and the **F–30** frequency is related to central integrations.

The points that have been detected can be treated either with frequencies or with semi-permanent needles (ASP).

In addition, the tragus points (area **D**) will also have to be checked and treated.

After treating, it is necessary to check that the **D** line reacts solely to **D**-Frequency.

### 26.4.2 Laterality Disorders

Most frequently, disorders related to laterality go unnoticed because they are of minor importance. If we systematically consider all the patients who come to our practice for problems as varied as joint pain or digestive, cardiac, or gynaecological disorders, we rarely come across patients well-balanced from the point of view of laterality. Very often, there are minor impairments for which the patient does not feel they should seek assistance.

In the field of laterality, the problems for which patients feel the need to consult us are of two kinds: thwarted left-handedness and right-hemisphere hyperactivity.

#### *26.4.2.1 Thwarted Left-Handedness*

This pathology has been known for a long time and is mainly observed in children. A right-handed person's language centre is located in the left hemisphere (96% of the population). A left-handed person has a language centre in the right hemisphere (4%). Normally, a right-handed person should have a directing right hand, a directing right foot, and a directing right eye. Whereas a true left-handed person has a directing left hand, a directing left foot, and a directing left eye.

For handwriting, 90% of the population statistically write with their right hand, and 10% with their left hand. This means that a significant proportion of those with their language centre in the left hemisphere write with their left hand. These patients suffer from impaired laterality and represent about 9% of the total population. They are also called left-handed or right-handed contrarians. These "dys-lateralised" subjects are prone to develop learning and behavioural disorders and should be treated. The left-handed person is more likely to be a boy than a girl.

Clinical signs of dyslaterality appear early in childhood: dyslexia, dysorthography, dyscalculia, speech disorders, and sometimes mirror handwriting. The child is generally shy and hyperactive. He will have difficulty following school and will need the help of a speech therapist. Each upgrade from one class to the next proves difficult. At the age of 18, what will always characterise the left-handed person may be difficulty in choosing, ordering, and obeying. They are a mediocre leader, a bad subordinate, and a frustrated spouse. At the age of 40, functional signs appear, such as eczema, stomach ulcers, sleep disorders, anxiety, and depression, which only few physicians will relate to dyslaterality.

When examined, the eye deviation test is impaired regardless of the subject and the question asked. The patient will look to the right, then to the left, then to the right again, without being able to really set the gaze.

It is the RAC that will give us the possibility of diagnosing impaired left-handedness. The frequency formula will consist of both **HF** and **BF** frequencies responding on both the right and left sides of the forehead (**Figure 26.9**). There is no frequency specificity.

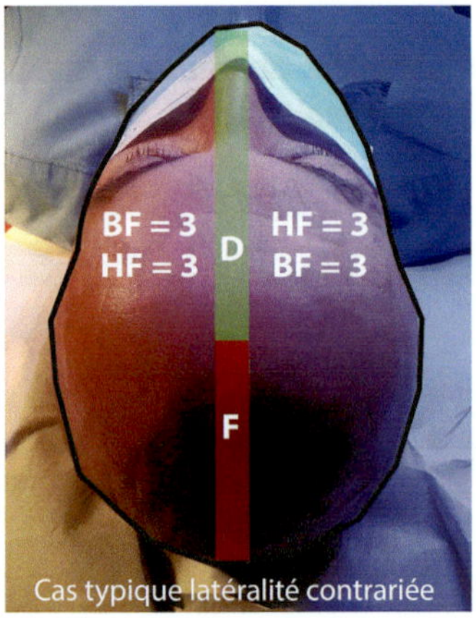


**Figure 26.9** Formula in thwarted left-handedness.

**Treatment** of this condition consists first of eliminating food hypersensitivities, which, in children, are responsible for numerous attention and laterality disorders. Then, the right and left L points on the anterior part of the tragus must be treated.

Treatment of impaired left-handedness takes a long time. It consists of monthly stimulation of the tragus points with ASP or **L**-frequency. It is necessary to restore a normal frequency laterality within the patient with either a right- or left-handed formula.

### *26.4.2.2 Right Hemispheric Hyperactivity*

Hyperactivity of the right hemisphere is a frequent condition. It may occur among perfectly well lateralized, right-handed or left-handed patients, following traumatic accidents, being exposed to multiple psycho-emotional problems, because of excessive exposure to television or indiscriminate playing of a musical instrument, after quitting smoking, or under hashish intoxication. In this type of situation, the activity of the two hemispheres is not 50/50; there is a 90% shift in favour of the right hemisphere. Information stagnates there and is not transferred to the left hemisphere because the corpus callosum does not fulfil its task properly.

The clinical symptoms due to this situation are:

- Morning fatigue
- Defeatism
- Memory problems, particularly for names
- Inability to concentrate
- Depression

In a right-handed person, the right/left blockage develops according to three stages (**Figure 26.10**).

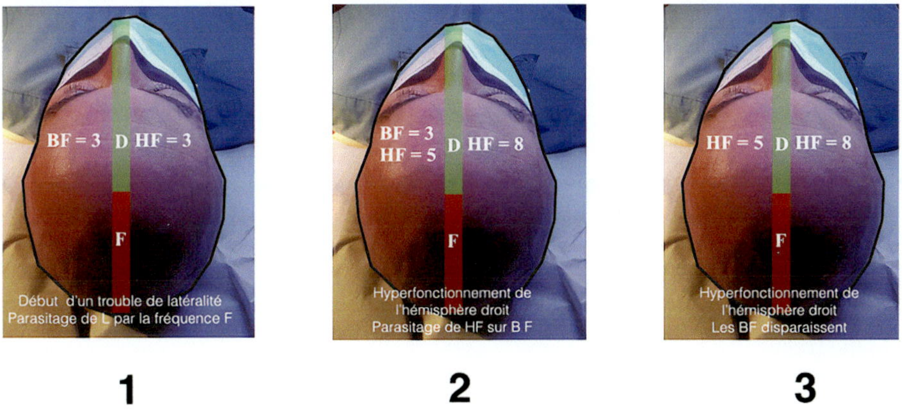


**Figure 26.10** The three stages of a right/left blockage.

- **The first stage** is characterised by parasite frequencies on the L line.
- **The second stage** consists of the appearance of **HF** on the left hemi-forehead.
- **The third stage** is characterised by the disappearance of **BF** on the left forehead.

During **clinical examinations**, the patient always deviates his eyes to the left side, regardless of the type of discussion. If asked to perform a mathematical operation, the patient cannot stabilise their gaze.

**Examination of the frequencies** will indicate the degree of blockage. Here again, there are three stages:

- **Stage 1 — HF** pulses increase on the right hemi-forehead front beyond 3 RACs and can reach as high as 30 RACs.
- **Stage 2 — HF** frequencies can also be found on the left hemi-forehead: this means parasitation by **HF**.
- **Stage 3 —** The **BF** frequencies disappear on the left hemi-forehead. In this case, the blockage is complete.

This procedure can evaluate the blockage by adding the **HF** pulse count and subtracting the **BF** pulse count. This is referred to as the **Right/Left score**. Normally, this score amounts to zero (3 – 3 = 0) (case n°1). Using the data from **Figure 26.8**, in case n°2, the score = 10 (8 + 5 – 3). In case n°3, the score = 13 (8 + 5). The higher the score, the greater the blockage. A score of 40 seems to be the maximum.

## 26.5 AURICULOTHERAPY: THE TRAGUS, SYMMETRY, AND LATERALITY

Auriculotherapy will help us considerably in treating symmetry and laterality disorders. Numerous ear points can be active, but the tragus points are mostly implied.

The tragus (Latin for *goat*) is a cartilaginous formation in front of the ear. It derives from the first mandibular bud of the first branchial slit. Its innervation is abundant:

- On the inner side of the tragus, above the foramen magnum, one can find the intermediary nerve, a branch of the facial nerve (VII bis).
- On the external side of the tragus, the glossopharyngeal nerve (IX) and the second cervical branch C2 are located (**Figure 26.9**).

On the tragus, we will find:

- Points that stimulate symmetry. They are located on the area innervated by the glossopharyngeal nerve **IX**.
- Points that stimulate laterality. They are located further forward on the area innervated by **C2**.
- A point situated in between the symmetry zone and the laterality zone. This is the zero prime or O′ point. It is located in the pre-tragal groove and has a balancing effect on symmetry and laterality. Contrary to the rule stating that symmetrical points should not be treated on both ears, it is, in fact, possible to treat this point symmetrically on the right and left ears (**Figures 26.11** and **26.12**).

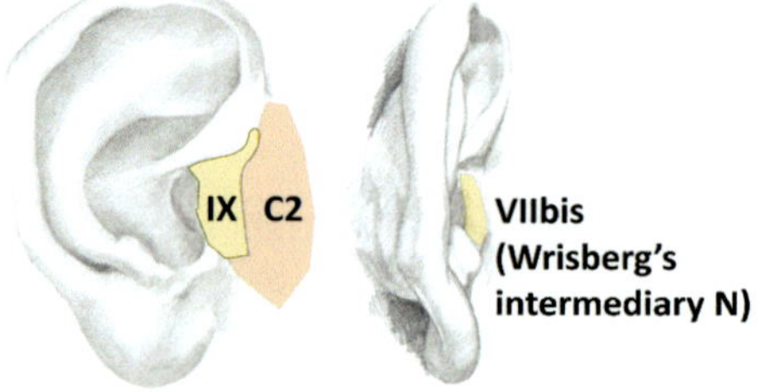


**Figure 26.11** Innervation of the external and internal tragus.

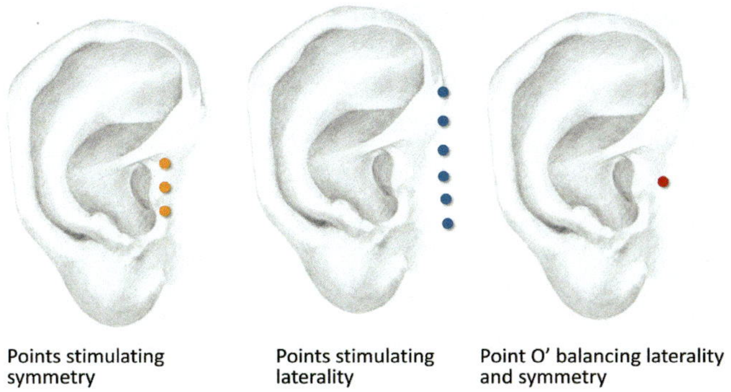


**Figure 26.12** Distribution of points on the tragus.

### 26.5.1 Detection and Treatment of Tragus Points

Tragus points are always detected with an electronic device. They cannot be found with a pressure probe. Painful tragus points do not seem to correspond to somatic pain.

Tragus points can be treated in several ways:

- **ASP** (semi-permanent needles)
- **D** frequency for symmetry disorders (**Figure 26.13**)
- **L** or **G** frequency for laterality disorders (**Figure 26.14**)
- Tragus points are first checked on the right ear and then on the left

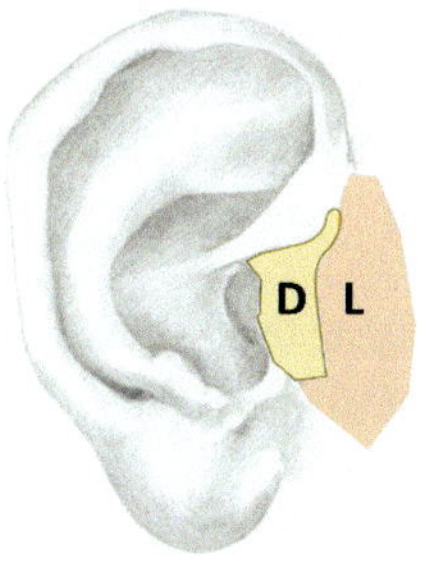


**Figure 26.13** Frequency zones on the tragus.

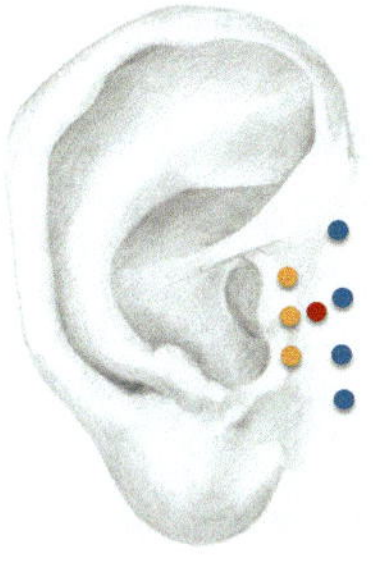

**Figure 26.14** Yellow: Points for symmetry Blue: points for laterality Red: 0' = zero prime point.

### 26.5.2 Indications for Treating Tragus Points

Before treatment, it is helpful to check for the issues below since they often involve treatment of the tragus points in auricular therapy (**Table 26.1**).

**Table 26.1 Indications for Treating Tragus Points**

| | | |
|---|---|---|
| ***Symmetry disorders*** | ***Laterality disorders*** | ***Memory problems*** |
| • Ocular convergence<br>• Lameness<br>• Scoliosis<br>• Postural disorder<br>• Rheumatic pain<br>• Low back pain<br>• Neck pain | • Dyslexia<br>• Dysorthography<br>• Dyscalculia<br>• Stuttering<br>• Mirror writing | • Loss of memory of names |
| ***Attention deficit*** | ***Reactive depression*** | ***Smoking cessation*** |
| • poor school results | | |
| ***Jetlag*** | ***Sleep disorders*** | ***Nychthemeral inversion (inversion of night and day)*** |
| ***Inflammatory attacks in autoimmune diseases*** | ***Multiple sclerosis MS*** | ***Ankylosing spondylitis*** |

## 26.6 SPECIFIC DISEASE MANAGEMENT

### 26.6.1 Multiple Sclerosis MS

#### *26.6.1.1 Clinical Overview*

- Demyelinating disease affecting the white matter of the brain and/or spinal cord.
- 80% women, 20% men.
- Average onset between 18 and 30 years.
- Almost no incidence below the equator, increasing as one approaches the north and south poles. More MS in Lille (Northern France) than in Marseille (Southern France). More in Marseille than in Algiers (North Africa).
- Often sudden onset with eye or visual problems, dysesthesia, paresis, etc.
- Evolves mainly by relapse attacks, rarely continuously.

#### *26.6.1.2 Causes and Predisposing Factors*

- Autoimmune disease
- Genetic predisposition?
- Hepatitis B vaccination involved?
- Insufficient or lack of breastfeeding?

#### 26.6.1.3 Conventional Treatments

- ***Treatment of acute attacks***: Cortisone. Cortisone treatments do not affect the long-term evolution of MS. They reduce the peri-lesional oedema and, therefore, the clinical signs without reducing the neuronal damage.
- ***Basic treatments for relapsing forms*** (all act on immunity)
  - Interferon beta (Avonex R)
  - Glatiramer acetate (Copaxone R)
  - Gilenya R
  - Tysabri R
  - Elsep R
- ***Treatments for progressive forms***
  - Endoxan R
  - Cellcept R

#### 26.6.1.4 Treatment by Way of Auriculotherapy

Treatment is based on three elements: learning to manage stress more efficiently, diet, and auriculotherapy.

1. **Diet**: Basically, the diet is simple. Since in MS, there is autoimmunity directed against myelin, the patient will be asked to eliminate all foods containing myelin. It is indeed most probable that eating myelin-like proteins stimulates the patient's lymphocyte count and increases autoimmunity. Myelin is composed of lipids and proteins. It wraps around most central nervous system axons, increasing the nervous impulse's propagation speed tenfold. In MS, the myelin proteins are the targets of T-lymphocytes.

   In terms of animal evolution, it is known that myelin appeared at the same time as the jaw. Only animals with jaws have myelin.

   In MS patients, the absorption of myelin or myelin-like proteins probably increases autoimmunity by a decoy effect. The patient must, therefore, avoid mammalian or poultry meat, avoid dairy products because some dairy proteins resemble those of myelin, and give preference to proteins from fish, the proteins of which are very different (if possible, without jaws, lamprey, for example), and shellfish. This diet simply proceeds from medical common sense. Having experimented with this diet on hundreds of MS patients, it seems evident to me today that remission of this disease can only be expected if there is a diet. It is a necessary, however not sufficient, step. It should be supplemented by auriculotherapy. Regrettably, treatment of MS does not include diet in neurology departments.

2. **Auriculotherapy**: While auriculotherapy alone cannot eliminate MS attacks, it can, in conjunction with a diet, reduce and space out attacks. It

seems that laterality disorders precede MS attacks, and that treatment of these disorders stops MS attacks. The treatment of MS by auriculotherapy is, therefore, closely linked to the treatment of laterality.

MS pre-attacks are always accompanied by a laterality frequency disorder, which can be measured with the GL+ (Micropad).

Normally, in a right-handed person, three reactionary pulses should be found using the radial pulse when a high frequency (8.74 Hz) is projected onto the right hemi-forehead and three when 3.75 Hz is projected onto the left hemi-forehead (**Figure 26.13**).

In a poorly balanced MS patient, this pattern is disturbed.

Before or during the crisis, no low frequencies can be observed on the left hemi-forehead. We are faced with a disturbed constellation of the type shown in **Figure 26.15**.

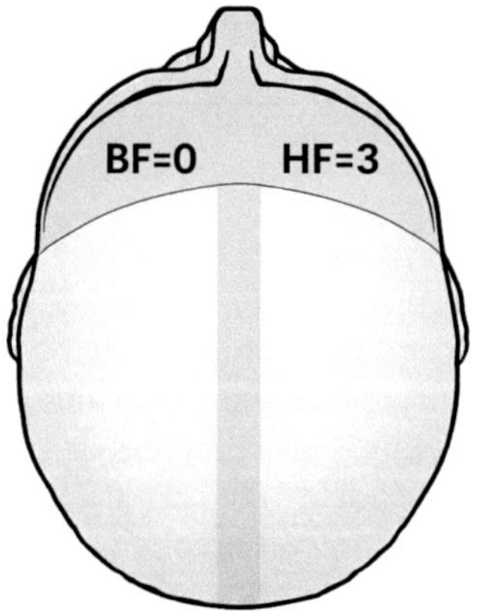


**Figure 26.15** Frequencies found on the forehead in unstable MS.

This constellation is not specific to MS and can be found in other pathological circumstances. Still, in an MS patient, it is a sign of instability that needs to be treated. This will help to stop the attack or postpone it.

The difficulty is maintaining this balanced *frequency laterality* over the medium and long term. This is where the need for a well-followed diet comes in. We know that when the patient does not follow a diet, frequency laterality will tend to go out of balance.

During a crisis, we see the patient twice or three times a week to check the frequency laterality and correct it if necessary. When it seems to have stabilised, we space out the visits while checking that it remains normal. First every week, then every month, then every two months, then every six months. The aim is to detect frequency laterality disorders and treat them with auriculotherapy if necessary. It is very rare (I have only seen it once out of more than a thousand patients) to observe an MS attack with a normal frequency constellation.

#### 26.6.1.5 Points for Restoring Laterality

1. *First, dental foci and scars* should be treated. Look for an exhaustion of the RAC, explore the edge of the ear with the black tip detector, and treat the reactive points with a semi-permanent needle. This first step is essential because it conditions the rest. It will be difficult to obtain a lasting result if there is a pathological focus. In women, it is necessary to check for a caesarean scar.
2. The *right and left tragus* should then be checked, and the O′ points treated if necessary.
3. *The point of the first cervical vertebra* should be treated on the external part of the right ear. This point is tiny and is sometimes difficult to find. It is this point that will ultimately restore the disturbed laterality. This point is usually treated with a Chinese needle, which is left for about two minutes. A semi-permanent needle can be used if the patient lives far from the practice. Why is this point so effective? It is difficult to explain. Paul Nogier used to repeat repeatedly: "MS is a problem linked to the first cervical vertebrae" and he often added: "To treat MS well, you have to work a lot on your patient".
4. After the needle is inserted, the frequency laterality is immediately checked with a **DB 165** or a **GL+** frequency generator. At this stage, it should have returned to normal.

If, despite treatment, the frequency laterality remains disturbed, it is necessary to detect the correct first cervical point once more. Sometimes it takes a while. This point is detectable with a white tip detector and an electric detector. It is very small and not necessarily painful. If the treatment is well conducted, laterality should stabilise (**Figure 26.16**).

#### 26.6.1.6 Protocol Summary Concerning MS

##### 26.6.1.6.1 In Case of Acute Crisis

When a patient has a seizure, they should be seen rapidly to be treated as soon as possible after a complete neurological examination. Then, plan the treatment. Personally, I do not propose cortisone at the first session. I only suggest it later if I have failed to control the crisis with auriculotherapy.

During the first session, laterality is restored, and a RAFT examination is performed to identify food sensitivities (see Chapter 27). This is an important step.

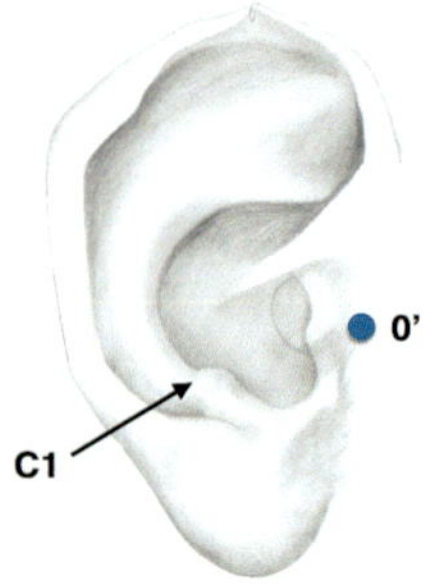


**Figure 26.16** Treatment of MS attacks.

The patient is then seen twice or three times weekly to check laterality. There should be 3 HF on the right hemi-forehead and 3 BF on the left. If this is not the case, the scars, dental foci, and first cervical should be treated again. Sessions can be spaced out as soon as laterality stabilises over time.

#### *26.6.1.6.2 Outside Crises*

The patient is monitored every month, then every two months, and then every three months.

In each case, the patient is examined neurologically to assess the course of the disease.

The RAFTs are checked mainly for meat and dairy tests. If these tests are positive, the patient is not following the diet properly. In this case, it is necessary to investigate, together with the patient, the various mistakes they may be making. It should not be forgotten that sandwich bread contains milk and that some sweets contain pork, etc.

The most important thing is to check the frequency laterality using a **GL+** or a **DB 165.** One must find three RACs for high frequencies on the right hemi-forehead and three RACs for low frequencies on the left hemi-forehead.

If the laterality is not disturbed, the sessions can be spaced out.

#### *26.6.1.6.3 The Specific Case of Pregnancy*

It is known that MS attacks are rare during pregnancy but frequent after delivery. This is why it is necessary to monitor MS patients within three months following delivery. Patients are asked to come immediately after discharge from the clinic.

It is important to inquire about the delivery process and treat scars, episiotomy, or caesarean section if necessary.

It is not uncommon to find laterality disorders, which are treated immediately and monitored twice a month for three months after delivery.

#### *26.6.1.6.4 Should the Current Chemical Treatment Be Changed? That Is the Question*

It is always difficult to withdraw a drug treatment that a fellow neurologist has started. This is why it is preferable to see the patient at the beginning of his illness, to treat him in the first instance. Here, a diet will be implemented, and auriculotherapy alone will be used. If the attacks cannot be controlled with auriculotherapy, it is essential to offer drug treatment. If, on the other hand, treatment by the ear is effective, chemical treatment should be avoided.

Most patients who come to us have already been treated with medication. Disappointed by conventional medicine because of unsatisfactory results, they turn to us. Nothing prevents us from treating them with auriculotherapy while keeping their chemical treatment. The way of proceeding will be the same for those who come to see us without medication. Above all, we pay attention to laterality disorders and treat them.

The question of continuing chemical treatment arises after several years of stabilisation of the disease. Should drug treatment be continued or not if, after ten years, the patient has not reported any attacks? There is no standard answer. Each case is different. It all depends on the age of the patient, the number of attacks before auriculotherapy, and their desire to stop taking medication.

#### *26.6.1.7 Conclusions*

- With auriculotherapy, we can help MS patients.
  The first crisis is always the most difficult to control. It is necessary to work hard on one's patient, work again and again until laterality is stabilised, which seems to allow the patient to get better.
- The most difficult patients to treat are men and patients with progressive forms of MS.

### 26.6.2 Inflammatory Rheumatic Diseases

Some inflammatory diseases, such as **ankylosing spondylitis**, develop in the form of attacks. Like MS, it is not uncommon to find laterality disorders before and during the attacks. In this case, as in MS, one must treat the tragus points and sometimes the C1 point of the right ear.

I have the opportunity of treating a young man having suffered from ankylosing spondylitis for several years with regular attacks of inflammation accompanied by near to unbearable pain. Under my advice, he follows a diet without red meat and dairy products, which does not prevent him from having occasional flare-ups. He usually calls me as soon as the pain returns. On each examination, I come up against a frequency laterality disorder. I noticed in this young patient that the C1 point in the right ear had a radical effect on him because, within a few hours, the inflammation and the pain subsided.

### 26.6.3 Liver Disorders

Sometimes, despite a normal white light test, stimulation of hemi-foreheads with HF and BF does not induce any RAC response.

Clinically, this situation is encountered in people who complain of fatigue and memory problems, especially in the elderly. In Norway, I have often observed this constellation in my Sunday morning class during practical work after late-night drinking of wine and aquavit on Saturday nights. That is why I called this constellation the Norwegian syndrome.

This corresponds to a liver disorder.

To return to a normal frequency constellation, the treatment must be performed on the right ear with one or two semi-permanent needles on the hepatic area representation.

It should be noted that the liver point is probably the most effective of all ear points for memory loss in senile dementia (**Figure 26.17**).

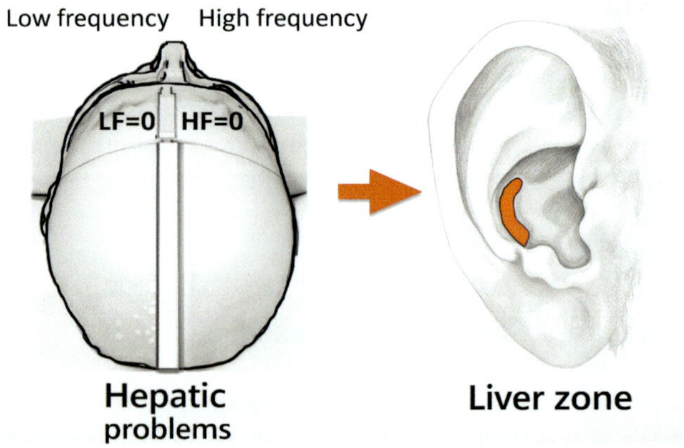


**Figure 26.17** Treatment of liver function disorders.

### 26.6.4 Conclusion

The clinical understanding and management of symmetry and laterality disorders through auriculotherapy represents a sophisticated approach to complex neurological and functional conditions. Through careful assessment using both clinical observation and RAC-based frequency testing, we can identify and treat disorders that conventional medicine often overlooks. The tragus points provide us with powerful therapeutic tools for addressing these fundamental aspects of human neurological function.

The success of these approaches, particularly in conditions like MS and inflammatory diseases, demonstrates the practical value of understanding the distinction between symmetry and laterality functions. While symmetry ensures our basic structural and functional balance, laterality enables the cognitive abilities that define human intelligence. The therapeutic challenge lies in maintaining an appropriate balance between these two essential functions.

As we continue to develop these techniques, it becomes increasingly clear that many chronic conditions may benefit from this perspective on neurological organisation and the targeted interventions that auriculotherapy provides.

## NOTE

1. Translator's note: the abbreviation BF, for low frequency, originates from the French term "Basse Fréquence".

## BIBLIOGRAPHY

1. Bourdiol René. *Elements of auriculotherapy.* Maisonneuve 1981.
2. Bricot Bernard. Study of the effectiveness of the treatment of the projection zones of the interhemispheric commissures in balance disorders and objectification in stabilometry. IIIe international symposium of auriculotherapy. Lyon. GLEM. France 2000.
3. Israel Lucien. *Cerveau droit, Cerveau gauche.* Plon 1995
4. Lazorthes Guy. *L'histoire du cerveau*, page 17 Editions Ellipses 1999
5. Lazorthes Guy. *Le Cerveau et l'Esprit.* Flammarion 1982
6. Nogier Paul. *A correction concerning the D and E frequencies.* Journal Auriculomedecine n° 7, page 45 April 1977
7. Nogier Paul. *From auriculotherapy to auriculomedicine.* Éditions Maisonneuve 1981.
8. Nogier Raphaël. *Introduction to auriculomedicine.* Haug 1993
9. Nogier Raphaël. *From displacement to laterality.* Annales du GLEM 2006–2007, pages 81 to 96
10. Nogier Raphaël. *Photo emission, photoperception, L frequency.* Les annales du Glem 2007–2008, pages 94 to 105

## CHAPTER 27

# Food Hypersensitivities and the RAC

**Raphaël Nogier**

## 27.1 INTRODUCTION

Food allergies cannot merely be reduced to the immune mechanisms triggered by the absorption of an allergenic foodstuff, followed in the next few minutes or hours by mast cell degranulation and release of histamine, leading to the impressive signs that we all know as physicians: urticaria, angioedema, diarrhoea, asthma, or shock. Indeed, many food allergies remain unnoticed because the physio-pathological mechanisms involved do not lead to mast cell degranulation but to the production of interleukins responsible for much less marked but nonetheless unpleasant chronic symptoms and signs, such as constipation, nervous breakdown, mood disorders, fatigue, migraines, and eczema, which at first glance do not necessarily suggest a possible link.

Whereas allergies with mast cell degranulation (IgE-dependent), known as type I, are relatively easy to diagnose (questioning, prick tests, specific IgE assay, transit test), the second type of non-IgE-dependent allergic hypersensitivity creates hopeless difficulties for allergologists, who have no means at their disposal to diagnose it. The delay between the absorption of the food allergen and the onset of clinical signs can be several days, and even with precise questioning, it is impossible to establish a link between the food intake and the signs and symptoms. Furthermore, stopping the food in question will only have effects at a later stage since it may be necessary to eliminate a foodstuff for several weeks before observing clinical improvement or healing of the pathology.

***In this context of diagnostic impotence in the field of allergology, the possibility of detecting food allergens utilising the RAC is obviously of great value.***

It comes as a surprising fact that, unlike in many other countries, the French medical profession has not really shown interest in non-IgE-dependent food allergy-type disorders.

One possible explanation is the following. Until the 2010s, many medical instructors had experienced wartime or post-war restrictions.[1] The illnesses they encountered had more to do with deficiencies than with overeating. Our consumer society is young, and disorders resulting from overeating have not been known for very long. Only twenty years ago, who would have thought of prescribing diets for chronic diseases such as MS or ankylosing spondylitis? Attitudes have changed, and now you can go to any restaurant and find on the menu indications such as "gluten-free" or "lactose-free", etc.

 DOI: 10.1201/9781003753629-27

Physicians are timidly beginning to show interest in this subject and are wondering about the deleterious systemic effects of an excessively rich and disordered diet. I have recently encountered a few rheumatologists advising their osteoarthritis patients to follow a dairy-free diet. This was unthinkable twenty years ago. The way physicians see things is changing. With recent discoveries, particularly concerning the microbiota, exciting perspectives on food hypersensitivity are appearing. Little by little, we are discovering the outlines regarding the main dietary principles and, consequently, the therapeutic possibilities offered by well-conducted diets. Nevertheless, even if general principles exist, we are now becoming aware that they cannot be indiscriminately applied to everyone because individual food sensitivities vary considerably. Let's sum up by saying that what is good for Peter is not necessarily good for Paul. Each person is unique, both in terms of genetic make-up and history. It would, therefore, be desirable and even necessary to promote the concept of personalised nutrition.

### 27.1.1 Proteins, the Building Blocks of Life: The Self

We are all composed of water, minerals, vitamins, carbohydrates, fats, and proteins. Among these components, the proteins specific to each of us differentiate us from each other. They are the expression of the genome since they are made from DNA.

The sum of all our proteins put together forms the "self". My "self" is different from the "self" of my neighbours.

Among the very numerous proteins that our cells produce, some are devoted to "signalling". Each cell of the organism expresses on its membrane specific signalling proteins, which are the same for each organism and which belong to one single individual, a kind of "protein tattoo" that allows our immune system to distinguish our own cells from those belonging to intruders. Foreign cells do not have the same protein tattoo on their surface.

Our immune system, which is made up partly of sedentary cells in the lymph nodes and partly of cells that patrol the body, can therefore discriminate between self and non-self proteins. When a foreign protein enters the body, it is immediately spotted and captured by patrolling cells, which then transport it to a lymph node for "processing" by the sedentary cells.

The food we eat is made up of proteins that are foreign to us. Under physiological conditions, they remain in the digestive tract without being able to pass the intestinal barrier and thus end up inside the body. However, it may occur that a food protein finds its way into the bloodstream due to certain pathological mechanisms. The immune system will then trigger a series of reactions that can lead to IgE- or non-IgE-dependent allergies.

### 27.1.2 The Intestinal Barrier

The intestinal barrier is an anatomical and chemical structure, the purpose of which is to prevent the entry of certain compounds into the body while allowing absorption of nutrients, water, and mineral salts. The digestive tract, which runs from the mouth to the anus, is about 9 metres long. From the stomach onwards, the tube is lined by an epithelium, the cells bound together by occlusive junctions. In the small intestine, there are finger-like projections called villi, which considerably increase the exchange surface of the intestine. The epithelial cells undergo permanent renewal, as 17 billion cells are replaced daily, and the entire epithelium is replaced in 5 days. As a result of this turnover, epithelial cells are particularly vulnerable to agents that inhibit cell division, such as anti-cancer drugs. The centre of the villi contains a lymphatic vessel and a capillary network.

Ingested proteins are split into peptide fragments, first in the stomach by *pepsin* and then in the small intestine by *trypsin* and *chymotrypsin* from the pancreas. These fragments are then split into free amino acids by pancreatic *carboxypeptidase* and *aminopeptidase* located on the epithelial cell membranes. The free amino acids can enter the epithelial cells by active sodium-bound transport. From these cells, they enter the bloodstream.

Normally, no food protein can or should pass the intestinal barrier.

### 27.1.3 Causes of Intestinal Hyperpermeability

The wall of the intestine can sometimes become hyperpermeable, thus opening the way to the passage of food proteins and generating possible sensitisation. These hyperpermeabilities can be encountered during physiological phenomena but are more often linked to various pathological circumstances.

#### *27.1.3.1 Physiological Causes*

- In newborns, the intestinal barrier is immature, so dietary proteins pass into the bloodstream. Maturation of the intestinal barrier can take several months.
- During intense or prolonged physical effort, blood supply to the intestinal compartments is limited in favour of the muscles. The barrier's functionality is then reduced, thus allowing the passage of proteins. This explains the frequent hypersensitivities to wheat observed among top athletes whose diet is mainly based on pasta, known to be a slow sugar.

#### *27.1.3.2 Pathological Causes*

- **Fever**: When the body temperature rises, the intestinal function is disturbed. The intestine no longer plays its role as a barrier, so food sensitisation can result. This is why it is necessary to adopt a light diet in case of fever. Our grandmother's recipe was common sense: a good hot broth.
- **Excessive alcohol intake**: Alcohol is a toxic agent that appears to inhibit the function and performance of the intestinal barrier.
    - Anti-inflammatory drugs, especially cortisone: It is not uncommon to observe signs of food allergies following cortisone treatments.

    - Chemotherapy or radiotherapy treatments.
    - Contraceptives.

- **Food hypersensitivities**: Food hypersensitivity is liable to create local intestinal reactions responsible for intestinal hyperpermeability, which in turn causes food proteins to pass through the intestinal barrier, causing additional food hypersensitivities.

- **Intestinal pathologies**: Coeliac disease.

Each of these items can promote the passage of proteins through the barrier and create allergic sensitisations. The problem of food allergy is basically linked to the functionality of the intestinal barrier.

### 27.1.4 What Happens If a Food Protein Passes the Intestinal Barrier?

When a dietary protein enters the bloodstream, it will be chased by the immune system, particularly by B-lymphocytes, which will first harpoon it and then bring it to the nearest lymph node containing T lymphocytes. There, the B-lymphocyte will present the intruding protein to the T lymphocytes. An immune reaction follows, leading to an immediate or delayed IgE-mediated allergy process, depending on the Th1 or Th2 response.

### 27.1.5 The Weakness of the Human Species: The Large Head

Man's intelligence is his strength, but also his vulnerability.

Man has a brain that has developed in the course of evolution. This phenomenon has been accompanied by a decrease in the gestation period in women due to the increasing size of the child's head. Whereas large mammals have gestation periods of 12, 13, 18, and up to 24 months, women's gestation period is only 9. This is because of the size of the child's head. A donkey spends 1/30 of its life in its mother's womb, whereas a child spends only 1/100. At birth, it would be no exaggeration to say that a child's gestation period is not yet completed. The newborn child, barely viable, needs appropriate nutrition. In the mother's womb, it was fed by the umbilical cord. Outside the mother's womb, it still needs the proteins—now to be found in the mother's milk. This is why the intestinal barrier is not functional in children. For several months, this barrier remains open. During the first few months of life, the child will be able to absorb the proteins contained in the mother's milk intact. These include immunoglobulins, which will protect the child against infections that the mother may have experienced and against which she has formed antibodies.

This temporary physiological permeability of the intestinal barrier, a true natural wonder, can become a weakness if the child is fed with proteins other than its mother's. They will, in fact, cross the intestinal barrier and end up in the child's bloodstream, which may then be permanently sensitised to these food proteins.

It is now clear that the lack of breastfeeding plays a significant role in the development of food sensitivity.

### 27.1.6 Role of the Microbiota

We now know that the microbiota composition plays a major role in triggering food hypersensitivities. Childbirth by caesarean section, lack of breastfeeding, antibiotics, or poor nutrition all modify the microbiota and contribute to the development of food allergies.

## 27.2 CLASSIFICATION OF DISEASES DUE TO DIET

See **Figure 27.1**.

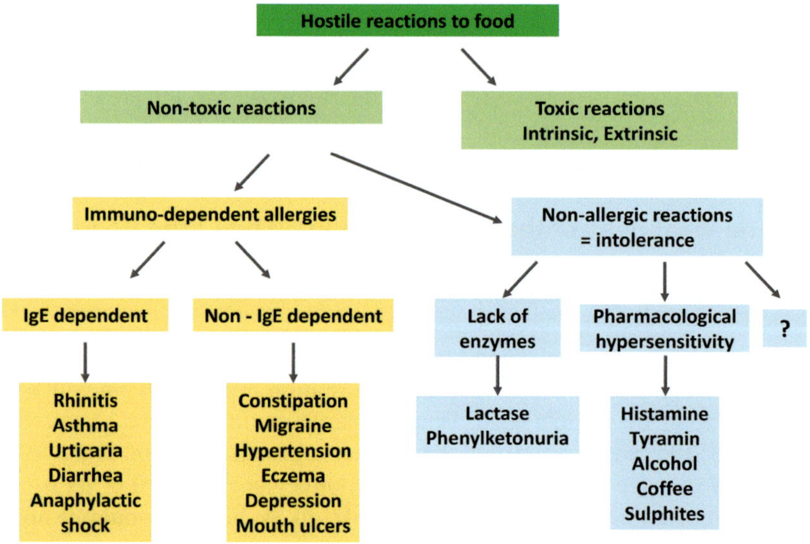


**Figure 27.1** Classification of food sensitivities.

### 27.2.1 Definitions

- **Food hypersensitivity**: a series of individual pathological manifestations of the body following the absorption of a food.
- **Food allergy**: food hypersensitivity that involves the immune system and concerns only proteins. A distinction is made between:
  - *Immediate IgE-dependent allergies* result in the mast cells' histamine release. The clinical signs can be impressive: diarrhoea, vomiting, urticaria, angioedema, and anaphylactic shock. The diagnosis is made by questioning, using a specific IgE assay, prick tests, and TPO.

  - *Non-IgE-dependent allergies* do not lead to mast cell degranulation but to a release of cytokines. The manifestations are delayed, and the signs are more discreet: constipation, fatigue, depression, eczema, asthma, sleep disorders, tachycardia…
- **Food intolerance**: a food hypersensitivity that does not involve the immune system and may concern sugars, fats, proteins, colourants, etc. There are several types of intolerance:
  - *Intolerances due to enzyme deficiency.* There are thousands of these: lactose intolerance due to lactase deficiency, phenylketonuria, etc.
  - *Intolerances due to non-allergic hypersensitivity to pharmacologically active products contained in foods: histamine, tyramine, alcohol, glutamate, and coffee.* They are called pseudo-allergies.
  - *Cultural intolerances.* A food can be associated with painful memories. If I am told that someone close to me has died, just at the moment that I am eating tomatoes, I may develop a hypersensitivity to tomatoes, which will always be associated with bad news.
- **RAFT (Radial Artery Food Test)**: food test performed by taking the pulse on the radial artery to detect an arterial response (RAC).
- **Test ring** (sometimes loosely referred to as "**food test**"): a transparent ring consisting of two lamellae between which the food is inserted under the form of a thin slice (see Chapter 12).

## 27.3 CLINICAL SIGNS OF FOOD ALLERGIES

***Food hypersensitivities* (Table 27.1) *are more common in children and women.***

**Table 27.1 Symptomatology of Food Hypersensitivities**

| Food allergy | Probable signs | Possible signs |
|---|---|---|
| Systemic | Anaphylactic shock | |
| Respiratory system | Rhinitis, asthma, alveolitis | |
| Eye | Conjunctivitis | |
| Digestive tract | Constipation, mouth ulcers, geographic tongue, gastritis, colitis | Ulcerative recto-colitis |
| Skin | Hives, eczema, angioedema | Dermatitis herpetiformis, alopecia, lucitis |
| Joints | | Pain, arthritis |
| Nervous system | Migraine, headaches, fatigue, sleep disorders | Mood disorders, anxiety, depression |
| Cardiovascular system | Arrhythmias, tachycardia, low blood pressure | |
| Gynaecological system | Mastodynia, infertility | |

Birth by caesarean section, lack of breastfeeding, the introduction of proteins too early in the infant's diet, the rise in oestrogen levels in adolescence, and the use of birth control pills are undoubtedly factors favouring the occurrence of food allergies.

To understand and diagnose delayed hypersensitivities, three elements need to be taken into consideration:

1. The delay between the time the food was consumed and the onset of the pathological signs may sometimes be more than seven or eight days. Neither the patient nor the physician can establish a precise relationship between the consumption of the food and the onset of symptoms. All the more so, if the food in question has been consumed daily all year round.
2. The removal of the food from the diet may have lasted for a long time, several weeks, or several months before the signs disappear. This increases the diagnostic difficulty. Sometimes, the patient spontaneously tries to suppress a particular food under the advice of family or friends for a few days. Still, as there are no convincing results in the short term, they mistakenly think that the food that has been suppressed is not linked to the symptoms.
3. The causative food is often highly appreciated and, therefore, frequently consumed by the patient. In the field of nutrition, it is said that "the patient is attracted by his enemy". However, even if the causal food is only eaten once every week or two, this is enough to cause serious problems in case of an allergy.

***Reasons for consultation that are suggestive of a possible food allergy.***

- **Constipation**: this is an almost constant sign of food allergy. It is rare to observe a delayed food allergy without a transit disorder. When a woman describes a problematic bowel movement with three, two, or one bowel movement per week, we must consider a food allergy after having eliminated a mechanical cause. In general, these types of constipation date back to childhood or adolescence and have significantly disrupted the patient's life. Let us not forget that a normal transit consists of at least one daily bowel movement.
- **Irritable bowel**: bloating, spasms.
- **Mood disorders**: mood disorders are also frequently related to food allergies. When a woman is sad, depressed, and cannot cope properly, she should, of course, be questioned and checked for objective causes. But if there are none, we must then check for food hypersensitivity. How many women take antidepressants and anxiolytics every day without being conscious of the fact that they are consuming the foods responsible for their misfortunes?
- **Sleep disorders**: they are encountered especially in young adolescents who, until then, had no problems and, at the time of puberty, develop typical

symptoms of fatigue and hypersomnia. The typical sentence repeated by helpless parents, "Our daughter is a great sleeper", often hides a medical reality that can be linked to dietary hypersensitivity.

- **Mouth ulcers** often occur in hypersensitivity to certain cereals, mainly wheat.
- **Eczema**: many eczemas labelled atopic can be solved by a diet suppressing one or two foods.
- **Hives**: some hives are dramatically improved by diet: chronic and solar hives. Chronic hives are those that occur every day for at least six weeks. This type of hives is challenging to treat and requires prolonged antihistamine treatment. Not all hives are food-induced, but food tests should be systematically performed. In the case of sun hives, some disappear if an allergenic food is removed.

## 27.4 FOOD TESTS WITH THE RAC

Food testing with the RAC is based on the work of Paul Nogier, who was the first to apply the vascular signal to this purpose. The protocols he used in the 1980s have evolved, and we no longer use the same ones today. We are now trying to produce protocols that consider current knowledge of allergies and intolerances.

When a chemical or biological compound, diluted in a solution and placed in a transparent test ring, is brought close to the skin, the radial pulse reacts if the subject is hypersensitive to the compound. This may be pollen, a chemically active product, or a thinly sliced food. For this to happen, it is imperative that photons can pass through the test ring. This is due to the fact that the skin is a photoreceptor. Light passing through the thinly sliced food is loaded with spectral information that is apparently recognised by the skin. The phenomenon disappears in total darkness.

With the RAC, the physician can test food for each patient.

RAC tests are subjective and must, therefore, be interpreted appropriately. They must be performed by trained medical practitioners capable of making diagnoses and sufficiently trained in the field of allergy to understand the test adequately.

RAC tests are no substitute for prick tests or patch tests. They bring an additional element to the physician's diagnostic arsenal.

### 27.4.1 How to Prepare Food Tests

The food should be cut into a very thin slice and placed between the slide and the coverslip so that light can pass through. Alternatively, the food may be diluted and placed in a neutral liquid, such as water. **The food should be tested**

**as it is consumed**. Wheat, for example, should be tested as bread or cooked pulp. Foods that do not keep well should be tested in dried or freeze-dried (lyophilised) form: dried tomato, dried banana, dried beef, powdered milk, and instant coffee.

Liquids can be tested: oils, fruit juices, commercial drinks, white wine, red wine, or other alcohols. A small blotter is sometimes used to absorb the liquid, specially made to fit inside the test ring between the slide and the coverslip. However, this can be avoided

Foods in powder form can also be tested, such as pepper, cinnamon, nutmeg, etc.

### 27.4.2 What Foods Should Be Tested?

**Animal proteins**

- **Meat**: beef, pork, mutton, chicken, duck, rabbit
- **Fish**: freshwater, seawater
- Shellfish
- **Eggs**: white and yellow; raw and cooked
- **Milk**: cow, goat, sheep, buffalo
- **Cheeses**: cow, goat, sheep

**Plant-based proteins**

- **Cereals**: wheat (soft wheat, hard wheat, spelt, small spelt, also called common wheat), oats, rye, barley, corn, rice
- Buckwheat, quinoa, manioc (tapioca)
- **Fruits**: citrus fruits (orange, lemon, grapefruit), olives, hazelnuts, walnuts, cashew nuts, dried grapes (sultanas), apples, pears, kiwis, bananas, pineapples, chestnuts, coconuts, dates, persimmon (khakis), apricot, figs, avocado, etc.
- **Vegetables**: carrots, potatoes, leeks, fennel, peas, sweet potato, aubergine (eggplant), courgette
- **Leguminous plants**: lentils, chickpeas, soybeans
- **Condiments (seasonings)**: garlic, onions, pepper, mustard, thyme, rosemary, bay leaf (laurel)
- Coffee, tea, chocolate, honey, and by-products
- **Oils**: olive, sunflower, corn, grape seed, sesame, walnut, rapeseed (colza)

### 27.4.3 Approaching the Food Test towards the Ear

This basic test will allow us to discriminate between intolerances and allergies (**Figure 27.2**). The examiner, while taking the patient's pulse with the left hand, will slowly approach the food test containing the food in the direction of the patient's ear with the right hand, starting at approximately 30 cm to measure the distance at which a RAC is triggered (see Chapter 12).

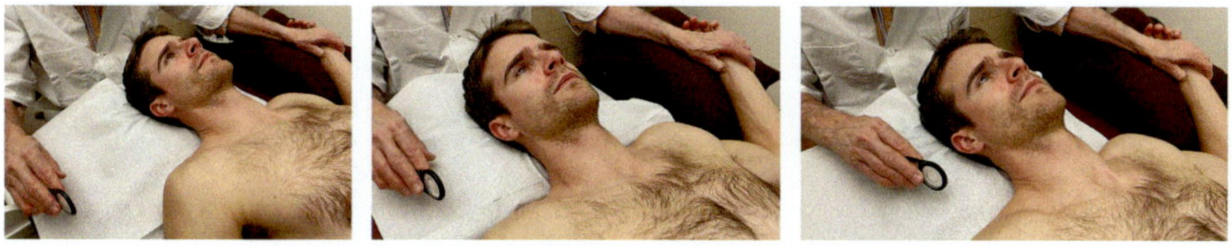

**Figure 27.2** Approach test for the detection of food hypersensitivity.

Usually, at 8–12 cm, the examiner will feel a positive RAC reaction. The pulse becomes stronger. This reaction is normal. It means the patient is neither intolerant nor allergic to the food they may consume normally. We call this RAC reaction the *recognition sign* and interpret it as an "adaptation" of the body to the tested substance. It seems that when the organism recognises a substance, it will not trigger a rejection process.

*In case of intolerance (non-allergic),* the recognition sign reacts much further away from the ear. More than 12 cm away, it can be observed up to 30 cm. The greater the recognition distance, the greater the intolerance. In this category, the patient will be asked to reduce the quantity of food consumed. As this is not an allergy, it is not necessary to eliminate the food entirely. This is often the case with foods that contain active chemical substances, such as coffee, alcohol, chocolate, and foods containing histamine (Sauerkraut, spinach, tomato, eggplant, avocado, citrus fruit, strawberries, bananas, etc.).

*In case of allergy,* the recognition sign does not exist. No positive RAC is observed when the test ring is approached towards the ear. There is even a collapse of the pulse, which can last for several seconds. For years, we believed that the sign of allergy was a positive RAC produced on approaching the food. This was a mistake due to confusion with food intolerances, which are much more frequent than allergies. In fact, in the case of allergy, it seems the body is fighting against a substance it does not recognise.

### 27.4.4 Contact Test

The purpose of this test is to identify food *allergies.*

The contact test consists of placing the test ring directly on the skin, not on the ear, but usually on the chest (**Figure 27.3**), to observe the reactions of the radial pulse following contact. During the test, the patient's chest must be exposed to a sufficiently powerful light. Normally, when a test ring containing food is placed on the skin, the pulse does not change. But in case of food allergy, the pulse will collapse after one, two, or three beats. This is an example of negative RAC (see Chapters 5 and 28): comparing the artery to the tube of a bicycle tyre, you get the impression that the tyre is deflated and no longer consistent. The test ring should then be removed and placed

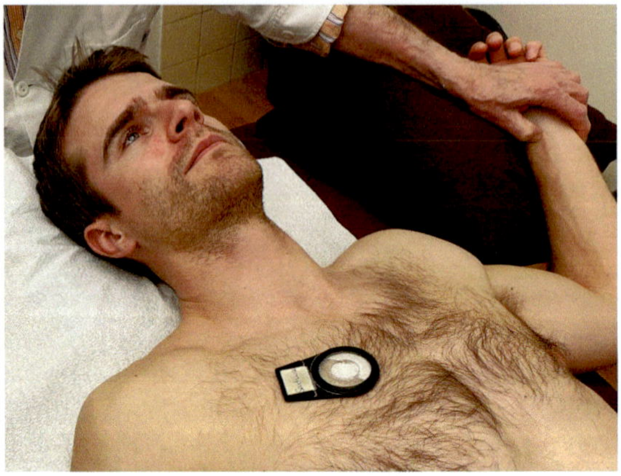

**Figure 27.3** Contact test for allergic hypersensitivity.

at a distance from the patient, if possible, behind the examiner, so that it no longer has any parasite influence on the patient. The number of pulses required to restore the pulse to normal must then be counted. The number of reactive pulses (negative RACs) will determine the importance of the allergy. In the case of a minor allergy, the pulse returns to normal in less than five beats. The maximum to have been observed so far is two hundred. Counting the pulses is essential for establishing the hierarchy of allergies in the event of several allergies within the same patient.

The phenomenon is less marked in children than adults; the pulse count (negative RACs) before returning to normal is lower. As few as two pulses before returning to normal in a child indicates an established allergy.

- Conditions for the food tests to be valid.
- Only foods consumed by the patient can be tested. If the subject does not eat a particular food for several weeks, testing this food results in the absence of reaction and, therefore, is uninterpretable. The patient must have consumed the food to be tested within a fortnight before the test session. This often raises a problem because today, it is common to see patients who, following questionable biological tests, have eliminated various foods from their diet.
- Some drugs may alter the tests, beta-blockers, cortisone, and antihistamines.
- The foods should be tested one by one. One must pay attention to keeping the test rings that are not being tested at a distance from the patient, so they do not influence the testing. I recommend putting the rings under a white cloth at a fair distance from the patient, behind the examiner. If the food is too near the patient, the light passing through it can create parasite RAC reactions.
- The RAC and the photogram must be of good quality, and there should be no RAC exhaustion. The white light test must be perfect.

## PROTOCOL 10: SCREENING FOR NON-IgE-DEPENDENT FOOD ALLERGIES

The tests require two or more sessions. The first session is the most important and will condition the rest of the patient's course.

### Questioning the Patient

Often, at the first session, we face a patient who comes to us after having tried other therapeutic methods. The question we often ask ourselves is: Are the symptoms exhibited by the patient related to food hypersensitivity? Several elements can guide us.

- Delayed food allergy is most often found in **women and children**. Men sometimes develop hypersensitivities, but less frequently.
- All chronic diseases, whatever the type, should lead to a food investigation. Whether in the psychiatric, rheumatological, immunological, digestive, or endocrine fields, from the moment an illness becomes chronic, it appears imperative to look for a food allergy: for instance, in the case of polyarthritis, autoimmune diseases, non-reactive depression, migraines, joint pain, or fibromyalgia, etc.
- The combination of several signs described as possible in food allergy should suggest a probable diagnosis of food hypersensitivity:
  - Migraine–hypotension
  - Depression–constipation
  - Depression–eczema
  - Joint pain–hypotension
  - Urticaria–disgust of pure milk
  - Constipation–arterial hypotension
  - Mastodynia–constipation
  - Infertility–urticaria–thyroiditis
  - Mouth ulcers, constipation, sleep disorders: This triad, which I call *Nogier's triad*, can often be the expression of hypersensitivity to wheat.
  - Etc.

### Consulting the Health Record

The health record, established during childhood, is a key element for diagnosing food allergy. What is the history referring to the patient's birth and early childhood?

- Delivery by vaginal route or caesarean section?
- Breastfeeding? Bottle-feeding?
- Abdominal pain?
- Eczema?
- Otitis?

What foods and drugs were introduced from birth to 12 months of age? Adults often show hypersensitivity to foods consumed during the first year of life. **Therefore, it is necessary to scrupulously consult and analyse the health record and question the parents**. If they are alive and not present at the consultation, the best thing to do is to try to reach them by telephone or mail, to gather the necessary information. One should also pay attention to the fact that some drugs given during early childhood contain food proteins and can trigger certain food sensitivities. This is the case with vitamin D, often given with olive oil as an excipient.

- What vaccinations did the child receive?
- Medical and surgical history
    - Tonsillectomy?
    - Infectious diseases?
    - Antibiotics?
    - Anti-inflammatory drugs?
    - Birth control pill?
    - Nervous breakdowns?
    - Mastodynia?
    - Sun hives (urticaria)?
    - Constipation?

All these items may point to food hypersensitivity. Some allergies occur after an episode of fever. It is important, for example, to know what diet followed a febrile infectious disease and if this disease led to food hypersensitivity. Tonsillectomy is often a sign that infections occurred during childhood, with a likelihood of allergy, etc.

## Physical Examination of the Patient

### At Inspection

#### *General condition of the patient*

- Slender?
- Well-developed thighs?
- Slender women with thin, muscular thighs often have high blood pressure, whereas women with large thighs ("saddlebags") tend to have low blood pressure. This can be easily explained. When there are food allergies, cytotoxins seem to be released, dilating the venous vessels. The blood then accumulates in the venous compartment, to

the detriment of the arterial compartment, which explains the drop in blood pressure. After some time, this venous dilatation tends to create a particular conformity in women: saddlebag thighs. It is sometimes believed that they suffer from water retention.

- Arterial hypotension and unattractive thighs usually disappear with a well-chosen and well-managed eviction regime (**Figure 27.4**).

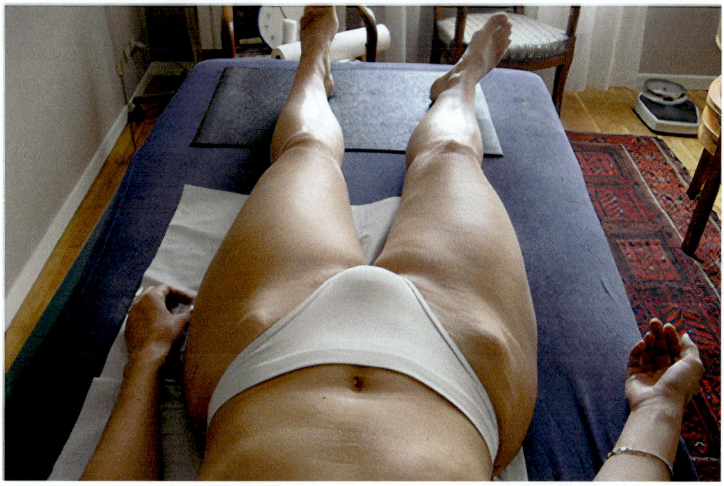

**Figure 27.4** Developed thighs in women with food sensitivities.

- Skin texture: A person suffering from a food allergy often has pale, translucent skin. In many cases, the skin can be detached from the deep planes. It is possible to observe a sign of skin folding (described by R. Nogier). This sign is to be looked for on the skin of the back. Between the thumb and forefinger of both hands, ten centimetres apart, the skin is pulled to detach it. Normally, the skin should remain attached to the deep planes. We have noticed that a fold appears in patients suffering from food allergy (**Figure 27.5**).
- One may also observe marbling on the thighs. Contrary to popular belief, a child with marbled thighs is less healthy than others. Livedo is very common in cow's milk protein allergies. It is rare in cereal allergies (**Figure 27.6**).

*Looking for suggestive clinical signs*

- **Pallor of the skin**: In a healthy individual, the complexion is fresh, and the cheeks are pink. In a person suffering from food allergy, the skin is pale, and the complexion is cloudy.

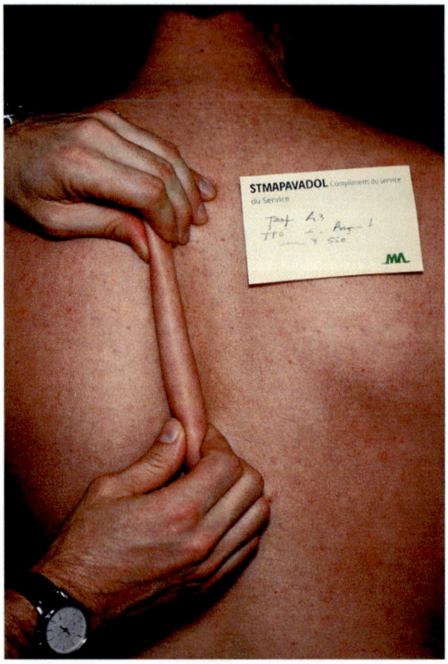


**Figure 27.5** The skin fold sign.

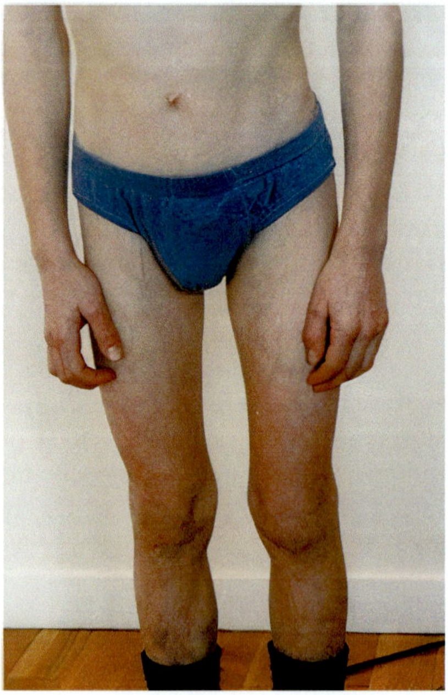

**Figure 27.6** Marbled thighs of a 14-year-old boy suffering from wheat allergy.

- **Low blood pressure**: Low blood pressure is a valuable sign pointing to possible food hypersensitivity. It had never been described in this condition, but I have observed it over many years. When we examine a woman having a systolic pressure of 90 mm Hg, we should always look for other signs that could similarly suggest a nutritional disorder, such as migraine, depression, or constipation. This type of hypotension can occur due to the action of interleukins secreted in delayed allergy and influencing vasomotor activity.
- A person not taking any chemical treatment, and whose systolic pressure is below 90 mm Hg suffers a priori from a food allergy until proven otherwise. It should also be noted that very low blood pressures are mainly observed in women. Men with a systolic pressure below 100 mm Hg are rare. Measuring the arterial pressure on both arms is advisable, with the patient first lying down and then standing. Orthostatic arterial hypotension should also be considered.
- **Sign of Chvostek**: The facial nerve is struck with a flick of the fingers (chiquenaude) against the cheek to observe whether this produces a contraction of the upper lip. If it does so, it means there is a neuromuscular hyperreactivity and, therefore, probably a mineral deficiency. This would suggest the possibility of digestive malabsorption and, therefore, the risk of food allergy (**Figure 27.7**). However, the Chvostek sign cannot be considered a sure sign of allergic hypersensitivity.

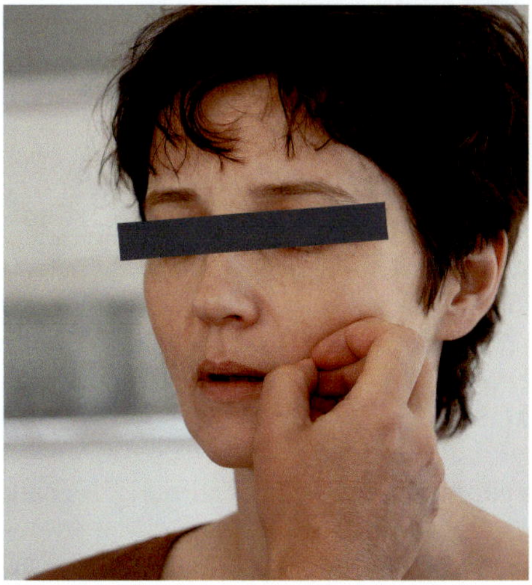

**Figure 27.7** Chvosteck's sign.

- **Dermographism**: Neither is dermographism a pathognomonic sign of food allergy. Usually, when one touches or lightly scrapes the skin of the patient's back with a foam tip, nothing will happen. In the case of dermographism, a red line, or more rarely a white line, will appear within seconds, up to a minute. This represents a localised pressure urticaria with local mast cell degranulation. Dermographism is present in many food hypersensitivities. It is important to note the delay in the onset of the skin reaction. There appears to be a correlation between the time of onset of the skin reaction and the duration necessary for the exclusion diet. The longer the delay of onset of the dermographism, the longer the diet should last (**Figure 27.8**).

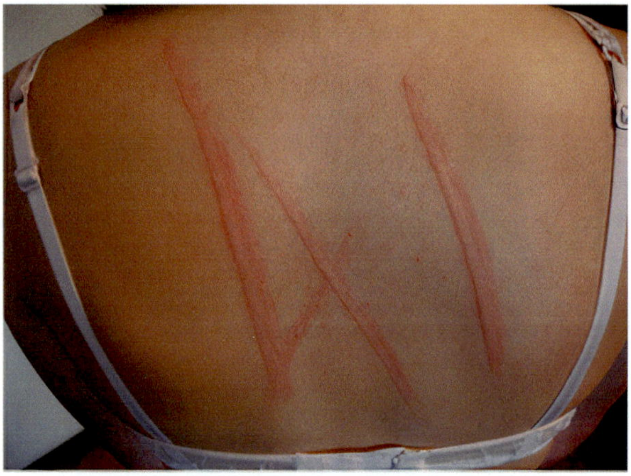

**Figure 27.8** Dermographism in a patient with potato allergy.

- **Alteration of hair and nails**: In case of food hypersensitivity, it is not uncommon to observe dry, dull, and brittle hair.
- **Oedema of the extremities**: In case of intestinal malabsorption, we can observe mild oedema of the extremities due to hypoproteinaemia. Malabsorption has many aetiologies, including food hypersensitivity.
- **Pallor of the conjunctiva**: A sign of anaemia, is common with gluten intolerance.
- **Tense abdomen and bloating**: A normal abdomen should be soft and not tense. It is not uncommon in food hypersensitivities to observe swollen, tense, painful abdomens, sonorous on percussion.

## How the Tests Are Conducted

### *The First Session*

Following the classical part of the examination, we will proceed to testing with the vascular reflex. This requires a good-quality RAC and a normal photogram. If this is not the case, return to Chapter 25.

It should be remembered that when the patient eliminates a food for more than four or five weeks, testing that food will become negative even if there is still a clinical hypersensitivity. Therefore, only foods presently consumed by the subject can be validly tested.

During this first session, all the types of foods that the patient consumes are tested. We generally use the contact test, which consists of placing each test ring on the patient's chest for a few seconds. We then wait for five or six pulses to see if the pulse remains stable or collapses (note that in this test, the RAC consists of a *collapsed* pulse, referred to as a *negative* RAC). Immediately after the onset of the negative RAC, one removes the test ring from the thorax and counts the number of negative RACs occurring before the pulse returns to normal.

We will often identify several foods that induce a pulse reaction. So, recording the number of pulse reactions will allow us to compare the importance of hypersensitivity for each food.

After having tested the types of foods, the patient will be instructed to eliminate those found to react from their diet, for four weeks (between three and five weeks), after which they must then return for a second test.

### *The Second Session*

During this session, we will test only the foods detected in the first session that were removed from the patient's diet. The aim is to identify primary and secondary allergens. Only the primary allergens will induce a pulse reaction in the second session. The others will not create any pulse change. On the practical level, only those foods found in both the first and the second sessions will be eliminated. Those who were "positive" only at the first session but not four weeks later can be consumed as normal again.

Following the second session, a strict diet can be implemented by excluding one or two foods.

***The Following Sessions***

Since diets sometimes take a long time to produce results, their validity should be assessed based on clinical signs that will have been noted at the first session. Only the improvement of the clinical signs will allow us to appreciate the validity of the diet.

At each session, we must ensure that the patient follows the diet correctly. To do this, we will test the foods the patient must eliminate at each session. If the tests remain positive after six weeks, it means that the patient is still absorbing the prohibited food. This happens frequently because patients often make mistakes through sheer ignorance, omitting to check the labels of the industrial products they consume.

If, after three months on the exclusion diet, the patient is not benefiting from it, do not hesitate to suspend the diet and start the tests again from scratch.

## What Foods Are Most Commonly Found in Food Allergies?

The following products are widely consumed:

- Wheat
- Dairy (cow, sheep, goat)
- Eggs
- Beef
- Potatoes
- Olives
- Pork
- Honey
- Tomatoes
- Oranges

However, delayed allergies can also be detected with foods consumed in small quantities.

### First Example

A 38-year-old man has been suffering from chronic urticaria for several years, treated with antihistamines four times a day. Hereafter is our correspondence.

6/12/2015

*Dear Doctor,*

*One year ago, your colleague, Dr Marc G., referred me to you to investigate a chronic urticaria (hives).*

*You detected a reaction to tomatoes, wheat, and pepper. I was taking four antihistamines a day at the time.*

*After a 6-month diet, I returned to see you in mid-June this year. At that time, I was not taking any medication.*

*Apart from a few spots of hives on my body, I haven't had anything since.*

*At our last meeting, you asked me to continue my diet and to contact you again at the end of the year.*

*I am writing this message to you to find out what I should do next.*

*With best regards,*

*M.*

17/12/2015

*Dear Sir,*

*Thank you for letting me know how you are doing.*

*Could you, in a first stage, start eating pepper again for a month, then tomatoes for a month, and finally start eating wheat again in the form of small spelt (einkorn), which you can find in organic food shops. Take care that it is small spelt and not spelt.*

*Then, after reintroducing the three foods one by one, I would like to see you again during springtime to repeat the tests.*

*Should the hives reappear, please do not hesitate to contact me.*

*Dr Nogier*

12/01/2016

*Hello Doctor,*

*I wish you a very happy New Year.*

*I have introduced pepper into my diet (in very limited amounts), and after a few days, I started to itch again and have some hives.*

*I did not retake any medication (antihistamine), but since then, I have stopped eating pepper, and I still suffer from itching.*

*What should I do now?*

*Sincerely*

*M.*

12/01/2016

*Dear Sir,*

*Do not use pepper again.*

*Usually, the itching should subside within two or three weeks.*

*If this is not the case, please call me.*

*Anyway, keep me informed.*

*Have a nice day*

*Dr Nogier*

12/03/2016

*Hello Doctor,*

*I'm back to give you an update on the course of hives.*

*I haven't had any itching or hives for about four weeks now.*

*I'm waiting to hear from you about what to do next.*

*Sincerely*

*M.*

12/03/2016

*Hello,*

*The pepper-free diet should be continued, and low-dose tomato consumption should be tried.*

*Take two tomatoes a week and see what happens.*

*Dr Nogier*

**Comments**:

This case is very representative of a delayed allergy.

1. It takes several weeks on a pepper-free diet before the hives disappear. Therefore, it is not an immediate allergy nor a non-allergic intolerance.
2. When pepper is reintroduced, it takes several days before the itching returns.
3. Returning to a pepper-free diet again requires several weeks before the signs disappear.
4. Normally, this patient should have returned 4 weeks after the first session to repeat the tests. This was not the case because he lived far away, and it was difficult to get him to return.

## Second Example

An informative case: Kathy K. Migraines. Age 30. Delayed onset of allergy to wheat only.

I first met this woman at age 30. She was suffering from severe attacks of migraine. Her first migraine attack occurred when she was 20 years old. For six weeks prior to this first attack, she had suffered from continuous headaches. A CT scan had been performed, and the neurologist, having no objective findings, had concluded it was a functional disorder.

Since then, the attacks had recurred regularly. Sometimes, the patient had two migraines per month, sometimes a single attack over two or three months, unrelated to the cycle.

The duration of the attacks was inconstant: between 12 and 72 hours. Sometimes, the attacks were mere headaches, accompanied by nausea; at other times, they were associated with a very strong aura or paresis of the right arm.

The patient had tried a non-corticoid anti-inflammatory drug, such as ibuprofen, but more frequently, paracetamol or aspirin.

Unfortunately, the medication usually led to a temporary reduction in pain, which returned after sedation. To such an extent that the medication prolonged the duration of the migraine attacks. So, the patient had decided not to take any more medication, to go to bed and to sleep, and to take an extra day off work just after the attacks had ended.

This woman had no notable personal history. However, her mother and grandmother, as well as her brother, also suffered from migraine.

I first saw Kathy at the age of 30 (January 2001), after ten years of migraine attacks. Her radial pulse tests revealed a hostile reaction to wheat and only wheat. Consequently, a wheat-free diet was prescribed.

Quite soon after starting the wheat-free diet, symptoms such as heartburn, less serious headaches and fatigue following meals disappeared.

The migraines became less severe, and the attacks shorter. In September 2001, the patient had her last migraine, eight months after starting the diet.

However, Kathy did consume rye. So, it was not a gluten-free diet. After two years on the diet, Kathy introduced small spelt, an ancient and rustic form of wheat. The migraines did not return.

During a holiday in 2008, the patient tried to resume normal wheat. The migraines reappeared after one week of consumption, resulting in more prolonged and more intense attacks than before. Moreover, the headaches reappeared frequently for two to three months (to the surprise of the patient, who had forgotten about them until then), even after the wheat was eliminated. The patient then took the final decision to eliminate wheat from her diet.

Kathy's case is fascinating. It is a case of wheat hypersensitivity without gluten intolerance. It is only wheat that causes the migraines. Kathy can consume other cereals containing gluten. Remember that cereals contain numerous proteins and that gluten only represents part of these proteins.

Furthermore, we are evidently in the presence of a delayed allergy. In 2001, it took several months from the time Kathy stopped eating wheat until the attacks disappeared. And in 2008, it took three months without any wheat before the migraine attacks disappeared. The same is true of the long delay in the onset of migraines when wheat was reintroduced. When Kathy returned to wheat after eight years of abstinence, the migraines only returned after consuming wheat for one week.

Finally, Kathy tolerates spelt (einkorn) but not soft wheat. True enough, the proteins are different in these two types of wheat. Soft wheat, commonly used today, has a genome with 42 chromosomes, whereas einkorn has only 14. The proteins are therefore different from one another.

## 27.5 PATIENT HANDOUT: ANSWERS TO YOUR QUESTIONS

**What is the meaning of RAFT** ***(RAC Assisted Food Test)*****?**

A RAFT is an examination carried out at your physician's office to screen adverse reactions to food.

**How is the examination conducted?**

The physician takes the patient's pulse while placing test rings containing the food onto the chest. By studying variations in the tone of the arterial wall (arterial reflex or RAC), the physician can detect abnormal reactions to individual foods.

**Is the examination painful?**

No

**Can RAFTs detect food allergies?**

Yes, with RAFTs, it is possible to diagnose food allergies.

**In what indications should RAFT be used?**

RAFTs are indicated in all chronic diseases and especially in autoimmune diseases. Here are the most frequently found diseases: migraine, constipation, irritable bowel syndrome, ulcerative colitis, Crohn's disease, mouth ulcers, chronic fatigue, nervous breakdown, sleep disorders, abnormal weight gain, chronic joint pain, eczema, urticaria, mastodynia, and fertility disorders in women.

**Are RAFTs 100% reliable?**

No, like any test, RAFTs are not 100% reliable. They must be interpreted according to the clinical context.

**Is one session enough?**

No, it usually takes two sessions at three to five-week intervals.

**Can RAFTs replace the classical examinations carried out by the allergologist: IgE assay, prick tests, re-introduction test?**

No, the examinations carried out by an allergologist can lead to valuable diagnoses. RAFTs should be considered as a complement.

**Are there any precautions to be taken prior to the tests?**

Yes, you should inform the physician about any medication you are taking before the RAFT is performed. Some medications may affect the results: cortisone or antihistamines. You should also know that eliminating a particular food before the RAFT will alter the results. You should, therefore, inform the doctor if you are already on a diet.

**Does Social Security reimburse the tests?**

No. Since health authorities do not currently recognise RAFTs in most countries (e.g. NHS in Great Britain, Medicare in the USA, Social Security in France, etc.), they are generally not reimbursed by social security.

### What is the cost of these tests?

Social Security does not reimburse these tests, so there is no standard quotation. The cost depends on the time spent, and the fees are at the practitioner's discretion. Some RAFTs are very time-consuming. Others take less time.

## NOTE

1. Until 1950, the French as well as the British were submitted to ration coupons.

## BIBLIOGRAPHY


1. Apfelbaum M, Romon M, Dubus M. *Dietetics and nutrition.* 7th edition. Collection Abrégés. Masson 2009
2. Bhombal S, Bothwell MR, Bauer SM. Prevalence of elevated total IgE and food allergies in a consecutive series of ENT pediatric patients. *Otolaryngology, Head and Neck Surgery* 2006 Apr, 134(4), 578–80
3. Bousquet J, Dhivert H, Michel *F. Immunological diagnosis of food allergy.* In Allergies alimentaires Navaro Shmitz. Doin 1993. pp. 193–207
4. Boyano-Martinez T, Garcia-Arac, *et al.* Validity of specific IgE antibodies in children with egg allergy. *Clinical & Experimental Allergy* 2001, 31, 1464–9
5. Caleb K, Venu G. Sex disparity in Food Allergy. Evidence from the PubMed Database. *Journal of Allergy* (Cairo) 2009 DOI: 10.1155/2009/159845.
6. Caffarelli C, Baldi F, Calzone L, Marani M, Pasquinelli P. Cow's milk protein allergy in children. A practical guide. *Italian Journal of Paediatrics* 2010, 36, 5
7. Campeotto F, Walligora-Dupriet AJ *et al.* Establishment of the intestinal flora of the newborn. *Gastroenterology Clinical and Biological* 2007, 31(5), 533–42
8. Carrocio A, Iacono G. Review article. Chronic constipation and food sensitivity – an intriguing relationship. *Alimentary Pharmacology and Therapeutics* 2006, 24, 1295–304. Journal compilation
9. Clark AT, Ewan PW. Interpretation of food tests for nut allergy in one thousand patients, in relation to allergy or intolerance. *Clinical & Experimental Allergy.* 2003, 33, 10141–5
10. Dahers, Tahan S, Sole D, *et al.* Cow's milk protein intolerance and chronic constipation in children. *Pediatric Allergy and Immunology* 2001, 12, 339–42
11. Delluc G, Delluc M, Roques Martine. *Prehistoric nutrition.* Editions Pilote 24. Périgueux 1995
12. Desroches A, Infante-Rivard C, Paradis L, Paradis J, Haddad E. Peanut allergy. Is maternal transmission of antigens during pregnancy and breastfeeding a risk factor? *Journal of Investigational Allergology and Clinical Immunology.* 2010, 20(4), 289–94
13. Diesner SG, Untersmayr *E et al.* Food allergy, only a pediatric disease? *Gerontology* 2011, 57(1), 28–32
14. Doussinaut G, Pavoine M-T, Jaudeau B, Jahier J. *Evolution of genetic variability in wheat.* INRA. Dossier de l'environnement n° 2001
15. Dupin H. *L'alimentation des français*, ESF Editions 1978

16. Dupont C. Les tests de perméabilité intestinale In *Allergies alimentaires* Navaro Shmitz. Doin 1993. pp. 209–23
17. Ebert CS Jr, Pillsbury HC 3rd. Epidemiology of allergy. *Otolaryngologic Clinics of North America* 2011 Jun, 44 (3), 537–48
18. Eigenmann P. Anaphylactic reactions to raw eggs after negative challenge to cooked eggs. *Journal of Allergy and Clinical Immunology* 2000, 105, 587–8
19. Fiocchi A. Assa'ad A., Adverse Reactions to food Committee; American College of Allergy, Asthma and Immunology. Food allergy and the introduction of solid foods to infants. A consensus document. *Annals of Allergy, Asthma, & Immunology* 2006 Jul, 97(1), 10–20; quiz 21, 77
20. Fougereau M. *L'immunologie*. PUF 1995
21. Genetet N. *Immunology*. 4th edition. Lavoisier 2002
22. Goulet O. *DIU Clinical Nutrition*. Hôpital Necker 2010
23. Greer F, Sicherer S, Burks A. Effects of early nutritional interventions on developing atopic disease in infants and children. The role of maternal dietary restriction, breastfeeding, timing of introduction of complementary foods, and hydrolysed formulas. *Paediatrics* 2008, 121(1), 183–191
24. Grevers G, Rocken M. *Atlas de poche d'allergologie*. Médecine-Sciences Flammarion 2002
25. Guandalini S, Newland C. Differentiating food allergies from food intolerance. *Current Gastroenterology Reports , Curr Gastroenterol Rep.* 2011 Oct;13(5):426-34.
26. Guariso G, Conte F, Presotto D, Basso D, Brotto F, Visona L, Pedini B, Haines ML, Anderson RP, Gibson PR. Systematic review. The evidence base for long-term management of celiac disease. *Alimentary Pharmacology & Therapeutics Aliment Pharmacol Ther.* 2008 Nov 1;28(9):1042-66
27. Hermier M, Lachaux A, Descos B. Intolerance to cow's milk proteins. *Pédiatrie T* 1986, 1, 71–81, 3, 251–261
28. Heyman M. Food antigens, intestinal barrier and mucosal immunity. *Cahiers de nutrition et de diététique* 2010, 17–23
29. Ikezono E, Ikezono T, Ackerman J. Establishing the existence of the active stomach point in the auricle utlizing Radial Artery Tonometry. *Am J Chin Med.* 2003;31(2):285–94.
30. Isolauri E, Turjanmaa K. Combined skin prick test and patch testing enhances identification of food allergy in infants with atopic dermatitis. *Journal of Allergy and Clinical Immunology* 1996, 97, 9–15
31. Kiefte-de J *et al.* Infant nutritional factors and functional constipation in childhood. The generation R study. *American Journal of Gastroenterology* 2010 Apr, 105, 940–5
32. Knekt P, Jarvinen R, Seppanen R, Pukkala E, Aromaa A. Intake of dairy products and the risk of breast cancer. *British Journal of Cancer* 1996, 73, 687–91
33. Lepine JP, Lelouch J, Lovell A, Teherani M, Pariente P. *Epidemiology of anxiety and depressive disorders in a French general population.* Groupe hospitalier Bichat-Claude Bernard, 1994
34. Maes M, Leunis JC. Normalisation of leaky gut in chronic fatigue syndrome is accompanied by clinical improvement. Effect of age, duration of illness and the translocation of PPS from gram-negative bacteria. *Neuro Endocrinology Letters* 2008 Dec, 29(6), 902–10
35. Maes M., Coucke F., Leunis J.C. Normalisation of the increased translocation of endotoxin from gram-negative enterobacteria (leaky gut) is accompanied by a remission of chronic fatigue syndrome. *Neuro Endocrinology Letters* 2007 Dec, 28(6), 739–44
36. Magnin P. *Des photons et de la vie*. Sauramps Médical Editions Montpellier 2010

37. Magnin P. *The forty-five years of the Glem. Les annales du Glem 2009–2010.* 49 rue Mercière 69002 Lyon
38. Marignan M. 1993. L'enregistrement du VAS in "La photoperception cutanée" by Raphaël Nogier. Haug, International Editions. Brussels
39. Marignan M. 2003. Vingt ans de recherche au Glem in "*Les actes d'Alba*". Éditions Sauramps Médical. pp. 87–112
40. Majamaa H, Moisio P, Holm K, Turjanmaa K. Cow's milk allergy. *Diagnostic Accuracy of Skin Prick and Patch Tests and Specific IgE*, 1999, 54, 346–51
41. Majamaa H, Moisio P, Holm K, Turjanmaa K. Wheat allergy. *Diagnostic Accuracy of Skin Prick and Patch Tests and Specific IgE*, 1999, 54, 851–56
42. Mccraken VJ, Lorenz RG. The gastrointestinal ecosystem. A precarious alliance among epithelium, immunity and microbiota.
43. Metchnikoff E. Studies on the intestinal flora. *Annales de l'Institut Pasteur Paris* 1910, 24, 755–770
44. Molkou P. *Food allergies. Current and future problems.* UCB Institute of Allergy 1995
45. Monneret-Vautrin DA, Andre C. *Immunopathology of food allergy and false alimentary allergies.* Masson 1983
46. Monneret-Vautrin. Guide du praticien en immuno-allergologie. Masson 1994
47. Miyake Y, Sasaki S, Tanaka K, Hirota Y. Consumption of vegetables, fruit, and antioxidants during pregnancy and wheeze and eczema in children. *Allergy* 2010 Jun, 65(6), 758–65. Epub 2010 Jan 22
48. Mullineaux CW. How do cyanobacteria sense and respond to light? *Molecular Microbiology* 2001, 41(5), 965–971
49. Navarro J, Faure C, Cézard JP. Manifestations digestives in *Allergies alimentaires.* Doin 1993. pp. 119–34
50. Nicolas JF, Thivolet J, Goujon C. *Les urticaires.* John Libbey Eurotext 2001
51. Nogier P. *Traité d'auriculothérapie.* Maisonneuve éditeur 1969
52. Nogier P. L'oreille voit - Possibilités d'un réflexe nouveau- *Revue Méridiens n°5- E.F.A-A.S.M.A.F.* -75007 Paris, 1969
53. Nogier P, Nogier R. The man in the ear. Editions Sauramps Médical 2009
54. Nogier R, Nogier P, Menezzo Y, Santini R, Khatchadourian C. Influence of skin illumination on plasma biogenic amines in the rabbit. *Acupuncture and Electro-Therapeutics* 1982, 7, 247–53
55. Nogier R. Ce lait qui menace les femmes. Le Rocher 1994
56. Nogier R. *From hidden allergies to breast diseases.* Sauramps Médical Montpellier 1997
57. Nogier R. Le bonheur est dans l'assiette. Ambre 2000
58. World Health Organisation. Quantity and Quality of Breast Milk. *Report on a* collective *study on breastfeeding.* 1987
59. World Health Organization. Diet, nutrition and prevention of chronic diseases. Report of a Working Group. *Technical Report Series 797*, Geneva 1990
60. Papageorgiou PS. Clinical aspects of food allergy. *Biochemical Society Transactions* 2002 Nov, 30 (Pt6), 901–6
61. Perrin L.F. Practical Allergology 3rd edition. *Collection abrégés.* Masson 1998
62. Rance F, Dutau G. Les allergies alimentaires. *Expansion scientifique française.* Institut UCB de l'allergie, 2004
63. Rancé F, Dutau G. Atopic dermatitis and food allergens in De la dermatite atopique à l'asthme. *Expansion Scientifique Française and UCB Institute of Allergy*, 2000. pp. 129–37

64. Rancé F, Dutau G. The multiple allergy syndrome. *Journal Revue Francaise d'Allergologie* 1998, 38, 267–74
65. Rance F, Kanny G, Dutau G, Monneret-Vauterin DA. Clinical aspects of food allergy. *Journal Revue Francaise d'Allergologie* 1998, 38 (10), 900–5
66. Rancé F. What is the optimal occlusion time for the atopy patch test in the diagnosis of food allergies in children with atopic dermatitis? *Pediatric Allergy and Immunology* 2004, 15, 93–6
67. Rapin JR, Wiensperger N. Possible links between intestinal permeability and food processing. A potential therapeutic niche for glutamine. *Clinics* (Sao Paulo). 2010 June, 65(6), 635–43
68. Reda SM. Gastrointestinal manifestations of food allergy. *Pediatr Health* 2009, (3), 217–29
69. Revillard JP. Immunology 2nd edition. De Boeck University Brussels 1995
70. Rivière-Wekstein. *Discovering the wheat genome, a challenge for the future.* Agriculture and Environment February 2011
71. Rouxeville Y. *L'acupuncure personnalisée.* Sauramps Médical Montpellier 2000
72. Ruemmele F. *Intestinal flora and immunity. Archives of Paediatrics* 2007, 14, 2–4
73. Santini R, Menezo Y *et al. Influence of skin illumination on blood glycemia of the rabbit.* Laboratory of Physiology. *INSA Villeurbanne* 1983
74. Sander, Sherman L. *Human Physiology.* 5e French edition Maloine 2009
75. Sausenthaler S, Heinrich J, Koletsko S. Early diet and the risk of allergy. What can we learn from the prospective birth cohort studies GINIplus and LISAplus? *American Journal of Clinical Nutrition. Am J Clin Nutr.* 2011 Dec;94(6 Suppl):2012S-2017S
76. Sekirov I, Finlay B. The role of the intestinal microbiota in enteric infection. *J Physiol.* 2009 Jun 2;587(Pt 17):4159–4167
77. Simeone D, Miele E, Boccia G, Marino A, Troncone R, Staiano A. Prevalence of atopy with chronic constipation. *Archives of Disease in Childhood* 2008 Dec, 93(12), 1044–7
78. Sousa de A. *The vascular signal.* Groupe Lyonnais d'Études Médicales 1996
79. Sousa de A. *The Auriculo Cardiac Reflex.* Groupe Lyonnais d'Etudes Médicales 2009
80. Syrigou E, Pitsios C et al. Food allergy-related paediatric constipation. The usefulness of atopy patch test. *European Journal of Pediatrics* 2011 Sep, 170 (9), 1173–8
81. Tatham AS, Shewry PR. Allergens in wheat and related cereals. *Clinical and Experimental Allergy* 2008, 38, 1712–26
82. Terral C. *Pain and acupuncture.* Sauramps Méical 2009
83. Tursi A, Giorgetti GM, Brandimarte G, Elisei W. High prevalence oc celiac disease among patients affected by Crohn's disease. *Inflamm Bowel Dis.* 2005 Jul;11(7):662–6
84. Vandenplas Y. Epidemiology in "*Allergies Alimentaires " Progrès en pédiatrie.* Doin éditeur 1993. pp. 17–23
85. Vermeil G, Dartois AM, Fraissex du M. *L'alimentation de l'enfant de la naissance à 3 ans.* Doin éditeur. 1987
86. Vincent D, Bienvenu J, Muller JY, *Hypersensitivity reactions*, in Immunology 4th edition. Coordinator Noëlle Genetet EMF Editions Paris 2002. pp. 491–553
87. Vulliez C. *Infrared lasers in odonto-stomatology.* Conference at the Groupe Lyonnais d'Études Médicales 2011

# CHAPTER 28

# Use of the RAC in Miscellaneous Pathologies

**Raphaël Nogier**

## 28.1 PSYCHO-EMOTIONAL TRAUMA

### 28.1.1 Avicenna's Observation

Avicenna was a physician and philosopher who lived in the Middle East around the year 1000 AD. Today, Iraqis say he was an Iraqi, while Iranians claim that he was Persian. Widely known, he was considered one of the great physicians of his time and left many works that inspired generations of physicians and philosophers after him. One of his observations, which has remained famous, can be considered relevant to the techniques we present in this book

One day, while travelling throughout Persia with a group of friends, Avicenna is called upon by a Sultan. Having heard of the physician's widespread reputation, the Sultan urges him to examine his nephew, a young man twenty years old, who has not uttered a word for several weeks, remains prostrate, and no longer answers any of the questions put to him. His worried uncle has already consulted many local doctors, but none of them had any idea of either diagnosis or treatment. After having been informed of the young man's story, Avicenna realises that he is faced with a seemingly impossible task, that he might well be falling into a trap, and end up making a fool of himself.

At this point, he would have considered leaving immediately had not one of his friends persuaded him to meet the challenge. Avicenna finally accepts but asks for relatives close to the young man to be fetched and brought in. After examining the young boy and finding no physical problem, Avicenna starts addressing questions to the young boy's relatives while taking the young man's pulse. How old is he? Where does he come from? How is he related to the Sultan? Where does he live, and who lives nearby? It appears that the young man, from an aristocratic family, lives in a village nearby.

In the presence of an impressive audience, Avicenna continues asking questions while taking the young man's pulse and, in the end, addresses the Sultan, saying: I know why your nephew does not speak. He suffers from an ailment everyone can suffer from, maybe even you, and this ailment is lovesickness. Your nephew is in love with a young girl living in the same village, but he cannot marry her because she is not of royal blood. The Sultan, believing this to be a farce, grows very angry and orders Avicenna to leave immediately. The other doctors present, jealous of Avicenna's fame, are already

DOI: 10.1201/9781003753629-28

rubbing their hands, only too pleased by his failure. But just as Avicenna and his friends are about to leave, coup de theatre, the young man suddenly rises and begins to speak. Addressing his uncle, he says: " Avicenna has told the truth".

This is a shock to everyone. The Sultan humbly apologises to his guest while everyone gathers around Avicenna to ask him how he had found the diagnosis. "I directed my questions according to variations of the pulse. Every time the patient had an emotion, the pulse changed" (**Figure 28.1**).

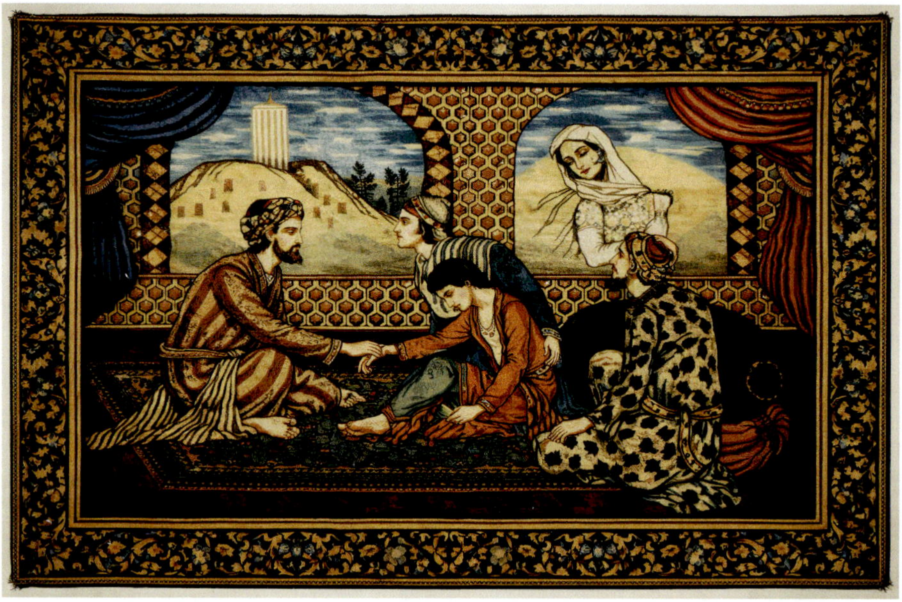

**Figure 28.1** Avicenna perceiving the young man's emotions by way of feeling the changes on his radial pulse. (Copyright © Raphaël Nogier.)

Today, of course, we do not know precisely what variations Avicenna perceived on the pulse. Nevertheless, this remarkable observation is in line with the method developed by Paul Nogier: what the patient feels emotionally elicits a response on the pulse. Note that this type of vascular response is not initiated by an external skin stimulation but internally by an emotional reaction (Section 2.1).

### 28.1.2 Searching for a Negative RAC

During the last thirty years, I have been practising and teaching the "Avicenna method", which consists of arousing emotions within a patient while at the same time analysing the pulse reactions. Observation of the radial pulse indeed makes it possible to measure the impact a trauma has had on the nervous system. A patient who has suffered psycho-emotional shock or has been exposed to some difficult situation is encouraged to speak about the problem while the examiner takes the radial pulse. When the patient comes to a painful part of the story, *negative RACs* will appear. The pulse collapses, deflating "as would the tube of a bicycle tire". The negative RAC will last for as long as the patient is recalling the painful situation. This method is very interesting because it can help detect a psychological problem that the patient may not be aware of.

Alternatively, the patient can be asked to look at photographs that have some link with the trauma. I do this with patients who do not speak my language or with those who find it difficult to express their suffering. At the following session at my practice, the patient is invited to bring photographs of landscapes, houses, or people related to the trauma. The patient looks at the photo for about fifteen seconds while I take the pulse, expecting to feel a negative RAC (collapse).

### 28.1.3 Treatment with Auriculotherapy

The patient is asked to concentrate on the traumatic event and to continue doing so for a while. This will induce a collapse of the pulse, which should last for as long as the patient maintains the mental representation of the trauma. During the time the collapse lasts, the examiner scans a black rod over the surface of the lobule, particularly over the line of sounds (see below), to detect a *positive RAC* on one or more points. These points can be found on either the right or left ear and should be confirmed with an electrical detector. They will then be treated either with needles or with **F** frequency. Treating the points should restore the pulse to normal. Usually, between two and three points can be found.

It is important to treat only one trauma per session and to see the patient again after a fortnight.

This method is very effective. It has inspired our colleague, Dr Daniel Asis, an anaesthesiologist from Argentina, who has modified the technique and proposed a structured protocol.

### 28.1.4 The "Line of Sounds"

The "line of sounds", or "sound line", is situated just below the antitragus (**Figure 28.2**). It was described by Paul Nogier in the 1970s. He had noticed that points were liable to appear on this line whenever a patient was suffering from a conflict with a person of the opposite sex: a man with his wife, a mother with her son, a brother with his sister, etc. He thought that points appearing on this line could be the expression of an unpleasant perception of either high or low tones, hence the name "sound line". To study this line, Paul Nogier even had his patients listen to piano notes and then describe the sensations they experienced. If a woman had a dislike of low tones, he would suggest a conflict with a man. If a male patient experienced

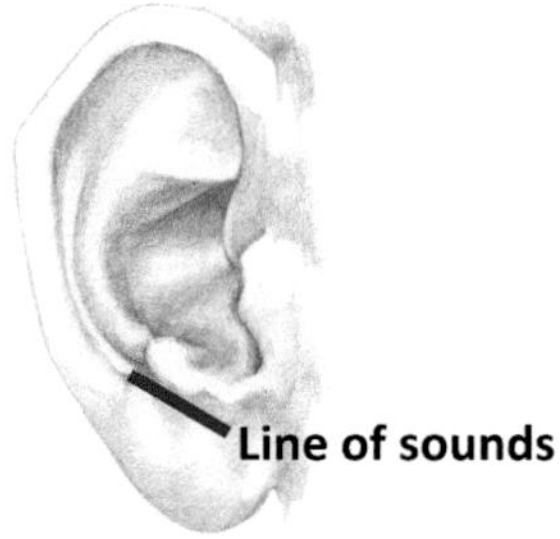


**Figure 28.2** The sound line.

high tones as unpleasant, he would suspect a conflict with a woman. He would then examine the points that would appear on the sound line.

This kind of process is typical of auriculotherapy: it can sometimes be necessary to (briefly) induce either physical or emotional suffering to elicit relevant points appearing on the ear.

## 28.2 VERTIGO

Vertigo is one of the most challenging pathologies to treat because we do not know how to tackle the problem. It is, of course, necessary to eliminate a pathological scar, a first rib, but after that, how do we proceed?

The method I use produces very good results. It is similar to the treatment applied to psycho-emotional trauma that we have just been discussing. Once again, the idea is to induce a collapse of the pulse (negative RAC) and then search for auricular points by scanning the ear with the black rod. To do this, the patient, lying supine on the examination table, is instructed to very slowly turn their head to the right, even forcing the rotation slightly, and then to turn the head back straight again and continue by turning the head towards the left. While the patient does this, the practitioner takes the pulse. If the patient is in good condition, the pulse should not vary. If the patient suffers from vertigo, the pulse usually collapses during head rotation. As long as this negative RAC lasts, one looks with the black rod for one or more points to appear (positive RAC) on the ear opposite to the direction of rotation. These points must be confirmed with an electronic detector. Normally, as soon as the point(s) are treated, the pulse ceases to collapse upon head rotation.

This phenomenon of pulse collapse upon head rotation in cases of vertigo can also be observed in the first rib syndrome (Section 9.4). A differential diagnosis must be made between these two conditions. When a first rib blockage exists due to compression of the stellate ganglion, the appropriate points for treatment will be found on the *mastoid aspect* of the ear (see Chapter 9), as opposed to vertigo, in which the points for treatment are to be found on the *external aspect* of the ear (**Figure 28.3**).

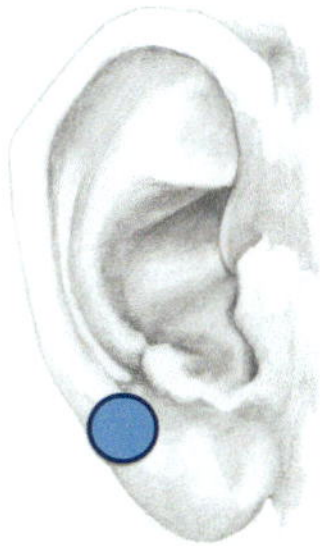

**Figure 28.3** Area to be explored in vertigo, on the *external* aspect of the ear, as opposed to a first rib syndrome, in which the points are to be found on the *mastoid* aspect of the ear.

## 28.3 THE NOTION OF FREQUENCY SIGNATURE

Using the RAC allows us to obtain a considerably better understanding of the pathologies we come across by analysing the frequencies to which an ear point (or any other portion of the skin surface) reacts. Whenever we detect a point on the ear, whether by measuring a lowered electrical resistance or using the RAC, we have the possibility of analysing to which frequencies this point reacts (see Chapter 21) and thus specify what we refer to as the *frequency signature* of that point. Practically speaking, while taking the pulse, we will project (in low or "diagnostic" mode) onto the point successively all the fundamental frequencies and find which one(s) trigger(s) a positive RAC. For example, suppose we find one point that reacts to frequencies **B** and **G**, and another that reacts to **A**. We then speak of a **B** and **G** frequency signature for the first point and an **A** signature for the second.

The same technique can be applied to a superficial skin lesion (mycosis, psoriasis, eczema, tendonitis, etc.) or to any location sufficiently accessible to define its frequency signature. We project each frequency onto the lesion in turn and note which one(s) respond(s), thus defining the lesion's frequency signature.

It is important to note that the frequency signature of a lesion is the same as that of the corresponding auricular point. Example: If we find an **A**, **C**, **F** signature on an inflamed knee, the corresponding ear point will respond to these same frequencies. It is interesting to note that the ear point can be the classical representation of the knee, but it can turn out to be a completely different point, such as a dental focus point.

Studying frequency signatures of various lesions will also enable us to establish relationships between different pathologies.

### 28.3.1 Clinical Example

Describing this technique reminds me vividly of one of my many teaching trips to Denmark. On that occasion, we were discussing frequencies. Following my presentation, just as I was about to illustrate the topic with a clinical demonstration, I was asked to examine a 37-year-old woman who had been suffering from chronic infectious otitis in her right ear for the last two years. She had consulted any number of specialists and been treated with all kinds of antibiotics without the slightest result. So, boosted by my audience, I chose to look for a frequency signature of the lesion she had in her ear. By chance, the tip of the frequency generator (GL+) happened to be just the right diameter to fit inside the external acoustic meatus (at the time, I did not know this).

So, I had the patient lie on the couch, took her pulse, and inserted the tip of the GL+ into her ear, while scrolling through the group of frequencies. The RAC response came out with three different frequencies. Consequently, the next step was to scan across the auricle in search of one or several ear points that bore the same frequency signature as the lesion. As a result, I found a point located on the ascending branch of the helix of the right ear, which turned out to be a representation of the uterus.

I then discreetly asked the patient if she was wearing an intrauterine device (IUD). She looked at me in a puzzled way that made me think she was aware of the importance of my question and replied that she had indeed been fitted with an IUD during the last two years. She added that it had been inserted just before the onset of the otitis. So, my prescription was simple: have the IUD removed. She had this done two days later, and shortly after, the otitis disappeared.

This case can be considered spectacular for two reasons. The first is that it raises the question of what possible link there can be between IUDS and otitis. The second is how the link has been identified. This leads me to a comment on intrauterine devices. They represent foreign bodies from which unexpected problems can sometimes arise. I remember a woman colleague from Argentina who was suffering from severe low back pain. The CT and MRI images showed no relevant explanation. However, considering the symptoms, a neurosurgeon had operated on her twice. I cannot recall exactly what the operations consisted of, but they apparently did not produce any improvement. When I examined this woman's ear, I was struck by the absence of pain when pressing the ear points corresponding to the lumbar region. Whereas the point corresponding to the uterus reacted with a strong positive RAC reaction when exposed to punctual light. This woman was wearing an IUD. I asked her to have it removed, and as a result, the pain disappeared immediately.

## 28.4 DEPRESSIVE STATES

A good deal of our patients are depressed. Not so long ago, the health situation, with fear of COVID-19 and confinement, has not made things any better. What symptoms could be more frequent in our practices than fatigue, lack of concentration or motivation, need to cry, gloom, or nutritional disorders? All these symptoms are expressions of inner suffering.

When we examine such patients with the RAC, we can come across different situations:

1. **Variation of the reactivity index** (see Chapter 9): Normally, this index is equal to 3. In some depressive states, it is considerably higher and can reach 15, sometimes even more. This reflects what could be referred to as a "struggle syndrome". In such cases, we will scan through the ear with a white rod or a white spotlight (Heine's lamp) to detect one or several points that react *with the same number of RACs as the reactivity index*. If the reactivity index is 15, we will find points that will induce 15 RACs. These are most likely to be ACTH points and are usually treated with semi-permanent needles.
2. **Exhaustion phenomenon**: This is the opposite situation: the RAC becomes exhausted after a small number of flashes. In this case, auricular points on the edge (rear border) of the lobule and helix should be examined by scanning the ear with a black rod, confirmed with an electric detector, and then treated with semi-permanent needles.
3. **Red colour photoreception disorder**: In some cases, the reactivity index is normal, but there is a photoreception disorder. The photogram (see Chapter 25) shows a gap concerning the red colour. This is generally observed in bipolar depressive states and can be treated with points on the rear border of the lobule on the *left ear* (**Figure 28.4**).
4. **Right/Left disorder** with Right/Left (see Section 26.5.2) scores above five, up to thirty, and more. This is usually corrected by points on the tragus.

In nervous breakdowns, as in many other diseases, it is important to normalise the disturbed tests.

## 28.5 PARKINSON'S DISEASE

Auriculotherapy can also be applied to Parkinson's disease. When possible, it is preferable to begin the treatment as early as possible after confirming the diagnosis and

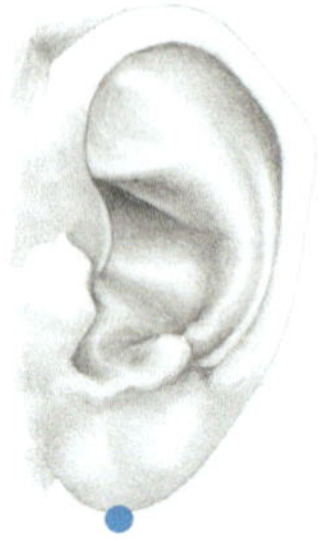

**Figure 28.4** Auricular treatment of red colour photoreception gaps.

avoid waiting for the disease to set in. Sometimes, the diagnosis is clear, particularly when the patient suffers from tremor. In other cases, the diagnosis can be uncertain. As we know, many patients have no tremor and see their physician for various other reasons, such as muscle pain, problems with walking, or nervous breakdown. Patients over sixty suffering from a nervous breakdown should particularly attract our attention because this condition often occurs as part of the prodromal stage of Parkinson's disease.

Another feature I have noticed is a rather unusual resting pulse, which feels abnormally ample and wide, probably due to the lack of dopamine, a vasopressive substance. It follows that the perception of the RAC can prove a little tricky with patients suffering from this condition.

**Treatment** of Parkinson's disease by auriculotherapy consists of scanning through the ear in search of points responding to **C** frequency. This frequency is attributed to movement and is typically that of Parkinson's disease. Using a frequency generator such as the GL+, we will scan **C** frequency (in low, "diagnostic" intensity) over the lobule, particularly the antitragus area (**Figure 28.5**). After finding a point that responds to **C**

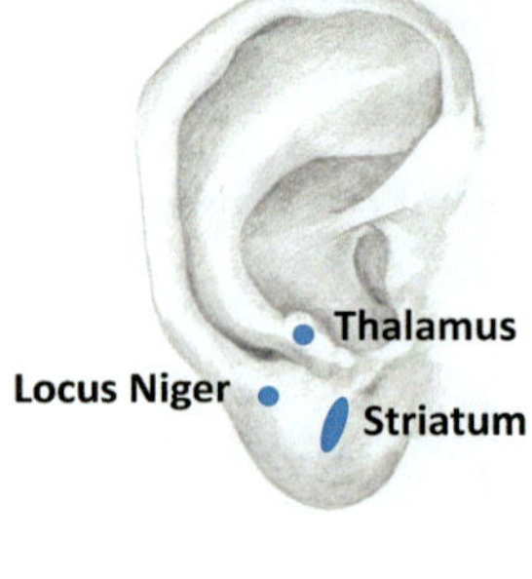


**Figure 28.5** Points frequently detected in Parkinson's disease.

frequency (positive RAC), we will treat it with the same frequency (in high, "therapeutic" intensity) and then add a semi-permanent needle to that same point.

Patients should be treated every month if possible, and of course, if auricular treatment alone proves insufficient, classical medication should be introduced.

## BIBLIOGRAPHY

1. Asis D. *Auricular chromotherapy in the treatment of psychological trauma.* VIIe International Symposium on Auricular Therapy. Lyon 2012
2. Bourdiol *R. Elements of auriculotherapy.* Éditions Maisonneuve. 1981.
3. De Leuze P-F., *The power of auriculotherapy on the emotional brain.* VIIe International Symposium of Auriculotherapy. Lyon 2012
4. Nogier P., with the collaboration of Bourdiol R. and Bahr F., *Loci auriculomedicinae.* Maisonneuve. 1975
5. Nogier P., in collaboration with R. Nogier. *The man in the ear.* Éditions Maisonneuve. 1979
6. Nogier P., *Auricular reflex points.* Maisonneuve 1987
7. Sinoue, Gilbert, *Avicenne ou la route d'Ispahan.* Gallimard 1990

CHAPTER 29

# The RAC Applied to Dentistry

## *A Brief Introduction to Auriculo-Dental Practice*

**Chantal Vulliez**

Medical research is increasingly focused on the dental organ, characterised by its genetic potential and specific innervation.

- *"We implant a fragment of tooth in the eye, which serves as support for a Plexiglas lens"*, explains Professor Louis Hoffart, head of the ophthalmic department of the Timone Hospital in Marseille in 2017— "Such an operation, which is extremely rare, is carried out on patients with bilateral blindness".
- Stem cells from dental pulp are used in plastic surgery.
- *"They allow the bones of the face and skull to be repaired"*, says Professor Catherine Chaussain during her award ceremony presentation of the Fondation des Gueules Cassées (Trust for Broken Faces) on 21 November 2018.
- The exploration of this organ is in full evolution: *"Human teeth emit an autofluorescence, the intensity of which is stronger in the dentin than in the enamel"*, writes Dr Stéphane Browet in June 2019 in the Prevention Tribune – French edition.

Moreover, in recent years, the oral sphere has come to the centre of medical pathology.

Indeed, many cardiovascular, digestive, and joint impairments find their origins in diseases of the osteo-gingivo-dental organ (OGDO) (**Figure 29.1**).

The septic environment of the oral region and the high reactivity of the dento-maxillary innervation network provide two explanations for these peripheral impairments (**Figure 29.2**).

The intimate interrelationship between the dental organ and the ears explains the interest of auriculotherapy in dentistry.

These intricacies are numerous: embryological, anatomical, neurological, or postural. This explains why the dental focus is a paramount source of therapeutic blockage in auriculotherapy.


DOI: 10.1201/9781003753629-29

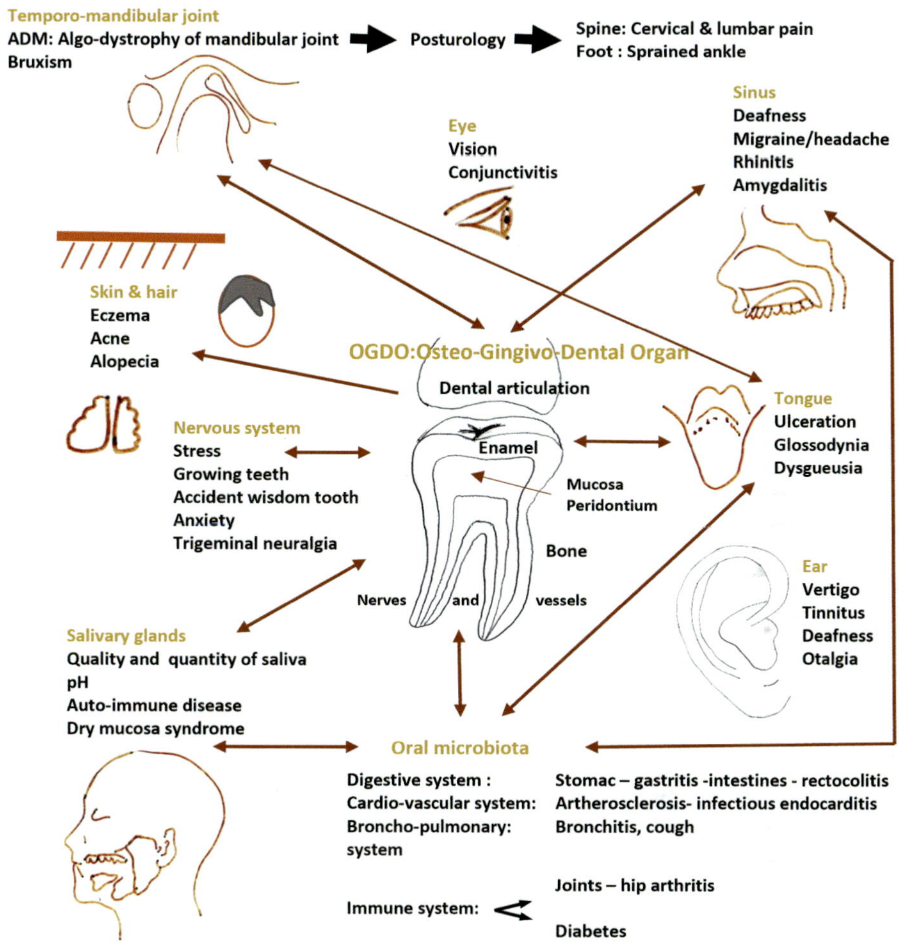


**Figure 29.1** OGDO – Information Centre.

## 29.1 DETECTION OF A DENTAL FOCUS

The dental focus can be defined in dental auriculotherapy as a specific hyperreactivity of an osteo-gingivo-dental organ (Chapter 10).

This reactionary state induces pathological information on the arterial pulse (RAC). There must be at least 5 RACs for an irritative dental focus to be diagnosed.

It can happen that several teeth are detected. The practitioner should very carefully note the number of RACs obtained for each tooth. The focus tooth is the one that gives the greatest number of RACs. It is not always painful (**Figure 29.3**).

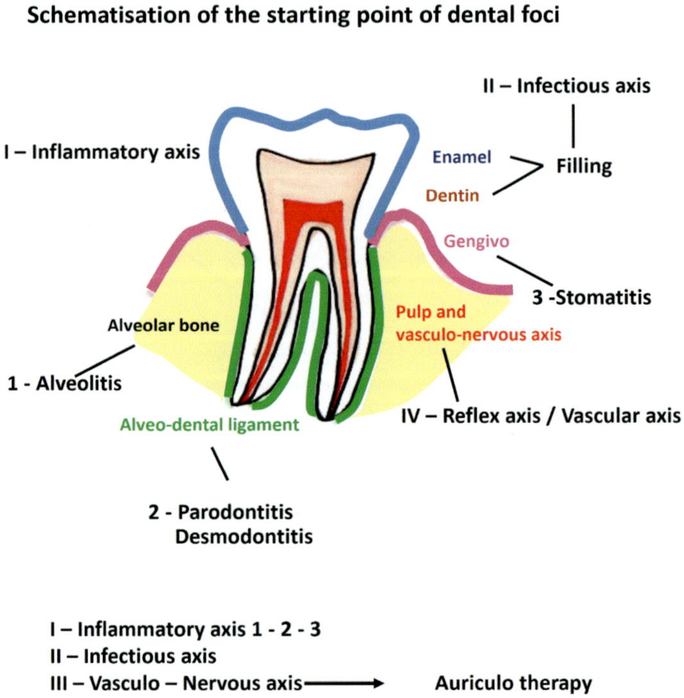


**Figure 29.2** Three etiological axes of a dental focus.

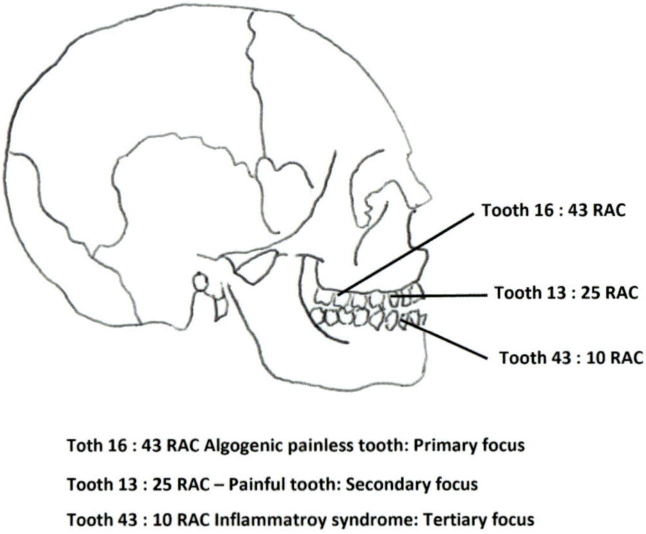


**Figure 29.3** Detection of an algogenic tooth.

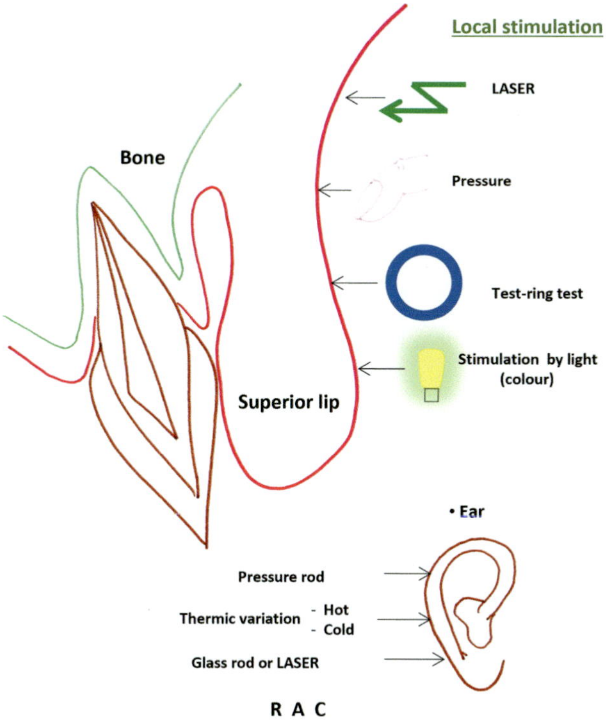


**Figure 29.4** Detection of a dental focus in Auriculodental practice.

The testing of these reactions can be performed both inside and outside the oral cavity (**Figure 29.4**).

The practitioner takes the patient's radial pulse to detect the RAC. Following this:

- The extra-oral examination can be carried out with various stimulations:
  - In a simple manner by lightly pressing the index finger consecutively on the cheek of the upper and lower jaws. Each tooth is tested (RAC) by lightly pressing the finger outside the mouth.
  - Lighting stimulation with Heine's lamp on the cheek allows us to be more precise in identifying an area containing a dental focus (RAC).
  - Stimuli with different frequencies acting on photoreception can be used with colour lamps. The Orange 21 Wratten Kodak determines the dental focus.
  - Photoemission tests, using various test rings, are also used, scanning them along the dental arches to locate the focal tooth.
  - The black and white rod can also be used on the black side for targeting a focus tooth.

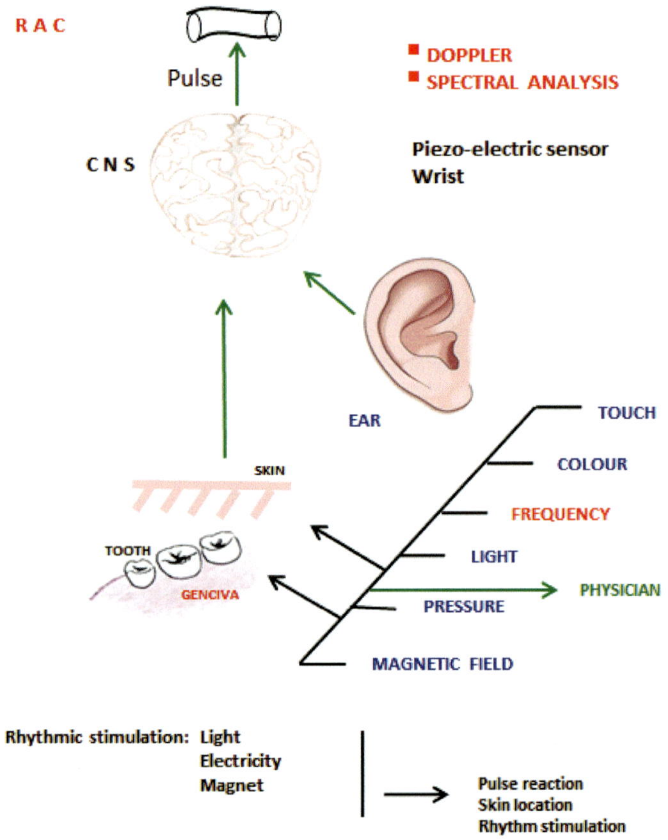


**Figure 29.5** Searching for the representation of a dental focus on the ear.

- The frequency infrared laser can be used inside and outside the oral cavity in search of one or more pathological frequencies (RAC) in the vicinity of one or several teeth.
- This search for a dental focus is to be completed by the detection of corresponding points or areas on the ear (**Figure 29.5**).

It is the number of RACs that allows us to find the causal tooth. Several teeth can yield RACs when examined. We will differentiate between the causal tooth and the secondary foci, which will not be treated in the first instance.

## 29.2 TREATMENTS IN AURICULO-DENTAL PRACTICE

Treatments are performed both in the oral cavity and on the ear.

First, a diagnosis is made to identify the primary dental focus and its possible incidence on the periphery. This OGDO must be assessed and treated by a specialist if it is confirmed to be a primary focus.

1. Stomatological treatment of the causative OGDO should be initiated as soon as possible. For example:
   - Solving the occlusal problem by setting up a perfect dental articulation.
   - Carrying out the eviction of a toxic substance (mercury) with all the usual precautions.
   - Remove any allergenic material from the root canal, which could have been introduced during root canal filling.
2. Auriculodental treatment is, as the name suggests, bipolar. A combined auricular and dental treatment can be started after a precise diagnosis of the dental lesion and the auricular reacting areas.

*Personally, I have been working most often with a frequency infrared laser for nearly 40 years with excellent results (see Bibliography 2). I have carried out work in electron microscopy, which led me to use this type of treatment, the summary of which I give here.*

This device can be used on the OGDO, both inside or outside the oral region and on the ear.

The pathological frequencies found on the reactive OGDO are mostly used in a so-called "homeopathic" mode. (This refers to the dental organ being treated with the same pathological *direct* frequency as found during diagnosis, as opposed to treating with the *complementary* frequency (see Chapter 22 on direct and complementary frequencies). Moreover, these same frequencies will also be detected on various ear points related to the OGDO pathology.

For example, neck pain occurring after dental treatment. We observe a reaction (RAC) on tooth 12, bearing frequencies A, C, and E, deviated at -30%. We then look for one or more areas on the ears that react to the same three frequencies, and find 3 points: the allergy point, a cervical point, and a dental point (**Figure 29.6**).

On questioning, the patient tells us that tooth 12 has been devitalized, and a root canal treatment was performed in the same session. We then think of an intolerance or allergy to the intra-canal product.

We will test the allergenic product that has been placed in the canal using the "approach and double contact" techniques used in auriculotherapy. The causal product is then extracted and replaced by a drop of Tea Tree Essential Oil (after being tested).

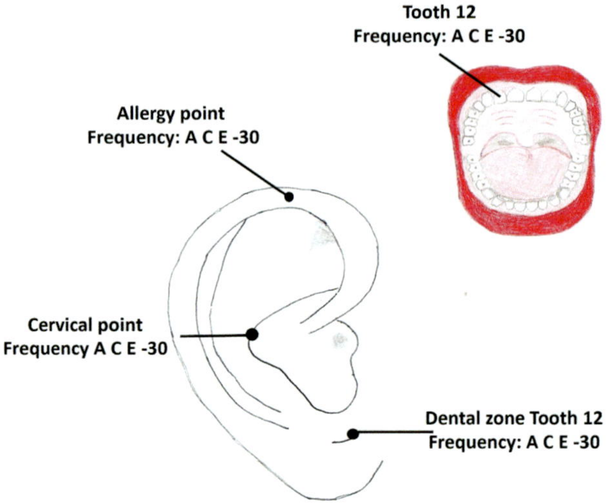


**Figure 29.6** Cervical pathology following intra-canal treatment of 12.

The patient is seen again one month later, after which the tooth no longer reacts (no RAC).

However, if it still does react, one or more laser sessions on the ear and the tooth will be necessary until the reaction is eliminated.

The neck pain gradually fades after the allergen is removed.

Other treatment techniques are also fix interest, such as massage or needles on the detected areas on the ear.

Chromotherapy can be used on the OGDO and on the ear. For example:

- A young woman is suffering from liver problems such as nausea, pain in the right hypochondrium, and weight loss. Intraoral examination reveals gingivitis focused on the area of tooth 15.
- The Kodak Wratten Red 25 colour gives a response (RAC) when projected near tooth 15 and on three ear points (**Figure 29.7**).
- The same colour, **Red 25**, is then projected for treatment (on the principle of chromotherapy), first intra-orally on tooth 15 and then on the ear, treating (separately) the 3 points found: liver, tooth, and V (trigeminal nerve).
- This light therapy treatment is combined with a stomatological treatment at a second stage.

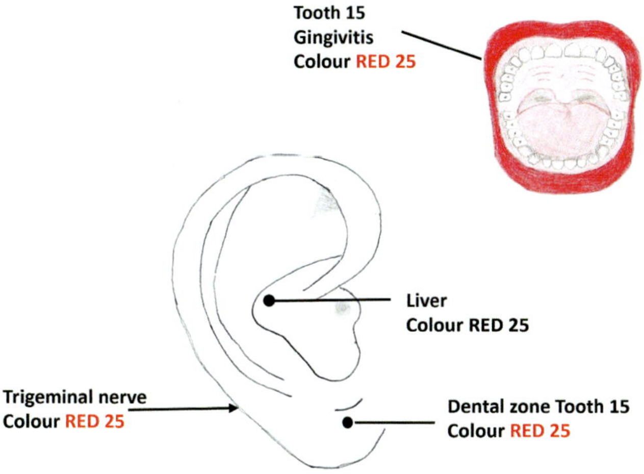


**Figure 29.7** Liver disorder in relation to gingivitis of 15.

## 29.3 CONCLUSION

The short summary above provides a better understanding of the diagnostic and therapeutic value of the Nogier Reflex in dentistry.

## GLOSSARY

**OGDO:** Osteo-gingivo-dental organ
**RAC:** Circulatory Autonomic Reflex (French acronym for Nogier's Reflex)
**TMJ:** Temporomandibular joint

## BIBLIOGRAPHY

1. Drews U. *Embryogenesis of the auricle: evolution of the 1er and 2e visceral arches.* Embryological Atlas (Flammarion). 1994
2. Vulliez Ch. Ajacques A., *Effect of the Infrared diode laser on the connective tissue–Study carried out in microelectronic copy.* Innovation and technology in Biology and Medicine–Lasers 11(1), 90. 1990
3. Vulliez Ch. *Auriculodentaire applied to dentistry.* Sauramps Médical. 2000.
4. Vulliez Ch. *Auriculotherapy and oral pathologie*s. Sauramps Médical. 2020

# Conclusion

**Anthony de Sousa**

Following the groundbreaking discovery of the arterial reflex by Paul Nogier in 1966, an understanding of the significance and the scope of this reflex has been a long, continuous, and highly fertile process, spread out over many years. Initially regarded merely as a new method for detecting ear points in the field of auriculotherapy, the arterial reflex RAC later broke partly free from this discipline. While being gradually recognised as intimately connected to the autonomous nervous system and, furthermore, as an especially well-adapted tool for exploring this system, the RAC became the key to brilliant new discoveries. Perhaps among the most prominent, *the skin* was found to elicit a specific pulse reaction when it was exposed to white light, coloured, or intermittent light. This led to the fascinating concepts of *photoreception* and *photoemission*, whereby the skin can be considered an interface for permanent exchanges of radiation and information between the internal organs and the outside world.

Clinically as well, the RAC has produced countless medical contributions; it has created a new approach to medicine and, as such, can virtually be considered a "universal reflex". It has greatly widened the scope of investigation into areas that are rarely taken into consideration by conventional medicine, for instance, measuring laterality, diagnosing food hypersensitivities, dental foci, or pathological scars.

Another remarkable example of what the RAC has made possible is analysing the way in which different but related pathologies develop over long periods of time, according to a dynamic process by which they interact with one another, adapting, influencing, or compensating one another. This we can readily observe through the sequence techniques using *colours or frequencies.*

We hope to have shown that these new techniques are in no way in opposition to mainstream medicine. On the contrary, we consider them as a fully integrated contribution to clinical medicine.

The object of this book is not only to give general information about the RAC, but to provide the reader with a method for learning the techniques and experiencing the pleasure of personally conducting a medical examination with the RAC. We hope that the preceding chapters may serve as an inspiration to the reader, both in exploiting the techniques described and in exploring the utility of the RAC for further research and clinical practice.


DOI: 10.1201/9781003753629-30

As we gradually draw this book to an end, I personally wish to pay a very special tribute to the memory of Paul Nogier, an exceptional physician and discoverer. I would also like to express my vivid gratitude for having been able to train with such a wonderful mentor, and more recently for the opportunity of experiencing the warm friendship built up while working together with Raphaël Nogier and Bo Kähler, on the preparation of this book.

# Epilogue

**Raphaël Nogier**

Before bringing this book to a close, let us explore some additional general considerations. It is the privilege of experience for an author to be granted the liberty of stepping aside from the main subject for the sake of addressing some-related topic.

The importance of language in the field of medicine cannot be overemphasised. Both words and syntax have a considerable influence on medical thinking.

1. Language is important as the vehicle of thought.
2. Language is important in the formulation of a diagnosis.
3. Language is important for communication among colleagues and scientists.

## 1 LANGUAGE AS THE VEHICLE OF THOUGHT

Socrates's saying: *Know thyself*, familiar to every philosopher, should also be highlighted in medical textbooks.

For ìf we are to make the most of the body's potential, we need to understand how the body functions.

Guy Lazorthes, a French professor of anatomy and neurosurgery, author of several publications, differentiates body, soul, and mind. According to him, the mind comprises not only knowledge but also the structure of thought.

It took me a long while to understand the meaning of this notion of "structure of thought". Without our knowing it, it determines our manner of grasping events, how we interpret them and how we react intellectually. A friend of mine, Dr Jean Goris, a German gynaecologist, has always insisted on this notion.

We have had thrilling discussions on this subject during the many trips I made to Hamm, a town in Westphalia, where I have been teaching for twenty-five years. When describing a person, Goris would talk about this person's structure, but despite my repeated questions, he never explained what he meant.

Our mind is constructed much like a book: on one the hand, we have *knowledge*, which will be backed up by the works cited. On the other hand, we have the author's path of thought, as it is laid out in the book's argument. We can think of that as an analogue to this notion of structure of thought. Or we could compare an individual's knowledge to the bricks of a house, and the path of thought to its architecture. A pile of bricks means nothing, but no house can be built without bricks. How the stones are arranged will determine the house's aspect, its functionality, and beauty.

The structure of thought, then, has its own architecture. As everyone knows, the plan for a house is essential and conditions everyday life. When a plan is poorly conceived, the life of the inhabitants can become an ordeal. The same applies to the architecture of thought, which should normally enable us to navigate a coherent system of knowledge. A pile of knowledge is nothing. The person who possesses this knowledge should be able to connect different aspects and select them when needed.

The mark of a satisfactory structure of thought is its capacity to unite all the existing data on a particular subject, to classify them by themes, and to express that subject's subtleties.

Today's society, because of its modes of education, privileges pure knowledge to the detriment of the structure of thought. Whatever the field, knowledge is easy to acquire. Everyone has access to a dictionary, an encyclopaedia, a computer or a smartphone linked to the Internet, capable of providing precise answers to specific questions. The answers obtained, however, will not lead to a coherent synthesis, as they are often fragmented and do not fit into an adequate thought process. We physicians observe this every day. Our patients will tend to interpret reports issued from biological assessments that they have undergone, merely by typing a keyword on the computer. But this will not lead to a correct diagnosis, because these patients do not possess the necessary structure of thought for this type of mental operation.

The illustrious French biologist Claude Bernard, in the last pages of his 1865 book *Experimental Medicine*, speaking of education, insisted on the idea that knowledge, which provides intelligence with its crucial tools, should not become a burden. The rules meant to support the weaker aspects of the mind should not hinder its more powerful and creative aspects.

## 2 LANGUAGE AS CRUCIAL TO THE FORMULATION OF DIAGNOSIS

It has taken me years of practice and discussions with foreign colleagues to understand the close relationship between the construction of language and the process of medical diagnosis. At first glance, these two notions have not much in common, but in fact, they are closely linked.

Inspired by numerous trips abroad, I have observed that medicine is not practised in the same way in all latitudes and on all continents. The attitudes towards patients differ in Paris, Algiers, Beijing, Tokyo, Buenos Aires, and Toronto. The standard of living partly explains these differences, but so does religion: "bedside manner" differs significantly among Buddhists, Shintoists, Muslims, and Christians. However, these factors do not explain everything. In addition, language—the style in which a sentence is constructed, and words are linked together—is decisive for shaping medical thinking. It is no coincidence that medicine originated in Greece and flourished in Mediterranean countries. Ancient Greece had an extremely precise language in which words were linked together in a structured and hierarchical manner. A language that made a clear difference between the subject (nominative) and the object (accusative). And complement (ablative), offered unlimited opportunities for fine-tuning thought. It is not by chance either that French medicine, practised by professionals who had been educated in Latin and Greek, reached such a high standard many centuries ago. Their education allowed them to practice a particular form of intellectual gymnastics, necessary for developing the art of diagnosis.

Studying Greek and Latin, beyond the words and roots to which it gives access, develops an ability to link words together and produce a constructed way of thinking. Latin and all highly inflected languages, such as Greek, German, Romanian, and Russian, have the property of stressing the word's function: nominative, genitive, dative, ablative, and accusative. Wherever a word is placed within the sentence, it is the case that will express the meaning, and a sentence changes its meaning if the words used change their ending.

Exercising a Greek or Latin version implies identifying the nominative (the subject), the accusative (the object), the verb, and the ablative (the means). This is what enables us to understand the meaning of the sentence. The location of a word within the sentence is not as important as the case. The meaning of the sentence is not defined by the position of the words but by the case of each word. This is not true of English or French, for example, where it is necessary to arrange the words according to a precise sequence, to give the sentence the intended meaning. The exercise of translating Greek or Latin makes it possible to link the words together, define their hierarchy, and give the sentence its true meaning.

Establishing a medical diagnosis, which requires specific skills and abilities, can be seen as similar. The examiner begins by asking the patient various questions to determine the subjective symptoms, such as pain, fatigue, and sleep disorders. After that, the patient will undergo a physical examination in search of objective signs, such as a skin rash, a white tongue, altered reflexes, and so on. Once we have determined the symptoms and signs, we must then link them together in a logical manner and establish a hierarchy. The diagnosis will depend on the examiner's ability to listen, examine, observe, and define the relationships and relative importance of each sign and symptom and to draw a coherent synthesis from this sum of information. This very specific approach requires a manner of thinking resembling a syntax exercise. One could almost speak of syntactic medicine. From a grammatical point of view, symptoms and signs can be compared to accusatives in the structure of a sentence. The next step will consist of finding the cause, or aetiology of the sign or symptom (nominative), in other words, the action by which the cause gives rise to the symptom (verb) and how this action is exerted (ablative).

**Example 1**

Ms. Smith comes to the office suffering from hives after falling amidst nettles. On questioning, she tells us that she has severe itching (accusative). On examination, what we see are hives. This is also the accusative.

What is the cause (nominative)? The nettles.
By what mechanism (ablative)? Nettles liberate histamine.
So, the nettles caused hives and itching due to the release of histamine.

**Example 2**

Mr Albert consults because of fatigue and paleness, which appeared over the last month.

There are several ways we can comment on this:

1. Mr. Albert's *pallor* was caused by *fatigue.*
2. The *pallor* caused Mr Albert to feel tired.
3. An unknown cause has resulted in Mr Albert's becoming pale and tired.

In this example, the words *fatigue* and *pallor* will produce a different diagnosis, depending on whether we interpret them as nominative or accusative.

Through these simple examples, we can see that language can either induce or prevent a deductive process of thought. There is no better exercise than the study of syntax to train a mind for the fields of science and medicine. Only through syntax can one learn to relate ideas to each other. Moreover, there is no better way to learn syntax than to study Latin and Greek.

Diagnosis is an art that requires not only knowledge but also a specific method for collecting symptoms and signs, establishing a hierarchy between them, and linking them together to define syndromes or diseases.

If the art of diagnosis depends on the art of language, it is easy to understand why acupuncture was born in China. Chinese writing, which utilises ideograms, has created a distinct way of thinking that differs from ours. A single ideogram designates each Chinese meridian point. It is difficult to imagine the concept of acupuncture without ideograms, to the extent that acupuncturists who are not Chinese often take the trouble to study Chinese to understand acupuncture and practice it at its best.

## 3 LANGUAGE AS CRUCIAL TO COMMUNICATION BETWEEN PHYSICIANS AND SCIENTISTS

Teachers are well acquainted with the way that words used indiscriminately distort discussion and create misunderstandings. Scientific discourse requires precise language. In a discussion, every word must have an exact definition to which all parties can refer. Today, science is evolving so rapidly that it is giving rise to new materials and new concepts, which require the creation of new words. They must be precisely defined to serve the purposes of those who use them. Choosing a new word is not insignificant. The root of the word, its ending, the number of its syllables, its sound, the ease with which it can be translated, everything must be carefully considered. Poorly chosen words can permanently destroy great hypotheses or concepts.

The term *auriculomedicine* has seriously harmed the work of Paul Nogier. Bringing together the terms *auricular* and *medicine* makes it tempting to suppose that such a method is solely concerned with the ear and that it can be practised only by physicians. Both assumptions are wrong.

The method, erroneously named auriculomedicine, consists of the examiner taking the patient's pulse to perceive an arterial variation resulting from stimulation of the organism. The stimulation can be either external, for instance, by exposing the skin to touch or light, or internal, by having the patient recall an emotional trauma. The auricle is therefore not necessarily involved, and the method is accessible to non-medical practitioners, depending on the indications. So, not only is the term *auriculomedicine* confusing but it also reduces the scope of action of Paul Nogier's method. The use of the arterial reflex (RAC) goes far beyond the auricle and reflex therapies. A new term must be found.

Four years ago, I gave a course in auriculotherapy at Johns Hopkins University in Rockville, Maryland, USA, to 150 colleagues. Before getting to the main subject for which I had been invited, I argued at some length on the importance of language in medicine, and on the necessity of being rigorous in the choice of vocabulary, to be understood and to get across. Although I expected to be criticised for this, it turned out that many attendees came to thank me, telling me that this had opened their horizons.

For many years, the French School of Medicine has been recognised worldwide for its capacity for innovation and efficiency. It has produced a considerable number of great physicians, biologists, scientists, and philosophers, such as René Leriche, Alexis Carrel, Claude Bernard, and many others. All of them had a mind structured by the study of classical literature, and this explains their exceptional thinking abilities. If we want to maintain such high standards in medical faculties worldwide, my advice would be that future doctors are given access to comprehensive training, not only focused on science but also on how to construct their thinking. I am in favour of creating a general preparatory approach before beginning medical studies. Selecting physicians essentially on scientific criteria deprives us of talents that are also needed. Naturally, the medical field requires scientists but let us not forget that medicine is an art, not a science. Medicine also needs writers, philosophers, and, why not, artists, musicians, and sportsmen. The medical profession calls for a wide range of skills that cannot be satisfied by scientific training alone. The aptitudes required for practising surgery, radiology, emergency medicine, or psychiatry are not the same. A Faculty of Medicine is equivalent to a school for engineers or musicians. Without delay, it must become open to other skills.

**Lyon, November 2021**

# Author Index

# Subject Index

For Product Safety Concerns and Information please contact our EU representative GPSR@taylorandfrancis.com Taylor & Francis Verlag GmbH, Kaufingerstraße 24, 80331 München, Germany

Batch number: 10777176

Printed by Printforce, the Netherlands

Also by Doug McCall:

*Harris County*

*By Proxy: A Final Good Deed*

*Blind Trust*

*Beneath Forbidden Ground*

*Pale Aftermath*

*Indiana Deaths: Questions of Greed*

*Only Darkness Every Day*

*Thickets*

Made in the USA
Monee, IL
08 November 2026

67383833R00151